Atlas of
Hair and Nails

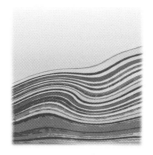

Atlas of
Hair and Nails

Maria K. Hordinsky, MD

Professor
Department of Dermatology
University of Minnesota Academic Health Center
Minneapolis, Minnesota

Marty E. Sawaya, MD, PhD

Principal Investigator Clinical Research
ARATEC Clinics
Ocala, Florida
Adjunct Professor of Biochemistry and Molecular Biology
University of Miami School of Medicine
Miami, Florida

Richard K. Scher, MD

Professor of Clinical Dermatology
Columbia University College of Physicians and Surgeons
Columbia-Presbyterian Medical Center
New York, New York

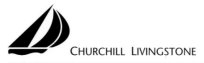 CHURCHILL LIVINGSTONE

A Division of Harcourt Brace & Company
Philadelphia London Toronto Montreal Sydney Tokyo Edinburgh

CHURCHILL LIVINGSTONE
A Division of Harcourt Brace & Company

The Curtis Center
Independence Square West
Philadelphia, Pennsylvania 19106

Library of Congress Cataloging-in-Publication Data

Atlas of hair and nails / [edited by] Maria K. Hordinsky, Marty Sawaya,
Richard K. Scher.—1st ed.

    p. cm.

  ISBN 0–443–07523–9

   1. Hair—Diseases—Atlases.   2. Nails (Anatomy)—Diseases—
Atlases. I. Hordinsky, Maria K.   II. Sawaya, Marty E.   III. Scher,
Richard K. [DNLM: 1. Hair Diseases—physiopathology
atlases.   2. Nail Diseases—physiopathology atlases.   3. Hair
Diseases—therapy atlases.   4. Nail Diseases—therapy atlases.
WR 17 A8819 2000]

RL 151.A86   2000

616.5′46—dc21

DNLM/DLC   98–53550

Atlas of Hair and Nails   ISBN 0–443–07523–9

Printed in the United States of America

Last digit is the print number: 9   8   7   6   5   4   3   2   1

CONTRIBUTORS

Philippe Abimelec
Nail Consultant, Hôspital Saint-Louis, Policlinique de dermatologie, Paris, France
Tumors of Hair and Nails: Tumors of the Nail Apparatus

Wasim Ahmad, MD, PhD
Department of Dermatology, Columbia University College of Physicians and Surgeons; Vanderbilt Clinic, New York, New York
Molecular Basis of Inherited Hair and Nail Diseases

Howard P. Baden, MD
Professor of Dermatology, Harvard Medical School; Dermatologist, Massachusetts General Hospital, Boston, Massachusetts
Developmental and Hereditary Disorders

Lynn A. Baden, MD
Instructor in Dermatology, Harvard Medical School; Associate Physician in Dermatology, Brigham and Women's Hospital, Boston, Massachusetts
Developmental and Hereditary Disorders

Ulrike Blume-Peytavi, MD
Senior Lecturer and Assistant Professor, Department of Dermatology, University Medical Center Benjamin Franklin, The Free University of Berlin, Berlin, Germany
Hair Shaft Abnormalities

Angela M. Christiano, MS, PhD
Assistant Professor, Department of Dermatology, Columbia University College of Physicians and Surgeons, New York, New York
Molecular Basis of Inherited Hair and Nail Diseases

Clay J. Cockerell, MD
Clinical Professor of Dermatology and Pathology, University of Texas Southwestern Medical Center at Dallas Southwestern Medical School, Dallas, Texas
Hair and Nail Histology: Histology of the Normal Nail Unit

Philip R. Cohen, MD
Clinical Associate Professor, University of Texas–Houston Medical School, Houston; Private Practice, The Woodland, Texas
Aging

Peter B. Cserhalmi-Friedman, MD
Associate Research Scientist, Department of Dermatology, Columbia University College of Physicians and Surgeons, New York, New York
Molecular Basis of Inherited Hair and Nail Diseases

Piet De Doncker, MD, PhD
Director, Dermatology/Medical Affairs, International Clinical Research and Development, Infectious Diseases–Dermatology–Allergy, Janssen Research Foundation, Beerse, Belgium
Fungal Infections

Zoe D. Draelos, MD
Clinical Associate Professor, Department of Dermatology, Wake Forest University School of Medicine, Winston-Salem; President, Dermatology Consulting Services, High Point, North Carolina
Cosmetic and Ethnic Issues: Nail Cosmetic Issues

Philip Fleckman, MD
Associate Professor of Medicine, Division of Dermatology, University of Washington School of Medicine, Seattle, Washington
Hair and Nail Physiology

Diana Garside, PhD
Supervisor, Quest Diagnostics, San Diego, California
Forensic and Medicolegal Issues

Bruce A. Goldberger, MS, PhD
Director of Toxicology and Assistant Professor,
    Department of Pathology, University of Florida
    College of Medicine, Gainesville, Florida
Forensic and Medicolegal Issues

Elke-Ingrid Grussendorf-Conen, MD
Senior Lecturer and Professor of Dermatology and
    Venereology, Faculty of Medicine; Head,
    Dermatohistology Laboratory, Department of
    Dermatology; and Head, Outpatient Dermatology
    Clinic, Universitat ders RWTH Aachen, Aachen,
    Germany; Consultant in Dermatology, Baksh Clinic,
    Jeddah, Saudi Arabia
*Tumors of Hair and Nails: Tumors of the Pilosebaceous
    Unit*

Christopher L. Gummer, DPhil(Oxon)
Research Fellow, Hair and Skin Research, Procter &
    Gamble, Egham, England
Cosmetic and Ethnic Issues: Hair Cosmetic Issues

Eckart Haneke, MD, PhD
Professor, Department of Dermatology, Clinical Health
    Center, Private University of Witten/Herdecke;
    Chairman, Department of Dermatology, Wuppertal
    Hospitals Ltd, Academic Teaching Hospital—
    University Düsseldorf, Wuppertal, Germany
Surgical Treatments

Mark Holzberg, MD
Assistant Clinical Professor of Dermatology, Emory
    University School of Medicine, Atlanta, Georgia
Nail Signs of Systemic Disease

H. Irving Katz, MD
Clinical Professor, Department of Dermatology,
    University of Minnesota Medical School—
    Minneapolis, Minneapolis; Courtesy Staff, Unity-
    Mercy Hospital, Fridley, Minnesota
*Adverse Effects and Drug Interactions of Medications
    Used to Treat Hair and Nail Disorders*

Harvey Lui, MD, FRCPC
Associate Professor, Division of Dermatology, University
    of British Columbia Faculty of Medicine; Medical
    Director, The Skin Care Centre, Vancouver General
    Hospital, Vancouver, British Columbia, Canada
Common Hair Loss Disorders

Nathalie Mandt, MD
Resident, Department of Dermatology, University
    Medical Center Benjamin Franklin, The Free
    University of Berlin, Berlin, Germany
Hair Shaft Abnormalities

Mary Gail Mercurio, MD
Assistant Professor of Dermatology, University of
    Rochester School of Medicine, Rochester, New York
Hirsutism and Hypertrichosis

Eva M. J. Peters, MD
Herbert A. Stiefel Fellow in Experimental Dermatology,
    Department of Biomedical Sciences, University of
    Bradford, Bradford, West Yorkshire, England
Pigment Disorders of the Hair and Nails

Gerald E. Piérard, MD, PhD
Professor, Department of Dermatopathology, Institute
    of Pathology, University of Liège, Liège, Belgium
Fungal Infections

Bianca Maria Piraccini, MD
Professor, Department of Dermatology, University of
    Bologna, Bologna, Italy
Dermatological Diseases That Affect the Nail

Elizabeth Reeve, MD
Assistant Clinical Professor, Department of Psychiatry,
    University of Minnesota Medical School—
    Minneapolis; Residency Training Director—
    Psychiatry, Hennepin County Medical Center/Regions
    Hospital, Minneapolis, Minnesota
Psychiatric Issues

Karin U. Schallreuter, MD
Professor of Clinical and Experimental Dermatology,
    Department of Biomedical Sciences, University of
    Bradford, Bradford, West Yorkshire, England;
    Institute for Pigmentation Disorders, Ernst-Moritz-
    Arndt University of Greifswald, Biotechnikum,
    Greifswald, Germany
Pigment Disorders of the Hair and Nails

Richard K. Scher, MD
Professor of Clinical Dermatology, Columbia University
    College of Physicians and Surgeons; Columbia-
    Presbyterian Medical Center, New York, New York
Aging

Jerry Shapiro, MD, FRCPC
Clinical Associate Professor, Division of Dermatology,
    University of British Columbia, Faculty of Medicine;
    Director, University of British Columbia Hair
    Research and Treatment Centre, Vancouver General
    Hospital, Vancouver, British Columbia, Canada
Common Hair Loss Disorders

Leonard C. Sperling, MD
Professor and Chair, Department of Dermatology,
    Uniformed Services University of the Health Sciences
    F. Edward Hébert School of Medicine, Bethesda,
    Maryland; Staff, Walter Reed Army Medical Center,
    Washington, DC
Cicatricial Alopecias

Kurt Stenn, MD, MA
Director, Skin Biology Research Center, Johnson & Johnson, Skillman, New Jersey
Hair and Nail Physiology

Melody Stone, MD
Resident in Pathology (University of Missouri–Kansas City School of Medicine), Truman Medical Center, Kansas City, Missouri
Hair and Nail Histology: Histology of the Normal Nail Unit

Angela R. Styles, MD
Assistant Clinical Professor, University of Arkansas for Medical Sciences, Little Rock; Staff, Johnson County Regional Medical Center, Clarksville, Arkansas
Hair and Nail Histology: Histology of the Normal Nail Unit

Desmond J. Tobin, BSc, CBiol, PhD
Lecturer in Biomedical Sciences, Department of Biomedical Sciences, University of Bradford, Bradford, West Yorkshire, England
Pigment Disorders of the Hair and Nails

Antonella Tosti, MD
Associate Professor, Department of Dermatology, University of Bologna, Bologna, Italy
Dermatological Diseases That Affect the Nail

David A. Whiting, MD, FACP, FRCP(Ed)
Clinical Professor of Dermatology and Pediatrics, University of Texas Southwestern Medical Center at Dallas Southwestern Medical School; Medical Director, Baylor Hair Research and Treatment Center, Dallas, Texas
Hair and Nail Histology: Histology of Normal Hair

PREFACE

Our goal at the initiation of this project was to produce an atlas on hair and nails that would benefit dermatologists in practice, physicians in training programs, and physicians in other specialties responsible for treating patients with hair and nail diseases. We wanted our book to be "user friendly." We also wanted the atlas to serve as a resource to industry, cosmetic, and pharmaceutical personnel and to others who had an interest in hair and nails.

The atlas is divided into four sections. The first discusses the basic principles of hair and nail physiology and histology, and the second presents hair and nail disorders. Medical and surgical treatments of hair and nail diseases are discussed within relevant chapters as well as in specific chapters in the third section, which is devoted to cosmetic and ethnic issues. The fourth section covers special issues—drug-induced changes, aging, forensic and medicolegal issues, and psychiatric issues in relationship to hair and nail diseases.

Experts in these areas and in the field of hair and nail biology were asked to contribute their expertise, knowledge, and clinical pictures to this atlas, and through their contributions a comprehensive atlas of hair and nails has been created. While the book was being prepared, significant advances in the therapy, pathophysiology, and molecular biology of several hair and nail disorders were made. We have incorporated these advances into this atlas. We believe this atlas will summarize for the clinician or individual with an interest in hair and nail disorders the state of each field as we enter the next century. We hope you enjoy our pictorial summary!

CONTENTS

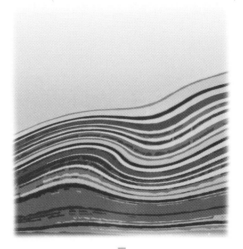

BASIC
PRINCIPLES

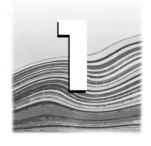

Hair and Nail Physiology

KURT STENN

—

PHILIP FLECKMAN

This chapter deals with the dynamics of the pilosebaceous apparatus and the nail unit–the controls of their development and growth. The purpose of this chapter is to review the biology of hair and nails broadly but with pertinent references to the literature so that the motivated reader can go further. Two major points are made: (1) nail and hair each forms from, and constitutes, a multicellular structure, and (2) the growth of hair, and probably of nail, is influenced and controlled by extensive cell-cell, cell-tissue, and cell-matrix interactions. Although these vicinal interactions are important, the growth of the hair follicle and of the nail is also affected by parameters of the body as a whole. Moreover, at least in the case of hair, the influence can be reciprocal: some aspects of follicular function affect the immunological and hormonal properties of the total body.

The dynamics of hair and nail growth control are related in several ways. Both are skin appendages serving protective functions. Both are epithelial products derived from a multicellular primitive epithelium. Both give rise to a differentiated epithelial product, which consists of tightly bound cells made rigid by special intermediate filament proteins, the hard keratins, and intermediate filament-associated proteins that bind and pack the filamentous proteins. Finally, in disease states when the hair is affected, the nail often is also (e.g., alopecia areata, lichen planus, monilethrix).

Hair Development and Physiology

The evident function of the hair follicle is to form a hair shaft. The function of the shaft is mainly protective (against trauma, insects, and temperature extremes), but it is also a means of interspecies and intraspecies communication. The follicle may participate in many other functions of the skin, including immune, neural, and reparative functions (discussed later). The follicle arises from the primitive integumental epithelium. With maturity it grows to adult size, forms a shaft, pigments itself, cycles, and, under the proper conditions, transforms from a small follicle to a large one. Each of these steps is considered in the following sections.

HAIR FOLLICLE EMBRYOGENESIS

Follicle formation is best understood in the context of the phylogeny of skin. In the invertebrate, the skin (integument) is covered by a simple epithelium. This single layer of epithelial cells usually is embellished by a secreted covering consisting of mucus (worms), calcareous deposit (mollusks), or chitin (insects). The epithelial covering of the skin changed dramatically with the development of vertebrates. The integumental epithelium became stratified, which allowed it to be embellished variously by secreted materials, and unlike simple epithelium, it could also amplify itself by upfoldings or downfoldings. The upfoldings led to the formation of scales in fish and feathers in birds; the downfoldings led to the formation of hair follicles, nails, and claws in mammals.

The phylogenic pattern is repeated in part during the formation of epidermis during gestation.[1] In the embryo, the skin cover initially consists of a single epithelial layer underlying the periderm. By 2 months, the epidermis is multilayered. Hair anlagen are seen first between the second and third months, when a bud appears on the lower epidermal surface; with time the bud grows into the developing dermis as a peg, and the column of epithelial cells differentiates into the multilayered hair follicle. What dictates the patterning, or placement, of hair follicles over the skin surface has been debated. Early workers suggested that the first signal for hair formation in the embryo arises in the dermis,[2] but more recent data suggest that transcription factors are expressed in the primitive epithelial cells at the site of follicle formation well before there is morphological evidence of that event in the primitive epidermis or dermis.[3] In addition, transcription factors associated with body patterning are found in follicles.[4-6] Regardless of where the first signal arises early in development, there is a dermal cell aggregate that forms below the epithelial bud. This aggregate precedes the peg into the deep dermis.

HAIR FOLLICLE FORMATION

Once the epithelial peg reaches the deep dermis, its constituent cells embrace the aggregate of dermal cells, referred to as the *follicular papilla,* and they begin to differentiate. Eight stages of hair follicle formation have been identified.[2] When the growing follicle is fully formed, it consists of three major embedded cylinders. The central cylinder of cells makes up the *shaft,* the only portion of the organized follicle that extrudes from the skin surface. The outermost cylinder, the multilayered epithelial *outer root sheath (ORS),* makes up the wall of the follicle separating it from the surrounding dermis. The third cylinder, between the shaft and the ORS, is the *inner root sheath (IRS).* The IRS molds and guides the shaft in its course outward. The IRS and the hair shaft move outward together, slipping along a plane at the innermost layer of the ORS. The IRS is tightly moored to the shaft by the intersecting cuticles of the shaft and the IRS: the cells of the cuticle point downward on the shaft and outward on the IRS.

Growth of the hair shaft and IRS arises from multiplication of cells in the follicular bulb. Most of the cell divisions occur in the lowermost cells of the bulb. In progressing outward, these cells give rise to the differentiated cell lineages that form the various follicular cylinders. The cells of the follicular bulb, along with those of the bone marrow and gut epithelium, are the most rapidly dividing cells of the adult body. For this reason a chemotherapeutic insult causes hair shedding along with anemia and gastrointestinal problems.

The centralmost cylinder of cells makes up the shaft. The shaft itself comprises three layers: cuticle, cortex, and, in some follicles, medulla. The cells making up these layers are for the most part vertically aligned along the axis of the shaft and filled with structural proteins that consist of or stabilize intermediate filament proteins. The intermediate filaments are made of more than 10 unique hard keratin proteins. A family of these proteins is now recognized, and their pattern of expression in the follicle is being characterized as to time and position.[7, 8] The filaments are packaged by intermediate filament-associated proteins, which are classified into those rich in sulfur amino acids and those rich in tyrosine/glycine amino acids.

The IRS actually consists of three cylindrical layers; from inside out, they are the cuticle of the IRS, Huxley's layer, and Henle's layer. The first layer to differentiate in the bulb is Henle's layer, followed by the cuticle and then Huxley's layer. As the cells of the IRS keratinize, they give rigidity to this sheath layer, supporting IRS function as a mold for the formative hair shaft. Racial differences in shaft cross-section (flat in Africans, round in Asians, and ellipsoidal in Europeans) are produced by the asymmetric formation of the IRS.

Embedded in the IRS, the hair shaft moves up the follicle toward the skin surface. Just below the level of the sebaceous duct, the IRS degrades and frees the mature shaft. Studies suggest that the sebaceous gland plays an active role in this shaft-sheath processing.[9] The tip of the newly formed shaft is pointed and not pigmented. The shaft courses through the pilary canal and then to the skin surface. Depending on the body site, the growth phase of the follicle may last from months to years; on the scalp, for example, hairs grow for 2 to 6 years, each hair growing about 0.4 mm/day.

CONTROL OF HAIR GROWTH

The growth of bulb cells depends on the stimulus and support of the follicular papilla. This structure consists of specialized fibroblastic cells with powerful hair follicle–inductive properties.[10] Follicular papilla influence is needed for follicular morphogenesis, for initiation of the new hair cycle, and for normal hair growth.[11] The character of the papilla influences the size, and presumably the properties, of the shaft.[10] The papilla has been associated with the production of a large number of growth factors and growth factor receptors, which may play a role in its supportive function of hair growth.[5]

HAIR CYCLE

Hair follicle growth is cyclical, manifesting periods of growth, regression, resting, and shaft shedding. The cyclical nature of hair growth allows an animal to shed its coat with the seasons and thereby adjust to environmental demands. Coat shedding also provides an opportunity to cleanse the body surface. In thinking about the hair cycle, it is important to distinguish the hair follicle cell cycle from the cycle of the hair follicle (the organ) itself. In the rapidly growing follicle, the cells of the bulb are undergoing rapid cell division and therefore rapid cell cycling. During this phase the follicle is not cycling but is committed to anagen. The hair follicle cycle involves the transition from one phase to the other. Although we recognize the morphological structure and the implications of each phase, we do not know which cell controls the cycle. The cycle could be controlled by the cells of the papilla, the epithelium of the follicle, the surrounding nerves, the surrounding vessels, or even the resident lymphoid cells in and about the follicle.

That it goes through a cycle at all underscores a unique feature of the follicle as the only structure in the normal human body that continually regenerates itself from birth to senility. Regeneration in any tissue implicates a population of cells with growth and differentiative plasticity. Because most cell divisions in the follicle occur in the bulb, it was long thought that the cells giving rise to the follicle, namely follicle stem cells, reside there. It has now been shown that cells with stem cell–like properties are found in the area of the follicle at the insertion of the arrector pili muscle.[12] This area, called the *bulge*, is prominent in the embryonic follicle and is irregularly obvious in the adult follicle.

The mature anagen follicle consists of two segments, or regions. The permanent portion is that which extends from the insertion of the arrector pili muscle to the skin surface. The transient portion is the cycling portion of the follicle, extending from the muscle insertion to the base of the bulb. What we have been describing heretofore is the anagen follicle, the actively growing phase that shows numerous dividing cells in the bulb, a well-defined IRS, nucleated cells progressing into the base of the generating shaft, and melanin-producing melanocytes.

At the end of the growth phase, the follicle receives an unknown signal, growth ceases, the papilla shrinks, and the proximal follicle withdraws to the level of the muscle. The mechanism of lower follicle retraction results, at least in part, from the process of controlled cell death (apoptosis) occurring in the cells of the ORS. It has been postulated that the retractive force drawing the lower follicle upward may be a result of the apoptotic process itself. A second hypothesis invokes the fact that the connective tissue sheath about the inferior portion of the follicle is rich in smooth actin-containing mesenchymal cells, which are envisioned to squeeze the follicle upward. Although the signal for catagen induction has not been defined, fibroblast growth factor 5 has been implicated in the process, because in the animal without this factor, catagen induction is delayed, resulting in the *angora* mutation.[13]

At the end of catagen, the follicle enters a resting phase, telogen. During this period, the shaft is held tightly within the bulbous base of the follicle, and few cell divisions occur in the follicular epithelium. The follicular papilla also retracts, but it rests as a cluster of cells associated with little extracellular matrix. At this point the follicle may enter another cycle without shedding the shaft, or it may shed the shaft and then enter another cycle. The shedding process, which has been

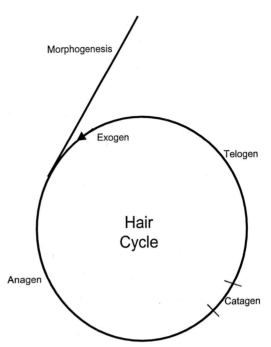

FIGURE 1–1 ■ Because follicle formation occurs only once in the lifetime of a mammal, the growth cycle of the follicle is best depicted in the configuration of the number 6; follicular morphogenesis differs from the repeating cycle of the follicle.

referred to as the exogen phase, occurs independently of follicle growth activity (i.e., anagen or continued telogen).

Because follicle formation occurs but once in the lifetime of a mammal, the growth cycle of the follicle is best depicted in the configuration of the number 6; follicular morphogenesis differs from the repeating cycle of the follicle. This concept is illustrated in Figure 1–1.

PATTERNING OF FOLLICLES OVER THE BODY

One of the major themes of follicular biology is that hair follicles, like the skin itself, show conspicuous morphological and functional heterogeneity. Excepting bilateral symmetry, follicles and their resultant shafts differ from site to site in shaft length, color, thickness, curl, and androgen sensitivity. This heterogeneity is supported in part by characteristics of the papilla.[14]

A significant element of follicle heterogeneity relates to the influence of androgens. Follicles over the body are either very sensitive (axilla and inguinal hair), mildly sensitive (beard hair), or insensitive to androgens (eyebrow). Androgen receptors have been most clearly demonstrated in the cells of the papilla,[15] and tissue culture studies have found that papilla cells from androgen-sensitive follicles respond to androgens. Such cells have been found to release insulin-like growth factor after exposure to androgen.[16, 17] This factor has been found to be an essential growth factor for follicles in culture.[18]

Most surfaces of the body are covered with hair. In the apparently hairless regions, the follicles are small, and the shafts produced may be microscopic. Such small, unpigmented follicles are referred to as *vellus follicles,* in contrast to the long, thick, pigmented *terminal follicles.* The powerful influence of androgens on follicle morphology is best illustrated by the conversion of vellus follicles to terminal follicles on the face of a pubescent boy. The event is dramatic in biology because there is a change from one highly differentiated small structure to an identical structure many times larger. The controls fundamental to this process implicate molecules found in other developmental systems, and such molecules are found to be expressed in the growing follicle.[5]

PIGMENTATION

In the anagen follicle, melanocytes are positioned above the papilla in the basal layer of the bulb. As cells forming the shaft pass by these resident melanocytes on their way up, they pick up melanin in a process thought to be similar to that seen in the epidermis. Follicular melanocytes, however, may differ from their epidermal counterparts.[19] Pigment is found in cells of the cortex and medulla but usually not in the cuticle or sheath cells.

Melanocytes become active in early anagen, but the initial shaft is unpigmented. The pigmentation cycle then, differs from the hair cycle, even though the cycles are coordinated. Toward the end of anagen, melanin distribution to hair cells ceases before hair growth stops, so that the base of the shaft (the club) is also not pigmented. In telogen it is not clear where the melanocytes or melanocyte precursors rest, because the usual markers of melanocytes are no longer expressed. Arguments for the presence of melanocyte precursors in either the mesenchyme or the epithelium of the resting follicle have been presented.

PERSPECTIVES IN HAIR FOLLICLE BIOLOGY

The hair follicle is a deceptively simple structure. It carries out a very complex function that is reflected, on close scrutiny, in its structure. The molecular basis of hair follicle growth control is only now being addressed. The major points of focus are the controls of follicle cycling, the switch from vellus to terminal follicles, the basis for follicular heterogeneity, and the control of pigmentation in relation to the hair cycle.

Nail Unit Development and Physiology

Nails protect the tips of the fingers and toes against trauma. They amplify fine touch and enable manipulation of small objects with the fingers. Nails are excellent both for scratching and as weapons. Like hair, nails are cosmetically important and serve as a means of sociosexual communication. The *nail plate* (also called the nail) is formed by the *nail unit.* In contrast to the follicle, the nail unit does not appear to function either immunologically or in epidermal repair. The nail unit arises early in embryogenesis from the epithelium, but its development is intimately related to the underlying bone. Unlike the follicle, nails neither grow cyclically nor pigment. The nail unit remains relatively unchanged throughout life.

NAIL UNIT EMBRYOGENESIS AND MORPHOGENESIS

Fingers and toes can be distinguished at between 6 and 7 weeks' estimated gestational age (toes lag behind fingers throughout this process). By 10 weeks a quadrangular area, the *primary nail field,* is delineated on the surface of the fingers by depressions in the epithelium; the distal depression defining the primary nail field is the *distal groove,* which persists in the fully developed nail unit. By 11 weeks, an area of epidermis just proximal to the distal groove thickens to form the distal ridge. This is the first area to keratinize in the embryo.

The distal ridge also marks the site of the *hyponychium,* the area that seals the undersurface of the distal nail plate to the *nail bed.* Concurrently, epithelium from the proximal part of the primary nail field, the matrix primordium, invaginates and migrates proximally and ventrally into the distal digit and differentiates into the *nail matrix,* forming the proximal nail groove in the process. The tissue dorsal to (above) the proximal nail groove becomes the *proximal nail fold.* The matrix begins to form the nail plate; by 14 weeks, the nail plate extends beyond the proximal nail fold, and by 17 weeks the nail plate has covered the entire nail bed and flattened the distal ridge to form the hyponychium.

During the formation of nail plate, keratinization proceeds proximally from the distal ridge, so that the nail bed is keratinized by the time the nail plate grows over it. Nail plate and bed keratinization initially includes formation of keratohyalin granules; however, as the nail plate grows over the matrix and nail bed, the granular layer is lost.[20] This process of keratinization of the nail bed with formation of granular and cornified layers also occurs throughout life when the nail plate is detached from the nail bed, either by disease or by surgery; as the regrowing nail plate reattaches, it "wipes" the granular and cornified layers off, repeating ontogeny.

STRUCTURE OF THE NAIL UNIT

The gross and microscopic anatomy of the nail unit is discussed and illustrated in Chapter 2. The nail plate is formed by the four structures that make up the nail unit: proximal nail fold, nail matrix, nail bed, and hyponychium.[21] The nail plate consists of anucleate keratinocytes oriented so that the cells are flattened in the plane of the plate. Intermediate filaments within nail plate cells are oriented perpendicular to the plane of growth of the nail plate. This orientation and the transverse and longitudinal curvature of the plate are thought to provide structural rigidity.[22]

Analogies have been drawn between the nail unit and the hair follicle on the basis of morphology and keratinization.[21, 23] To this may be added the patterning of the nail unit, which undoubtedly is important in development and is analogous to the patterning seen in follicle development. This patterning is manifest early in fetal development (it is, after all, easy to distinguish the little finger from the thumb, and fingers from toes), and it has been studied in the mouse.[6, 24] The resemblance of nail plate to hair shaft, both being hard structures formed by tricholemmal keratinization, is obvious.

The nail bed may be compared with the IRS. Both contribute little to the substance of the structure because they grow out with the hard, keratinized product. However, beyond this, similarities break down. No cuticles of the nail bed or nail plate exist, no layers resembling those of Huxley or Henley have been identified, nor does the nail bed mold or guide the nail plate as it grows out. The underlying bony phalanx plays a critical role in development of the nail unit.[25] Other than their origin from mesenchyme, it is difficult to relate this function to that of the cells in the hair papilla, and although the importance of the papilla for follicle development and growth is clear, the need for underlying bone once the nail unit has formed has not been demonstrated.

Components of the nail unit serve vital functions necessary for maintaining the integrity of the nail plate. The matrix makes the nail plate. The proximal nail fold protects much of the matrix and newly forming nail plate. The cuticle seals the proximal nail fold to the nail plate; disruption results in formation of a real space from a potential space, allowing irritants to enter and produce the inflammation seen in chronic paronychia. The hyponychium acts in a similar but inverted pattern, sealing the undersurface of the nail plate where it lifts off the tip of the digit; disruption of this area results in creation of a "cave" between the nail plate and the nail bed, as seen as onycholysis. The nail bed attaches the nail plate to the nail unit.[26]

As with hair, both epidermal and "hard" keratins are expressed in the nail unit, along with a number of intermediate filament-associated proteins, containing high sulfur or high tyrosine/glycine,[27] and trichohyalin.[28] Keratin expression in the proximal nail fold and fingertip epidermis is that of normal interfollicular epidermis. Keratins K5 and K14 are expressed in basal keratinocytes, K1 and K10 are expressed in suprabasal keratinocytes, and K2E is expressed by keratinocytes high in the spinous layer. (Note that the site of onset of K9 and K16 expression, seen in palmoplantar epidermis,[29] has not been defined; whether these keratins are seen in fingertip epidermis is unclear.) Nail matrix expresses normal interfollicular keratins; in addition, the hard keratins are expressed sporadically in the suprabasal layers of the matrix. Nail bed epithelium expresses the basal keratins, K5 and K14; K6, K16, and K17 are expressed in the suprabasal layers of the nail bed (I. Leigh, personal communication St. Bartholomew's and Royal London School of Medicine and Dentistry, London England, 1996). Trichohyalin, an intermediate filament-associated protein found in hair, is also found in the suprabasal layers of the nail matrix.[28]

CONTROL OF NAIL PLATE GROWTH

The cells of the nail matrix produce most of the nail plate; the nail bed contributes a few cells to the under-

surface of the plate. Despite arguments to the contrary, radioautographic studies support these conclusions.[26] Unlike the cells in the hair follicle, growth of the nail plate is constant rather than cyclical. When normal growth is interrupted, as in times of severe systemic stress, depressions in the surface of the nail plates result that are recognized as Beau's lines. The ultimate Beau's line is onychomadesis, shedding of the nail plate beginning from the proximal nail fold. An analogy could be drawn between Beau's lines and telogen effluvium, but it would be a stretch. How rapidly nail matrix cells divide in relation to hair, gut, or bone marrow is unknown. The rate of nail plate growth varies as a function of age, sex, season, and many other factors.[26]

The nail unit has no structure analogous to either the papilla or the bulge of the follicle. The limited number and distribution of nail units and the constant growth of the nail plate suggest that nails serve a more limited function than hair. Certainly nails are not involved in epidermal regeneration, as hair may be. One interesting aspect of nail development is its intimate association with development of the underlying bone. This has long been recognized clinically.[25] More recent studies of the developmental aspects of bone and nail may help to define this association.[24] Whether the underlying phalanx is necessary for continued health of a developed nail unit, as the follicular papilla is for the bulb, is unknown. The growth factors involved in development of the bone and nail unit are undefined.

Another unexplained aspect of nail growth and nail unit physiology is the relation between the lungs and the nail unit. First described by Hippocrates, the effects of lung parenchymal disorders on edema in the connective tissue beneath the lunula that result in clubbing have long been recognized but remain unexplained.[30] Even less well understood is the mechanism underlying decreased nail plate growth in the yellow nail syndrome, which is also frequently associated with pulmonary disorders.

PERSPECTIVES IN NAIL UNIT BIOLOGY

Even compared with follicle growth and development, understanding of the nail unit has far to go; descriptive science is lacking, and molecular mechanisms are for the most part unknown. Scientific tools available today suggest that several questions, clinical and more basic, can now be addressed at a more molecular level: (1) What genes and gene products control development and growth of the nail unit? What is the molecular basis for the relationship between the nail unit and the underlying bone? What is the molecular basis for brittle nails? (2) What is the molecular basis underlying the relation between nail growth and systemic metabolism, and what role does the lung play in this relation? What is the molecular basis for Beau's lines, clubbing, and the yellow nail syndrome? (3) What role does the immune system play in nail homeostasis? What is the molecular basis for the localization of psoriasis, alopecia areata, and lichen planus to the nail unit as well as the hair follicle? Does a systemic immunological defect underlie onychomycosis? The answers to these questions will lead to better understanding of the controls of nail development and growth and to more logical treatments for nail disorders.

REFERENCES

1. Holbrook KA, Fisher C, Dale BA, Hartley R: Morphogenesis of the hair follicle during the ontogeny of human skin. In: Rogers GE, Reis PJ, Ward KA, Marshall RC (eds): The Biology of Wool and Hair. London, Chapman & Hall, London. 1989, pp 15–35.
2. Hardy MH: The secret life of the hair follicle. Trends Genet 8: 55–61, 1992.
3. Zhou P, Byrne C, Jacobs J, Fuchs E: Lymphoid enhancer factor directs hair follicle patterning and epithelial cell fate. Genes Dev 9:570, 1995.
4. Bieberich CJ, Ruddle FU, Stenn KS: Differential expression of Hox 3.1 gene in adult mouse skin. Ann N Y Acad Sci 642:346–354, 1991.
5. Stenn KS, Combates NJ, Eilertsen KJ, et al: Hair follicle growth controls. Dermatol Clinics 14:543–558, 1996.
6. Godwin AR, Capecchi MR: *Hoxc13* mutant mice lack external hair. Genes Devel 12:11–20, 1998.
7. Rogers MA, Langbein L, Praetzel S, et al: Sequences and differential expression of three novel human type-II hair keratins. Differentiation 61:87–94, 1997.
8. Winter H, Siry P, Tobiasch E, Schweizer J: Sequence and expression of murine type I hair keratins mHa2 and mHa3. Exp Cell Res 212:190–200, 1994.
9. Williams DD, Stenn KS: Transection level dictates the pattern of hair follicle sheath growth in vitro. Dev Biol 165:469–479, 1994.
10. Jahoda CAB, Horne KA, Oliver RF: Induction of hair growth by implantation of cultured dermal papilla cells. Nature 311:560–562, 1984.
11. Link RE, Paus R, Stenn KS, Kuklinska E, Moelmann G: Epithelial growth in cultured rat vibrissae follicles requires mesenchymal contact via native extracellular matrix. J Invest Dermatol 95:202–207, 1990.
12. Cotsarelis G, Sun T-T, Lavker RM: Label-retaining cells reside in the bulge area of pilosebaceous unit: implications for follicular stem cells, hair cycle, and skin carcinogenesis. Cell 61:1329–1337, 1990.
13. Hebert JM, Rosenquist T, Goetz J, Martin GR: FGF5 as a regulator of the hair growth cycle: evidence from targeted and spontaneous mutations. Cell 78:1017–1025, 1994.
14. Jahoda CAB: Induction of follicle formation and hair growth by vibrissa dermal papillae implanted into rat ear wounds: vibrissa-type fibres are specified. Development II5:1103–1109, 1992.
15. Choudhry R, Hodgins MB, Van der Kwast TH, Brinkmann AO, Boersma WJA: Localization of androgen receptors in human skin by immunohistochemistry: implications for the hormonal regulation of hair growth, sebaceous glands and sweat glands. J Endocrinol 133:467–475, 1992.
16. Itami S, Kurata S, Takayasu S: Androgen induction of follicular epithelial cell growth is mediated via insulin-like growth factor-I from dermal papilla cells. Biochem Biophys Res Commun 212: 988–994, 1995.
17. Thornton MJ, Thomas DG, Jenner TJ, Brinklow BR, Loudon ASI, Randall VA: Testosterone or IGF-1 stimulates hair growth in whole organ culture only in androgen-dependent red deer hair follicles. In: VanNeste D, Randall VA (eds): Hair Research for the Next Millennium. Amsterdam, Elsevier Press 1996, pp 311–314.
18. Philpott MP, Sanders DA, Kealey T: Effect of insulin and insulin-like growth factors on cultured human hair follicles: IGF-I at physiologic concentrations is an important regulator of hair follicle growth in vitro. J Invest Dermatol 102:857–861, 1994.
19. Tobin DJ, Colen SR, Bystryn J-C: Isolation and long-term culture of human hair-follicle melanocytes. J Invest Dermatol 104:86–89, 1995.
20. Holbrook KA: Structure and function of developing skin. In: Goldsmith LA (ed): Physiology, Biochemistry, and Molecular Biology of the Skin, 2nd ed. New York, Oxford University Press, 1991, pp 63–110.
21. Zaias N: The Nail in Health and Disease, 2nd ed. Norwalk, CT, Appleton & Lange, 1990, p 1–255.
22. Forslind B: Biophysical studies of the normal nail. Acta Derm Venerol 50:161–168, 1970.
23. Gonzalez-Serva A: Structure and function. In: Scher RK, Daniel CR (eds): Nails: Therapy, Diagnosis, Surgery, 2nd ed. Philadelphia, WB Saunders, 1997, pp 18–19.
24. Loomis CA, Harris E, Michaud J, Wurst W, Hanks M, Joyner AL: The mouse engrailed-1 gene and ventral limb patterning. Nature 382:360–363, 1996.
25. Baran R, Juhlin L: Bone dependent nail formation. Br J Dermatol 114:371–375, 1986.
26. Fleckman P: Basic science of the nail unit. In: Scher RK, Daniel CR (eds): Nails: Therapy, Diagnosis, Surgery, 2nd ed. Philadelphia, WB Saunders, 1997, pp 37–54.
27. Powel BC, Rogers GE: Differentiation in hard keratin tissues: hair and related structures. In: Leigh IM, Lane EB, Watt FM (eds): The Keratinocyte Handbook. Cambridge, Cambridge University Press, 1994, 401–436.
28. O'Keefe EJ, Hamilton EH, Seung-Chul L, Steinert P: Trichohyalin: a structural protein of hair, tongue, nail, and epidermis. J Invest Dermatol 101(Suppl):65S–71S, 1993.
29. Moll I, Heid H, Franke WW, Moll R: Distribution of a special subset of keratinocytes characterized by the expression of cytokeratin 9 in adult and fetal human epidermis of various body sites. Differentiation 33:254–265, 1987.
30. Dickinson CJ: The aetiology of clubbing and hypertrophic osteoarthropathy. Eur J Clin Invest 23:330–338, 1993.

Hair and Nail Histology

...

HISTOLOGY OF NORMAL HAIR

DAVID A. WHITING

The human hair follicle consists of a permanent upper segment, comprising the infundibulum and the isthmus, and an impermanent lower segment, comprising the lower follicle and the hair root. The follicular apparatus almost continuously extrudes hair in a cyclical fashion.[1-3] The single hair fiber is a cellularly derived, tubular structure composed of keratin fibers embedded in sulphur-rich material and enclosed in a protective cuticle. The growing hair is generated by the hair bulb, which consists of the dermal papilla surrounded by hair matrix cells and root sheaths.

The rapidly dividing matrix cells differentiate into central medullary cells and many surrounding cortical cells, which are invested by hair cuticle cells. Mature medullary cells are seen only in terminal hair, and their significance is not clear. Cortical cells constitute the major portion of hair and are responsible for its mechanical properties. The cuticle cells bind the cortical fibers together.

Other components of the follicular apparatus include the inner and outer root sheaths. These mold the hair and allow outward migration of the developing hair shaft. The cuticular cells of the inner root sheath interlock with the cuticular cells of the hair shaft to ensure that the growing hair is not easily dislodged. The inner root sheath is present only in the inferior segment of the hair follicle; in the isthmus, it disappears and is replaced by trichilemmal keratin. The follicular infundibulum links the isthmus to the skin surface from the entrance of the sebaceous duct. It is lined with keratinizing epidermis continuous with surface epithelium.

Hair Development and Growth

The embryological development of hair follicles begins by the end of the second month of pregnancy.[1-4] Initially, an increased density of nuclei in the basal layer of the epidermis of the eyebrows, upper lip, and chin is seen. Other hair follicle precursors develop on the scalp and elsewhere, and the initial population is complete by 22 weeks of gestation. Fine, lanugo hair grows from these developing hair follicles and is shed by the end of the eighth month of gestation in an advancing wave from the frontal to the occipital scalp. A second coat of lanugo hair appears and is shed in a more or less synchronized wave pattern by the third or fourth month of life. By the end of the first year of life this synchronization is lost. After that, random distribution of follicles in all stages of the growth cycle is maintained. This produces an ever-changing mosaic pattern of growing follicles on the scalp.

The growth or anagen phase lasts from 2 to 6 years, 1000 days on average; and the resting or telogen phase lasts 2 to 4 months, an average of 100 days. The end of telogen is signaled by shedding of the telogen hair and development of the anagen hair. Assuming an average of

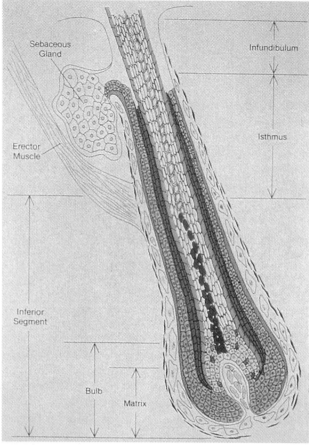

FIGURE 2-1 ■ Normal hair follicle. The hair follicle comprises the infundibulum, isthmus, and inferior segment. (From Whiting DA, Howsden FL: Color Atlas of Differential Diagnosis of Hair Loss. Fairfield, NJ, Canfield Publishing, 1996.)

100,000 hairs on the human scalp, with approximately 10% in telogen at any one time, then up to 10,000 hairs are shed every 100 days, an average loss of 100 hairs per day.

Large hairs, often pigmented and medullated, have a diameter exceeding 0.03 mm, grow to more than 1 cm in length, and are classified as terminal hairs. Small hairs, with no pigment or medullary cavity, a diameter less than 0.03 mm, and a length of less than 1 cm, are classified as vellus (downy) hairs. Depigmented hairs that are less than 0.03 mm in diameter and have been miniaturized by androgenetic alopecia, alopecia areata, or any other cause can be classified as vellus-like hairs. The designation *vellus hairs* in this chapter includes both true vellus and vellus-like hairs. Terminal hairs are rooted in the subcutaneous tissue, but vellus hairs are rooted in the dermis. The ratio of terminal to vellus hairs therefore denotes the proportion of large to small hairs, and in a normal scalp the average ratio is 7:1.

The termination of anagen is signaled by the onset of catagen.[1, 3-5] Catagen is the short intermediate phase between anagen and telogen; it indicates the onset of telogen, because it irrevocably commits the growing follicle to a resting phase. In catagen the hair shaft retracts upward, accompanied by shrinkage of the outer root sheath or trichilemma. This leads to progressive disappearance of the lower or impermanent part of the hair follicle, so that in telogen the resting hair root is seen near the insertion of the arrector pili muscle, the so-called bulge area containing stem cells,[6] where the permanent follicle begins.

The telogen bulb lacks pigment and both internal and external root sheaths and is surrounded by trichilemmal keratin. An angiofibrotic strand extending down from

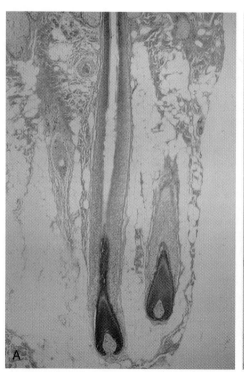

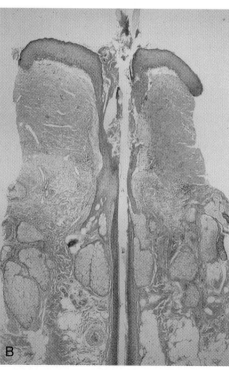

FIGURE 2-2 ■ Vertical section of a biopsy of scalp skin. *A*, The lower follicle, showing the hair bulb enclosing the dermal papilla and the hair shaft surrounded by internal and external root sheaths. *B*, The overlapping upper follicle comprising the infundibulum and isthmus. (Hematoxylin and eosin stain, original magnification 30×.)

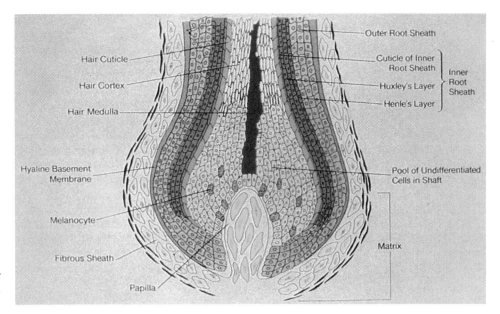

FIGURE 2-3 ■ Normal anagen hair root. The hair bulb surrounds the dermal papilla. It contains matrix cells that give rise to the medulla, hair cortex, cuticle of the hair shaft, inner root sheath (consisting of the cuticle of the inner root sheath, Huxley's layer, and Henle's layer), and outer root sheath (invested by hyaline membrane and fibrous sheath). (From Whiting DA, Howsden FL: Color Atlas of Differential Diagnosis of Hair Loss. Fairfield, NJ, Canfield Publishing, 1996.)

the permanent follicle indicates the former position of the retracted follicle. As a new anagen hair develops and grows, the club hair is shed and the cycle repeats.

Histology of Terminal Anagen Hair

In vertical sections the terminal anagen hair (Fig. 2-1) is seen to extend upward from the hair root in the

subcutaneous tissue, through the lower follicle, isthmus, and follicular infundibulum (Fig. 2-2), to exit the epidermis.[1-3, 5] The root (Fig. 2-3) consists of the hair bulb, which surrounds a conical dermal papilla that is composed of connective tissue cells, nerves, and blood vessels. The papilla is surrounded by undifferentiated, actively dividing, hair matrix cells (Fig. 2-4).

At the apex of the dermal papilla there are usually some melanocytes present, and the hair matrix cells in this area may give rise to medullary cells. Most of the hair matrix cells surrounding this central area give rise to elongated hair cortical cells, which stream upward to

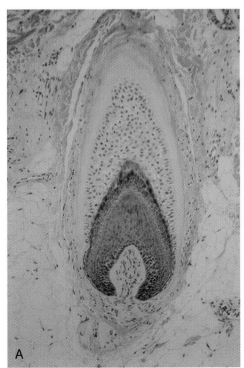

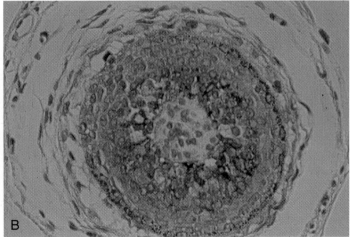

FIGURE 2-4 ■ A, Vertical section of hair root. The dermal papilla is surrounded by matrix cells and enveloped by the inner and outer root sheaths, hyaline membrane, and fibrous sheath. (Hematoxylin and eosin stain, original magnification 100×.) B, Horizontal section of hair bulb. The dermal papilla in the center contains connective tissue and fibroblasts. It is surrounded by melanocytes and hair matrix cells and then the inner root sheath, outer root sheath, and fibrous sheath. (Hematoxylin and eosin stain, original magnification 400×.)

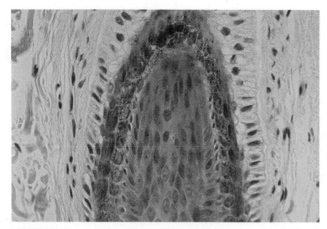

FIGURE 2–5 ■ Vertical section of lower follicle near bulb. The developing cortex is surrounded by cuticle cells, which point upward, toward the distal end of the hair, and which interdigitate with cuticle cells of the inner root sheath, which point downward. These are invested by Huxley's layer, Henle's layer, the outer root sheath, hyaline membrane, and fibrous sheath. (Hematoxylin and eosin stain, original magnification 400×.)

form the developing hair shaft. As they progress higher they enter into a keratogenous zone and later become compacted into hard keratin. The outer fringe of matrix cells forms the cuticle of the hair shaft, which invests the hair with 6 to 10 overlapping layers of cuticle cells. These later become keratinized and project outward and forward to interlock with the inwardly projecting cuticular cells of the inner root sheath (Fig. 2–5).

The inner root sheath develops around the cuticle of the hair shaft and is composed of three layers. The inner layer forms the cuticle of the inner root sheath; it consists of a layer of elongated cells that in due course slant downward. Surrounding the cuticle of the inner root sheath is a layer of three or four cells, somewhat cuboidal, which is known as the *layer of Huxley*. Surrounding them is a single layer of elongated cells known

as the *layer of Henle*. The layer of Henle is invested by one or more layers of cells of the outer root sheath, which are covered in turn by a hyaline or vitreous membrane and finally by the connective tissue or fibrous sheath of the hair follicle. A pad of elastic tissue, known as the *Arao-Perkins body*, may develop under the dermal papilla.[7]

Proceeding upward from the bulb, the various layers surrounding the hair shaft become more obvious. Inner and outer root sheaths become thicker and well demarcated. The first layer to show keratinization is the outer layer of the internal root sheath, Henle's layer (Fig. 2–6). Trichohyaline granules become visible, and Henle's layer gradually becomes keratinized into a distinct, pinkish, keratinized band. Keratinization then commences in the cuticle of the inner root sheath and in the cuticle of the hair shaft. The last layer to develop trichohyaline granules and become keratinized is Huxley's layer (Fig. 2–7).

Keratinization of the inner root sheath is completed halfway up the lower follicle (Fig. 2–8A). Proceeding up through the lower follicle, the keratinization is maintained (Fig. 2–9A) until the isthmus is reached at the level of insertion of the arrector pili muscle (i.e., at the bulge). From this point upward, the crumbling inner root sheath is replaced by trichilemmal keratin from the trichilemma or external root sheath that lines the isthmus (Fig. 2–10A). This trichilemmal keratin persists upward through the isthmus until the point of entry of the sebaceous duct. From here, the trichilemmal keratin is supplanted by ordinary basketweave keratin with an underlying granular layer that lines the infundibulum (Fig. 2–11) and is continuous with the surface epidermis of the scalp (Fig. 2–12A). The infundibulum funnels outward and allows the hair shaft some freedom of movement. The hair shaft has no secure attachments to the isthmus or infundibulum, in contrast to the interlocking cuticles in the lower follicle.

The horizontal sections of the lower portion of the

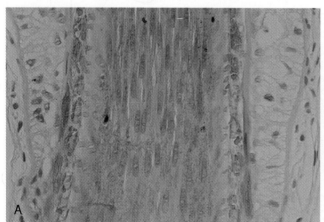
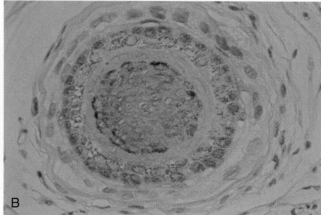

FIGURE 2–6 ■ Terminal anagen hair near bulb. *A*, Vertical section. Hair cortex is surrounded by its cuticle, the cuticle of the inner root sheath, Huxley's layer, Henle's layer (which is beginning to keratinize), the outer root sheath, hyaline membrane, and fibrous sheath. (Hematoxylin and eosin stain, original magnification 400×.) *B*, Horizontal section. The hair matrix cells are differentiating into central cortical cells, surrounded by the cuticles of the hair shaft and inner root sheath, Huxley's layer, the keratinizing Henle's layer with trichohyaline granules, the external root sheath, and the fibrous sheath. (Hematoxylin and eosin stain, original magnification 400×.)

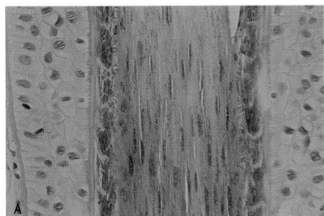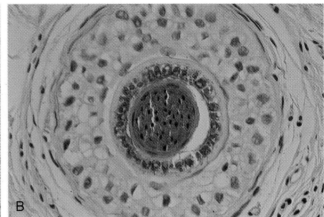

FIGURE 2–7 ■ Terminal anagen hair, lower segment. *A,* Vertical section. The central hair shaft is surrounded by its keratinized cuticle interdigitating with the cuticle of the inner root sheath. Trichohyaline granules are visible in the keratinizing Huxley's layer, which is invested by keratinized Henle's layer, the external root sheath, hyaline membrane, and fibrous sheath. (Hematoxylin and eosin stain, original magnification 400×.) *B,* Horizontal section. The central hair is surrounded by its keratinized cuticle and the keratinized cuticular layer of the inner root sheath. Huxley's layer is beginning to keratinize; Henle's layer outside it is completely keratinized and is invested by the external root sheath, hyaline membrane, and fibrous sheath. (Hematoxylin and eosin stain, original magnification 400×.)

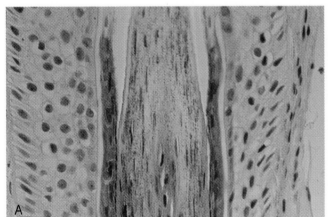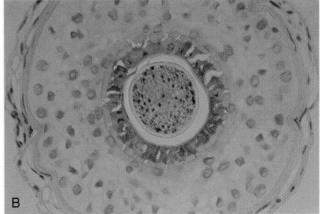

FIGURE 2–8 ■ Terminal anagen hair, mid-lower segment. *A,* Vertical section. The central hair shaft is surrounded by keratinized cuticle, keratinized internal root sheath cuticle, the keratinizing Huxley's layer, the keratinized Henle's layer, the external root sheath, hyaline membrane, and connective tissue sheath. At the upper end of the section the keratinization of the root sheath has become complete. (Hematoxylin and eosin stain, original magnification 400×.) *B,* Horizontal section. The hair shows a keratinized cortex and cuticle. The internal root sheath shows keratinization of the cuticle with advancing keratinization of Huxley's layer. Henle's layer is fully keratinized and is surrounded by the external root sheath, hyaline membrane, and fibrous sheath. (Hematoxylin and eosin stain, original magnification 400×.)

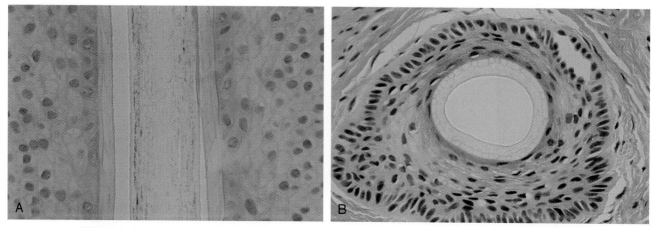

FIGURE 2-9 ▪ Terminal anagen hair, lower segment, middle to upper portion. *A,* Vertical section. The keratinized hair shaft and cuticle are surrounded by the totally keratinized internal root sheath, invested by the external root sheath. (Hematoxylin and eosin stain, original magnification 400×.) *B,* Horizontal section. A fully keratinized internal root sheath is surrounded by the external root sheath and fibrous sheath. (Hematoxylin and eosin stain, original magnification 400×.)

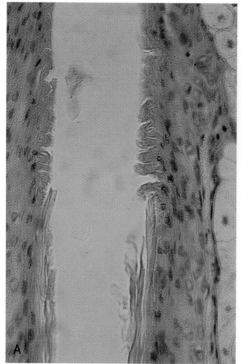

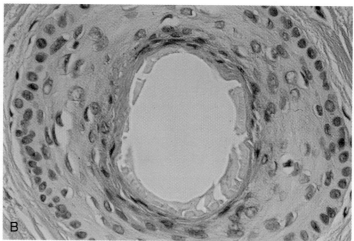

FIGURE 2-10 ▪ Terminal anagen hair, follicular isthmus. *A,* Vertical section. In the lower end of the section, the internal root sheath is seen entering the isthmus. It disappears and is replaced by trichilemmal keratin from the external root sheath, which is lining the isthmus. Sebaceous gland is present on one side of the section. (Hematoxylin and eosin stain, original magnification 300×.) *B,* Horizontal section. The clear, pinkish-gray fragments of internal root sheath are being replaced by reddish, trichilemmal keratin produced by the trichilemmal or external root sheath. (Hematoxylin and eosin stain, original magnification 400×.)

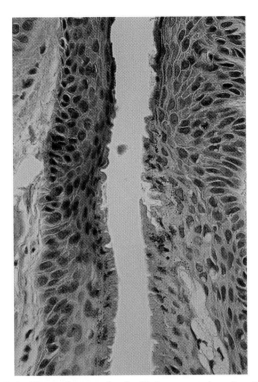

FIGURE 2-11 ■ Isthmus and infundibulum, vertical section. The sebaceous duct is seen entering the follicular canal in the middle of this section, and beneath it the canal is lined by trichilemmal keratin from the external root sheath. Above the level of the sebaceous duct, the trichilemmal keratin is replaced by keratin lining the infundibulum, which is generated by epidermis, which shows a granular layer that is continuous with surface epidermis. (Hematoxylin and eosin stain, original magnification 100×.)

hair bulb show a central dermal papilla containing connective tissue, fibroblasts, and blood vessels.[8–10] This is surrounded by a circular area of matrix cells that is covered by an inner and outer root sheath and then by a hyaline layer and a fibrous layer of connective tissue (Fig. 2–4B). Higher in the bulb, the dermal papilla is supplanted by matrix cells that may or may not show developing medullary cells in the center, in addition to melanocytes. Higher sections proximal to the bulb show the commencing keratinization in Henle's layer (Fig. 2–6B), and further up keratinization is seen in the cuticles of the hair shaft and inner root sheath. The last layer to keratinize is Huxley's layer (Fig. 2–7B), in which keratinization is complete by the middle of the lower segment of the follicle (Fig. 2–8B).

From the middle of the lower segment of the follicle to the level of arrector pili insertion, a fully keratinized, inner root sheath is characteristic of the anagen hair as seen in horizontal sections (Fig. 2–9B). Horizontal sections of the lower isthmus show that the inner root sheath is crumbling and is being replaced by trichilemmal keratin from the trichilemma (Fig. 2–10B). At the upper end of the isthmus, at the level of the sebaceous duct where the infundibulum commences, the trichilemmal keratin is replaced by basketweave keratin with an underlying granular layer (Fig. 2–12B).

Horizontal sections of scalp biopsies at the level of the sebaceous ducts show the presence of the so-called follicular units.[8, 9] These roughly hexagonal packets of tissue surrounded by a loose network of collagen contain several terminal and vellus hair follicles as well as sebaceous glands, sebaceous ducts, and arrector pili muscles

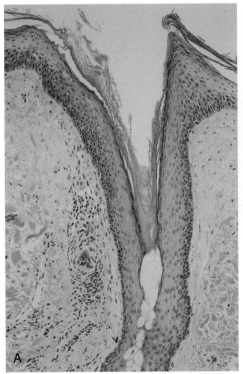

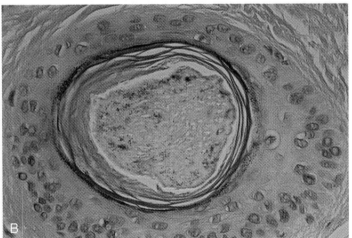

FIGURE 2-12 ■ Follicular infundibulum. *A*, Vertical section. The follicular infundibulum extends from the level of entry of the sebaceous duct up to the skin surface. It is lined by basketweave keratin, which is continuous with the keratin on the skin surface and under which the epithelium shows a granular layer. (Hematoxylin and eosin stain, original magnification 100×.) *B*, Horizontal section. A fully keratinized hair is seen surrounded by loose basketweave keratin, epidermis with a granular layer, and a connective tissue sheath. It is impossible to tell whether the hair shaft here represents an anagen hair, a catagen hair, or a telogen hair. (Hematoxylin and eosin stain, original magnification 400×.)

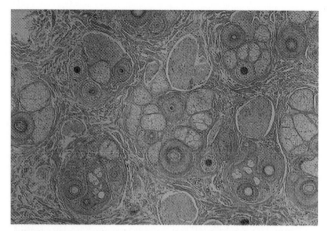

FIGURE 2–13 ■ Scalp biopsy. Horizontal section at the level of the sebaceous ducts displays roughly hexagonal follicular units surrounded by loose collagen. Each unit contains terminal and vellus follicles, sebaceous glands, sebaceous ducts, and arrector pili muscle. (Hematoxylin and eosin stain, original magnification 40×.)

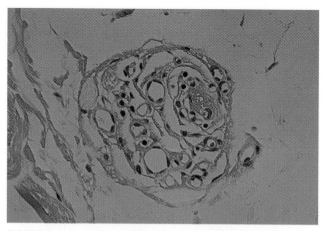

FIGURE 2–14 ■ Follicular stella, streamer, or fibrous tract, horizontal section. This angiofibrotic whorl, variously named a follicular stella, streamer, or fibrous tract, represents the former position of the hair shaft, which has retracted upward from its original position. (Hematoxylin and eosin stain, original magnification 400×.)

(Fig. 2–13). The average number of follicular units per 4-mm punch biopsy is 13, and each represents about 1 mm² of tissue.

(Fig. 2–15).[8–10] Follicular stellae in the reticular dermis are indicators of catagen, telogen, and vellus hairs and appear as round or oval islands of angiofibrotic tissue.

Histology of Vellus and Vellus-like Hair

Vellus hairs are rooted in the upper half of the skin in papillary or upper reticular dermis.[1, 3, 5] Vellus hairs are less than 0.03 mm in cross-section, and the diameter of the hair is usually less than the diameter of its accompanying inner root sheath.[8] By virtue of their small size, vellus hairs cycle through growth and rest far more frequently than terminal hairs. It is not always possible to differentiate between true vellus hairs and vellus-like hairs, which may result from miniaturization caused by conditions such as androgenetic alopecia and alopecia areata.

Terminal hairs exceed 0.03 mm in cross-section, and the diameter of the hair shaft exceeds the thickness of the accompanying inner root sheath. It is sometimes useful to differentiate intermediate hairs, between 0.03 and 0.06 mm in diameter, which may represent early miniaturization of terminal hairs as seen in androgenetic alopecia. Vellus hairs usually contain no pigment and do not contain medullary cavities. As a rule, arrector pili muscles are not seen. Vellus-like hairs resulting from miniaturization show a more substantial external root sheath than do true vellus hairs. An angiofibrotic strand extending down from the vellus follicle, known variously as a follicular stella, streamer, or fibrous tract, indicates the former position of the retracted follicle. This fibrous tract is also seen below catagen and telogen hairs that are retreating upward in the resting stage of the hair cycle (Fig. 2–14).

Vellus hairs are usually clearly demonstrable in horizontal section, with a shaft diameter obviously smaller than the thickness of the surrounding inner root sheath

Histology of Catagen and Telogen Hair

With termination of the anagen or growing cycle, the hair goes into a temporary stage known as catagen for the next 10 to 14 days.[1, 3, 11] At that point the hair and hair bulb start to retract upward, leaving behind a fibrous streamer or stela. As the hair shaft retracts upward, it takes the inner root sheath with it and leaves behind an elongated mass of external root sheath or trichilemma. A volumetric shrinkage of this tissue en-

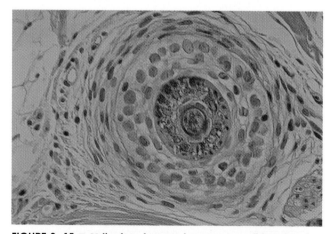

FIGURE 2–15 ■ Vellus hair, horizontal section. A small hair, less than 0.03 mm in diameter, is surrounded by an internal root sheath, the thickness of which exceeds the diameter of the vellus hair. The keratinizing internal root sheath is invested by the external root sheath, hyaline layer, and fibrous layer. (Hematoxylin and eosin stain, original magnification 400×.)

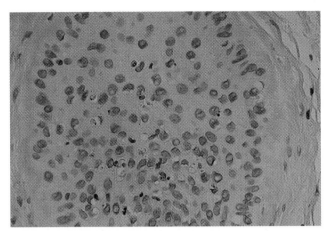

FIGURE 2–16 ■ Catagen hair. This horizontal section taken below the hair shaft shows trichilemmal keratin containing apoptotic cells. It is surrounded by a thickened and wrinkled hyaline layer. (Hematoxylin original magnification 400×.)

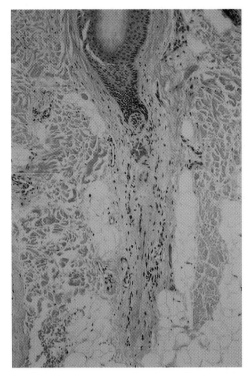

FIGURE 2–17 ■ Telogen follicle and stella. At the top of this vertical section a telogen follicle is seen retreating up the hair follicle above the root, beneath which is a follicular stella or angiofibrotic streamer. It extends down into the subcutaneous tissue to the level of the former position or the bulb. (Hematoxylin and eosin stain, original magnification 100×.)

sues. This is accomplished by individual cell death or apoptosis of trichilemmal cells. As this shrinkage occurs, there is a concomitant thickening and wrinkling of the hyaline layer that surrounds the trichilemma.

Catagen hairs show a characteristic appearance on horizontal section below the level of the hair shaft (Fig. 2–16).[8–10] Here trichilemmal keratin is surrounded by a thickened hyaline layer of connective tissue of the sheath. Many of the trichilemmal cells show apoptosis.

As the hair shaft retreats further upward, its base becomes club-shaped, rooted in a pocket of trichilemmal keratin and surrounded by trichilemma (Fig. 2–17). The vestigial dermal papilla trails below. As the telogen hair develops, it eventually retracts to the level of the bulge at the insertion of the arrector pili muscle. There a telogen germinal unit is formed below the telogen club. This consists of trichilemma that is somewhat convoluted and surrounded by palisading basal cells. This has a characteristic appearance and shows no apoptosis. This is the resting stage of the hair cycle; it lasts some 3 months until a new hair follicle grows below it.

The resting hair follicle or telogen germinal unit is an irregular island of basaloid cells, with some peripheral palisading, situated beneath the telogen club root (Fig. 2–18). When sectioned below the proximal hair shaft, the telogen hair shows a star-shaped central mass of trichilemmal keratin surrounded by trichilemma, hyaline sheath, and fibrous sheath; no apoptosis is seen (Fig. 2–19). Examination of horizontal sections of the impermanent or inferior portion of the hair follicle shows the differences between terminal anagen hairs, catagen hairs, and telogen hairs. The terminal anagen hair is characterized by the presence of intact, fully keratinized inner and outer root sheaths. Catagen hair shows retraction upward with volume shrinkage, and the lower portion of the hair follicle consists of trichilemmal keratin with apoptotic cells. As this turns into a telogen hair, there is a mass of trichilemmal keratin beneath the ascending hair follicle surrounded by trichilemma, but apopto-

sis is no longer visible and no inner root sheath is seen. In the permanent or upper portion of the hair follicle, there is no internal root sheath, and only a keratinized hair shaft can be seen. It is not possible to tell

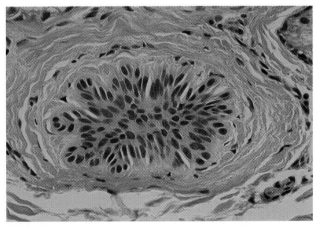

FIGURE 2–18 ■ Telogen germinal unit, horizontal section. This irregular island of basaloid cells with peripheral palisading represents the resting stage of the hair follicle. It remains here in telogen for 2 to 4 months at the lower end of the permanent follicle in the region of the bulge, where the arrector pili muscle inserts into the follicle. When telogen ends and anagen commences, a new anagen bud will grow down the original follicular tract to produce a new hair. (Hematoxylin and eosin stain, original magnification 400×.)

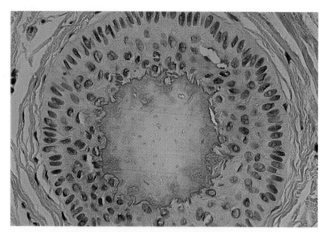

FIGURE 2–19 ■ Telogen hair. Horizontal section through the club-shaped bulb below the actual hair shaft. A central star-shaped area of trichilemmal keratin is seen. This is surrounded by external root sheath or trichilemma, hyaline membrane, and fibrous sheath. (Hematoxylin and eosin stain, original magnification 400×.)

on horizontal section from that level upward whether this represents an anagen hair, catagen hair, or telogen hair.

After 2 to 4 months of telogen, a new anagen hair

bud develops beneath the germinal unit and grows down the existing follicular tract to form an anagen hair.

Follicular Counts

It is sometimes useful to have an accurate count of the hair follicles in a section and to know what proportion are in anagen, catagen, and telogen.[9] It is also useful to determine the ratio of terminal to vellus hairs and the counts of follicular stellae and follicular units. Accurate follicular counts can be obtained on horizontal sections, and here it is important to bisect a punch biopsy 1 to 1.5 mm beneath the dermoepidermal junction and mount the two sections together face down in the block. Serial sectioning progresses upward into the papillary dermis and down into the reticular dermis and subcutaneous tissue. In this way all terminal hairs and follicular stelae in the reticular dermis and all vellus hairs in the papillary dermis can be counted.

With a 4-mm punch biopsy from the average normal control patient, the mean follicular count of a total of 40 hairs comprises 35 terminal and 5 vellus hairs, a ratio of 7:1; 93.5% anagen and 6.5% telogen hairs; and a follicular density of approximately 3/mm[3].[12]

■ ■ ■

HISTOLOGY OF THE NORMAL NAIL UNIT

MELODY STONE

ANGELA R. STYLES

CLAY J. COCKERELL

The nail apparatus is a specialized keratinous appendage whose functions in humans include protection of the terminal phalanx, contributions to fine touch and skilled hand movement, and the ability to pick up small objects.[13] It is produced by the germinative epithelium of the matrix in much the same fashion as the basal epidermal cells produce the stratum corneum. Nail cornification is similar to cornification of the epidermis and hair; however, in contrast to the soft keratin of the epidermis, nail and hair keratinocytes form a hard keratin. The hardness of the nail is caused by the high concentration of sulfur matrix protein.[14] Unlike hair, the nail continues to grow continuously, without a resting phase, by the addition of new cells from the matrix. Contrary to popular belief, the matrix cells cease DNA synthesis and cell division shortly after death, and therefore the nail is incapable of further growth. What is commonly thought of as nail growth after death is due

to retraction of periungual skin and soft tissue, which results in an apparent lengthening of the nail plate.

The anatomy of the human nail is defined by a complex set of structures collectively known as the *nail unit*. The nail unit as defined by Zaias[15] is composed of four epithelial components: the nail bed, the hyponychium, the proximal nail fold, and the matrix (Fig. 2–20). The nail plate is the horny end product of the most important epithelial component, the matrix. Like skin and hair, the nail unit is made up of an epithelial component with a "live" germinative cell layer that differentiates and cornifies, producing an end product that is considered to be "dead."[15] The nail plate is roughly rectangular and flat but demonstrates considerable variation. Although it is translucent, it appears pink as a consequence of the rich underlying vascular network (Figs. 2–21 and 2–22). A white, crescent-shaped lunula is seen projecting from under the proximal nail fold. It

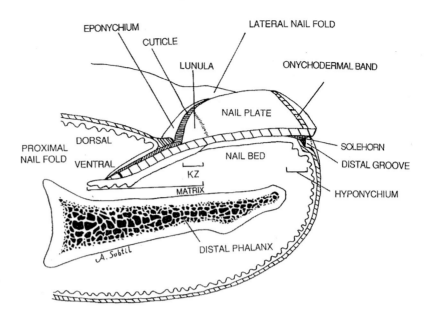

FIGURE 2-20 ■ Schematic illustration of a sagittal section of the nail unit. KZ, keratogenous zone. (Courtesy of Dr. Antonio Jubtil-DeOlivera.)

is the most distal portion of the matrix and determines the shape of the free edge of the nail plate.[14] Its color is caused by scattering of light by the nucleated cells of the keratogenous zone of the matrix.

As the nail plate emerges from the matrix, its borders are enveloped by three normal skin structures, known as the two lateral nail folds and the single proximal nail fold. The proximal nail fold is the most important of the three because it has a fundamental role in the formation of the nail plate. Approximately one fourth of the total surface area of the nail plate is located under the proximal nail fold.

Biopsy of the nail unit is the method by which etiologic, diagnostic, and prognostic information is obtained. However, knowledge of the histopathology of nail disease is more limited than that of disease of the glabrous skin because of a greater reluctance to biopsy the nail unit. In order to fully understand the numerous disease processes that affect the nail and to establish a correct

diagnosis from a biopsy specimen, it is essential to know in detail the normal histology of the nail plate and the four epithelial components that constitute the nail unit.

Microscopic Anatomy and Histology of The Nail Unit

NAIL PLATE

Microscopically, the nail plate consists of closely packed, cornified cells that lack nuclei and organelles.[16] The onychocytes of the dorsal nail plate are normally irregular, polyhedral, and anucleate. There are many intercellular links between cells, including tight, intermediate, and desmosomal junctions.[14] The cells on the surface of the nail plate overlap, slanting from proximal-dorsal to distal-volar.[17] As a result, the dorsal aspect of the nail plate

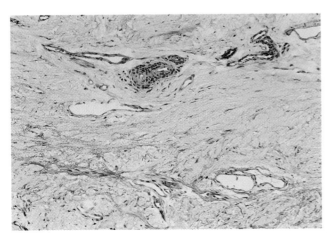

FIGURE 2-21 ■ Subepithelial stroma of nail unit. There is a loose fibromyxoid stroma containing numerous blood vessels. (Hematoxylin and eosin stain, original magnification 200×.)

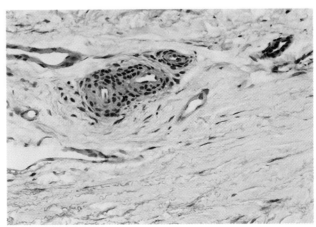

FIGURE 2-22 ■ Higher magnification of nail unit stroma demonstrates the presence of dilated blood vessels and glomus body. (Hematoxylin and eosin stain, original magnification 400×.)

reveals a smooth surface while the palmar aspect is irregular, as seen by scanning electron microscopy.[18] The lunula is composed of epithelial cells with flattened nuclei and eosinophilic cytoplasm with retained keratohyaline granules. This corresponds to the keratogenous zone of the nail matrix. These cells eventually lose their nuclei and form the nail plate cells, or onychocytes, which are devoid of keratohyaline granules.

The formation of the nail plate involves a progressive flattening of the basal cells from the matrix as they mature to form nail plate cells, with fragmentation and lysis of basal-cell nuclei and retention of nuclear membranes in the onychocytes.[15] The nail plate varies in thickness from 0.5 mm in women to 0.6 mm in men.[17] The length of the nail matrix determines the thickness of the nail, based on autoradiographic data.[15]

PROXIMAL NAIL FOLD

Three potential spaces would become apparent if the nail plate were not present; these are the single proximal and the two lateral nail grooves. Folds of skin known as the proximal and lateral nail folds wrap around the nail plate and form these grooves. The proximal nail fold is an invaginated, wedge-shaped fold of skin on the dorsum of the distal digit (Fig. 2–23). It consists of both a dorsal and a ventral surface epithelium (Fig. 2–24). The keratinization process in both portions is the same as that of the epidermis elsewhere, with a granular layer that is absent in all parts of the nail matrix (Fig. 2–25) (Table 2–1).

The dorsal surface of the proximal nail fold is a continuation of the epidermis and dermis of the digit and contains sweat glands but no follicles or sebaceous glands. The epidermis includes all the layers found in normal skin, including a granular layer and a rete ridge–dermal papilla pattern.

At the distal tip of the proximal nail fold the skin reflects proximally and ventrally, then extends approximately 5 mm toward the distal interphalangeal joint. The skin of the ventral portion is very thin and has all of the layers of normal epidermis, including a granular

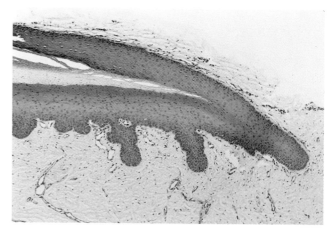

FIGURE 2–24 ■ Higher magnification of proximal nail matrix. Note the forming nail plate with parakeratotic nuclei. (Hematoxylin and eosin stain, original magnification 40×.)

layer; however, it lacks both a rete ridge–dermal papilla pattern and appendages. The stratum corneum of the dorsal tip and the ventral walls extends onto the dorsal surface of the nail as the cuticle; this provides a protective barrier to the entry of infectious organisms into the germinative matrix. Deep to the edge of the cuticle and continuous with the ventral wall dorsally is the eponychium. It has been demonstrated[15] that the eponychium results from cuticular desquamation occurring on the nail plate, although this theory has been the source of some controversy.[19] Diseases that affect the ventral portion of the proximal nail fold may affect the newly formed nail plate and lead to pits and grooves.

NAIL MATRIX

The nail matrix, the most important component of the nail unit, is the germinative epithelium that gives rise to the nail plate through differentiation of its basal cells. It is bordered proximally by the ventral proximal nail fold

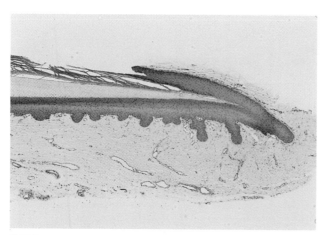

FIGURE 2–23 ■ Histology of the proximal nail matrix, scanning magnification. Note the elongated, thin epithelial retia. (Hematoxylin and eosin stain, original magnification 20×.)

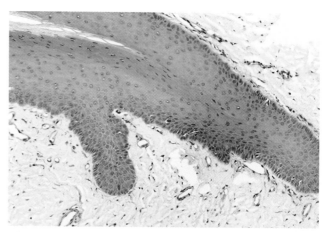

FIGURE 2–25 ■ Further magnification demonstrates the junction of the invaginated matrical epithelium with the incipient nail plate. There is no granular cell layer. (Hematoxylin and eosin stain, original magnification 400×.)

TABLE 2-1 ■ Epithelial Components of the Nail Unit

Epithelial Component	Histological Features	Horny End Product	Mitotic Activity
Proximal nail fold	Similar to skin or slightly acanthotic, with a granular layer	Cuticle	Active
Matrix	Acanthotic, without a granular layer	Nail plate	Very active
Nail bed	Flat, without a granular layer	Few horny cells added to underside of nail plate as it moves distally	Very inactive
Hyponychium	Acanthotic, with a granular layer	Few horny cells added to underside of nail plate distally, similar to cuticle	Active

and distally by the nail bed. The matrix is composed of a thick epithelium that is continuous with the epithelium of the ventral portion of the proximal nail fold. Because the matrix is devoid of a granular layer, the transition from the ventral part of the proximal nail fold to the matrix is seen easily. The matrix epithelium is acanthotic and demonstrates small villous structures that project downward from the basal layer and interdigitate in a finger-like fashion with the underlying papillary dermal counterpart (Figs. 2–26 and 2–27). From these projections, anchoring filaments extend from the basal cells to collagen fibers in the dermis.[15] This provides a firm attachment of the matrix to the subepithelial connective tissue and can be seen only for a few millimeters before the matrix flattens itself. Like the epidermis of the skin, the matrix contains a very actively dividing basal layer of keratinoblast-producing keratinocytes that differentiate, harden, die, and contribute to the nail plate.[14]

The epithelial differentiation process is similar to that seen in the hair matrix. The end product is a horny layer, the nail plate, which is a hard keratinous structure. The nail plate, as previously described, is formed by a process that involves flattening of the basal cells of the matrix, fragmentation of their nuclei, and condensation of the cytoplasm to form horny, flat cells.[15] The keratogenous zone corresponds to the lunula and is the region of the matrix where the cells begin to flatten and

develop eosinophilic cytoplasm. The nuclei are retained in this zone. Important histological features of the matrix include the lack of a granular cell layer, acanthosis, and papillomatosis. Papillomatosis is also found distally in the hyponychium but not anywhere else in the nail unit. There are few melanocytes in the nail matrix of Caucasians, but nail pigmentation is quite common in dark-skinned persons. Occasional Merkel's and Langerhans' cells are identified in the matrix.

The question of where the nail plate is formed is disputed. Some researchers believed that the nail plate is the product of three different matrices. However, Zaias, using autoradiography in monkey nail and the incorporation of ³H-labeled glycine and thymidine in human toenails, concluded that the matrix is solely responsible for the formation of the nail plate. Portions of the matrix that are proximal form the most superficial portions of the nail plate, and the distal matrix (lunula) cells form the deepest, or most ventral, portions of the nail plate. Zaias concluded that the deep part of the nail plate formed by the distal matrix (lunula) is "ahead of," or more distal to, the more superficial part of the plate, which is made by the proximal matrix area. This supports the theory that the shape of the nail is related to the shape of the lunula.[15] Accordingly, shortening of the distal matrix results in a thin nail plate, whereas focal

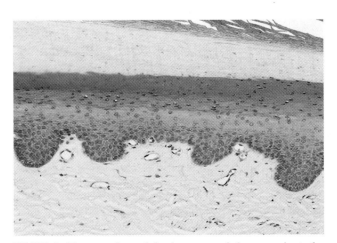

FIGURE 2-26 ■ Histology of distal matrix epithelium reveals similar changes to those seen proximally but with less elongation of epithelial retia. (Hematoxylin and eosin stain, original magnification 400×.)

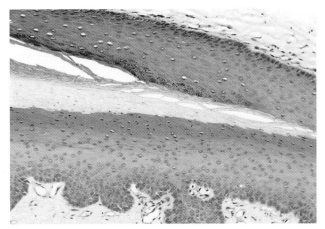

FIGURE 2-27 ■ Histology of a section of nail unit taken at level just distal to distal matrix including the proximal nail fold. Note the two distinct patterns of epithelial differentiation, with changes similar to those of distal matrix on the bottom and changes similar to those of normal skin with a granular cell layer on the top. (Hematoxylin and eosin stain, original magnification 400×.)

loss or scarring of the matrix results in a linear absence of nail plate with formation of "pterygium." Obviously, complete loss of the matrix results in complete absence of the nail plate.

NAIL BED

The nail bed begins where the distal matrix or lunula ends; it extends to the hyponychium near the end of the finger, where the free edge of the nail separates. Like the matrix, the nail bed epithelium cornifies without a granular layer. However, unlike the matrix, the nail bed consists of a thin epithelium that lies beneath the nail plate, and it is less active and has a longer turnover time than either the matrix or the skin (Figs. 2–28 and 2–29).[14] Therefore, histological differentiation between the matrical epithelium and that of the nail bed is a simple matter. The cornified layer of the nail bed is scant, and few cornified cells are added to the underside of the already formed nail plate. The transition zone from living keratinocytes to dead ventral nail plate cells is abrupt and is very similar to what occurs in the Henle layer of the internal root sheath of the formative hair shaft.[14]

The nail bed is firmly attached to the underlying dermis by a unique longitudinal, tongue-in-groove spatial arrangement of papillary dermal papillae and epidermal ridges.[15] These ridges are almost parallel to one another and are readily demonstrated after avulsion of the nail plate or in transverse histological sections. Fine capillaries traverse the parallel dermal ridges, and disruption results in the splinter hemorrhages commonly seen in normal and disease states.[15] The nail plate is firmly attached to the nail bed, more so than to the matrix, and this seems to be accomplished by interdigitation of the same longitudinal ridges of the nail bed with the undersurface of the nail plate.

Under normal conditions,[15] the nail plate is formed exclusively by the matrix. The thin, parakeratotic keratin that the nail bed produces is apparently dragged forward by the nail plate that is growing over it, rather than

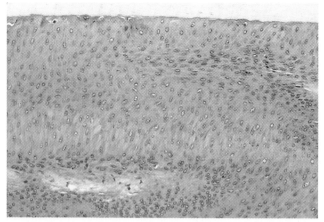

FIGURE 2–29 ■ Higher magnification of the nail bed reveals the maturation of the keratinocytes within the nail bed epithelium. Note the absence of the granular cell layer. (Hematoxylin and eosin stain, original magnification 400×.)

becoming incorporated into the nail. In addition, the nail bed cells stain eosinophilic, in contrast to the nail plate cells. This theory is apparently at variance with the observation that a splinter hemorrhage, located between the nail plate and the nail bed, grows out with the plate. Zaias[15] suggested that the growth rate and movement of the matrix and of the nail bed cells is identical as the sloughed nail bed epithelial cells progress distally toward the hyponychium. However, Samman[13] suggested that in certain pathological conditions the nail bed adds a ventral component to the undersurface of the nail plate. Future studies are required to clarify these issues.

HYPONYCHIUM

The hyponychium is a narrow zone of epidermis between the nail bed and the distal nail groove beneath the free edge of the nail plate. Like the volar skin of the finger, the hyponychium cornifies with a granular layer and produces a thick, compact, cornified layer (Fig. 2–30). The epithelium demonstrates marked acanthosis and papillomatosis with the crests oriented horizontally, an architecture that is similar to that seen in normal skin appendages.[14] An important feature of this zone is the accumulation of cornified debris under the distal nail plate, which renders the nail bed impermeable to external insults. Some authors have identified that part of the hyponychium that is most intimately attached to the undersurface of the nail plate as the "sole horn," a ventral "cuticle" lying between the plate and the distal bed epithelium.[18] The hyponychium is the initial site of invasion by dermatophytes in the most common type of onychomycosis, distal subungual onychomycosis.

The intermediate zone between the nail bed and hyponychium has been termed the *onychodermal band*. It varies in width from 0.5 to 1.5 mm and has a paler color than the pink nail bed because it has a different blood supply than the remainder of the nail bed has.[14]

The most distal boundary of the hyponychium and nail unit is marked by the distal groove. This area marks the demarcation of the "nail field," the earliest external change in the development of the nail.[17]

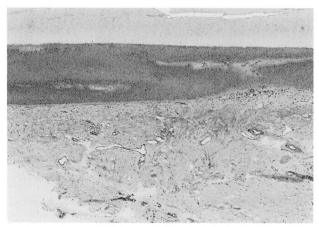

FIGURE 2–28 ■ Histology of nail bed tissue. Intact nail plate overlies a flat stratified squamous epithelium. (Hematoxylin and eosin stain, original magnification 200×.)

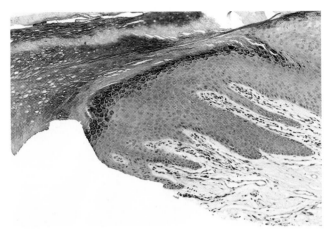

FIGURE 2-30 ■ Histology of the hyponychium. There are features similar to those of volar skin, with acanthosis, hypergranulosis, and hyperkeratosis. (Hematoxylin and eosin stain, original magnification 200×.)

LATERAL NAIL FOLDS

The lateral nail folds are structurally similar to the adjacent skin but are devoid of dermatoglyphical markings and pilosebaceous glands. As in the hyponychium, acanthosis and papillomatosis of the epithelium as well as a granular layer are present. The lateral nail folds do not contribute to the formation of the nail plate.

REFERENCES

1. Abell E: Embryology and anatomy of the hair follicle. In: Olsen EA (ed): Disorders of Hair Growth, Diagnosis and Treatment. New York, McGraw-Hill, 1994, pp 1–19.
2. Ackerman AB, de Viragh PA, Chongchitnant N: Neoplasms with Follicular Differentiation. Philadelphia, Lea & Febiger, 1993, pp 21–102.
3. Whiting DA, Howsden FL: Color Atlas of Differential Diagnosis of Hair Loss. Cedar Grove, Canfield Publishing, 1996, pp 4–17.
4. Pinkus H: Embryology of hair. In: Montagna W, Ellis RA (eds): The Biology of Hair Growth. New York, Academic Press, 1958, pp 1–32.
5. Montagna W, Parakkal PF: The Structure and Function of the Skin, 3rd ed. New York, Academic Press, 1974, pp 172–258.
6. Cotsarelis G, Sun T, Lavker RM: Label-retaining cells reside in the bulge area of pilo-sebaceous unit: implications for follicular stem cells, hair cycle and skin carcinogenesis. Cell 61:1329–1337, 1990.
7. Arao T, Perkins EM: The interrelation of elastic tissue and human hair follicles. In: Montagna W, Dobson RL (eds): Advances in Biology of Skin, vol 9: Hair Growth. Oxford, Pergamon Press, 1969, pp 433–440.
8. Headington JT: Transverse microscopic anatomy of the human scalp: a basis for a morphometric approach to disorders of the hair follicle. Arch Dermatol 120:449–456, 1984.
9. Whiting DA: The value of horizontal sections of scalp biopsies. J Cutan Aging Cosmet Dermatol 1:165–173, 1990.
10. Sperling LC: Hair anatomy for the clinician. Am J Acad Dermatol 25:1–17, 1991.
11. Kligman AM: The human hair cycle. J Invest Dermatol 33:307–316, 1959.
12. Whiting DA: Diagnostic and predictive value of horizontal sections of scalp biopsy specimens in male pattern androgenetic alopecia. J Am Acad Dermatol 28:756–763, 1993.
13. Samman PD: The Nails in Disease, 4th ed. Chicago, Year Book Medical Publishers, 1986.
14. Conejo-Mir JS: Nail. In: Sternberg SS (ed): Histology for Pathologists. New York, Raven Press, 1992, pp 399–420.
15. Zaias N: The Nail in Health and Disease, 2nd ed. Norwalk, CT, Appleton & Lange, 1990.
16. Jerasutus S: Histology and Histopathology. In: Scher RK, Daniel CR III (eds): Nails: Therapy, Diagnosis, Surgery. Philadelphia, WB Saunders, 1990, pp 52–75.
17. Fleckman P: Anatomy and physiology of the nail. Dermatol Clin 3: 373–381, 1985.
18. Gonzalez-Serva A: Structure and Function. In: Scher RK, Daniel CR III (eds): Nails: Therapy, Diagnosis, Surgery. Philadelphia, WB Saunders, 1990, pp 11–30.
19. deBerker DAR, Baran R, Dawber RPR: Handbook of Diseases of the Nails and Their Management. Oxford, Blackwell Science, 1995.

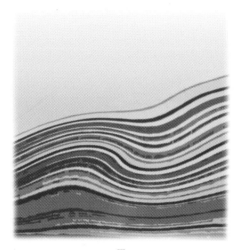

HAIR AND
NAIL
DISORDERS

Developmental and Hereditary Disorders

HOWARD P. BADEN

—

LYNN A. BADEN

Genetic disorders of hair and nails may affect only those tissues or may involve the skin itself, including other appendages. Furthermore, additional organ systems may be involved, and hair and nail changes may be a minor feature of the disease. The disorders covered in this chapter are the more likely to be encountered in the practice of dermatology. Lists of the rarer diseases may be found in texts on hair,[1] nails,[2] and genetics[3–4] and on the World Wide Web at the Online Mendelian Inheritance in Man (OMIM) site maintained by the Center for Medical Genetics, Johns Hopkins University (Baltimore, MD) and the National Center for Biotechnology Information, National Library of Medicine (Bethesda, MD). The OMIM entries cited in this chapter were accessed in 1996.

Hair shaft disorders represent a major category of genetic disorders of hair; they are discussed in Chapter 8. Although the morphology is well characterized and in some cases there are specific chemical markers, data on the genetic bases of the disorders described here (e.g., Menkes' kinky hair syndrome, lamellar ichthyosis) are limited. With the accumulation of more complete data on the human genome and more effective techniques for gene mapping, it is likely that the genetic basis for many of the hereditary diseases affecting hair and nails will be elucidated.

Darier-White Disease

The disease is inherited in an autosomal dominant fashion and is linked to chromosome 12.[5–7]

The nail changes of Darier-White disease are multiple subungual red and white longitudinal streaks, wedge-shaped subungual hyperkeratosis, and breaks of the free end of the nail (Fig. 3–1). Patients complain of nail fragility with minimal trauma. Secondary invasion with bacteria, yeast, or fungi may occur and may result in discoloration of the nail. Keratotic red plaques may be present in the scalp, and partial alopecia may be present (Fig. 3–2). The hair loss rarely causes a significant cosmetic problem.

The synthetic retinoids etretinate and isotretinoin are helpful for marked hyperkeratosis of the skin but do little for the nail changes. Systemic antibiotics are useful for flares resulting from secondary infection.

Pachyonychia Congenita

The disorder is inherited most commonly in an autosomal dominant manner and has been found to be associated with mutations of keratins K6A, K16, and K17.[8–12]

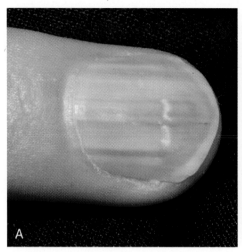
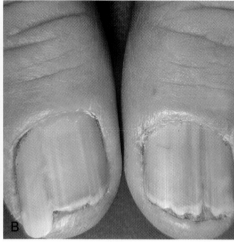

FIGURE 3-1 ■ Darier-White disease. *A,* Longitudinal red and white bands and lines. *B,* A wedge-shaped break in the nail with subungual hyperkeratosis.

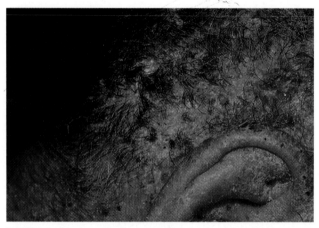

FIGURE 3-2 ■ Darier-White disease. The scalp shows loss of hair and thick scale crusts.

TABLE 3-1 ■ Anonychia: Selected Entries from Online Mendelian Inheritance in Man

Code	Topic
206800	Anonychia
107000	Anonychia-onychodystrophy
106995	Anonychia-onychodystrophy with hypoplasia or absence of distal phalanges
106990	Anonychia-onychodystrophy with brachydactyly type B and ectrodactyly
106900	Anonychia-ectrodactyly
106750	Anonychia with flexural pigmentation
188200	Thumbnails, absent

Online Mendelian Inheritance in Man. Baltimore, Johns Hopkins University. Available at: http://www3.ncbi.nim.nih.gov/omim/. Accessed 1996.

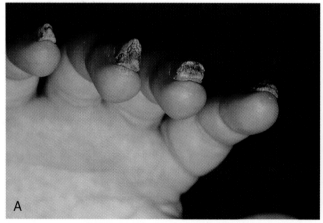
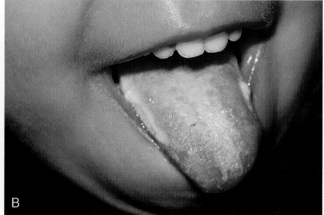

FIGURE 3-3 ■ Pachyonychia congenita. *A,* Subungual hyperkeratosis and lifting up of the nail. *B,* Leukokeratosis of the tongue is prominent.

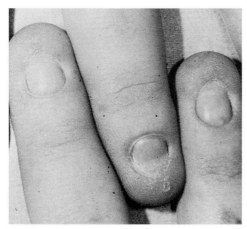

FIGURE 3-4 ■ Total absence of the nail. The nail bed is shining in this isolated case with no other epidermal or appendage abnormalities.

Pachyonychia congenita is a hereditary disorder manifesting as marked subungual hyperkeratosis resulting in lifting up of the nail (Fig. 3–3A). The disorder is classified into several types. Type I is most common; these patients have palmoplantar and follicular hyperkeratosis as well as oral leukokeratosis (Fig. 3–3B). Type II is like type I, but blisters of the palms and soles, early dentition, and steatocystoma multiplex are also observed. Type III (12% of those affected) produces, in addition,

angular cheilosis, corneal dyskeratosis, and cataracts. Type IV (7%) has the features of type III plus laryngeal lesions, hoarseness, mental retardation, and hair anomalies.

Treatment is grinding down of the nails.

Anonychia

Inheritance can be autosomal dominant or autosomal recessive.[13, 14]

Total absence of all nails is uncommon. More commonly there is a mixed picture of anonychia and hyponychia (Fig. 3–4). With isolated anonychia, an abnormality of the underlying bone is often found. Absent nails may also be observed with other defects (Table 3–1).

Trichothiodystrophy

The disease has an autosomal recessive form of inheritance and results from a mutation of the *XPB/ERCC3* DNA repair transcription gene in at least one of the several types that have been described.[15–17]

The nails in trichothiodystrophy are fragile and show thinning, splitting, and broken free ends (Fig. 3–5A). Patients have hairs of uneven lengths that break easily

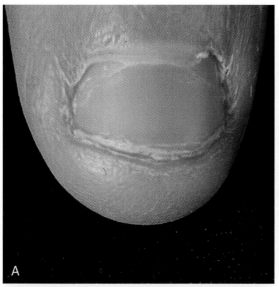

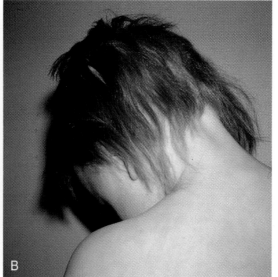

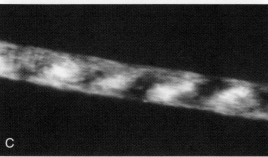

FIGURE 3-5 ■ Trichothiodystrophy. *A*, The nails break easily and are short. *B*, This patient with only skin changes showed hair of irregular length. *C*, Banding of the hair by polarizing microscopy.

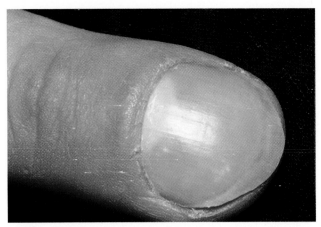

FIGURE 3-6 ■ Nail clubbing. The nail has a bulbous shape with exaggerated longitudinal and horizontal curvatures.

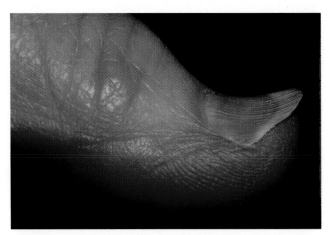

FIGURE 3-8 ■ Koilonychia. The nail is thin and concave.

(Fig. 3–5*B*). In some families intellectual impairment, decreased fertility in males, short stature, ichthyosis, and photosensitivity may be observed.

A characteristic finding is alternating black and white bands when a hair is examined by polarizing microscopy (Fig. 3–5*C*). Amino acid analysis of hair shows a 50% reduction in cystine content.

Clubbing

Autosomal dominance is the mechanism for the inherited disease.[18–20]

Clubbing of the nails is most commonly acquired but may have a genetic basis. It involves fingers and toes and most commonly starts at puberty. There is bulbous enlargement of the nail, with horizontal and longitudinal curvature (Fig. 3–6). The angle formed by the dorsum of the plate and the surface of the proximal digit (Lovibond's angle) is greater than 180 degrees.

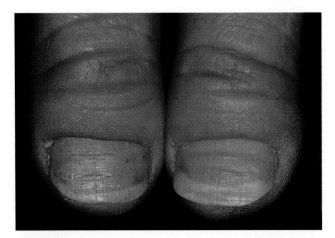

FIGURE 3-7 ■ Broad nail. The thumb nails are shorter and wider than normal.

Broad Nails

Broad nails may occur alone as an autosomal dominant disorder or in association with a variety of other syndromes with varying modes of inheritance.[21]

The condition, which is also known as racquet nails, manifests as a broad, short nail (Fig. 3–7). One or both thumbnails may be involved.

Koilonychia

The inheritance is autosomal dominant.[22, 23]

Koilonychia manifests at birth or appears in early childhood as thin nails that have a concave, smooth or rough surface (Fig. 3–8). It may be associated with other cutaneous changes and even with abnormalities of other organs.

Ectopic Nail

An ectopic nail is a developmental defect that is apparent at birth.[24] It can occur anywhere on the hands or feet and has the appearance of a nail plate without folds (Fig. 3–9).

It can be confused with a rudimentary digit or a fibrokeratoma.

Excision and histological examination allow the diagnosis to be established and eliminate the nail. If there is any doubt, analysis of the fibrous protein can distinguish between nail and epidermis.

Congenital Onychodysplasia

Autosomal dominant inheritance has been reported in a number of cases.[25–27]

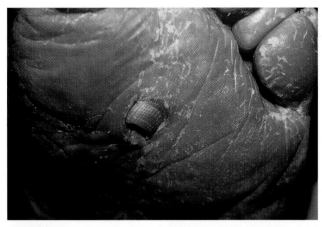

FIGURE 3–9 ■ Ectopic nail. A nail plate is growing out of the sole of the foot. (Courtesy of Dr. R.J. Aylesworthy.)

TABLE 3–2 ■ Leukonychia: Selected Entries from Online Mendelian Inheritance in Man

Code	Topic
151600	Leukonychia totalis
149200	Knuckle pads, leukonychia, and sensorineural deafness
151550	Leukonychia maculata
184500	Steatocystoma multiplex
124500	Deafness, congenital, with keratopachydermia and constrictions of fingers and toes
234580	Hearing loss, sensorineural, with enamel hypoplasia and nail defects
236300	Hooft disease
260130	Pachyonychia congenita, recessive

Online Mendelian Inheritance in Man. Baltimore, Johns Hopkins University. Available at: http://www3.ncbi.nim.nih.gov/omim/. Accessed 1996.

Congenital onychodysplasia is an uncommon disorder that almost exclusively involves the index fingers and manifests as anonychia, micronychia, polyonychia, and hemionychogryphosis (Fig. 3–10). The affected nail is most commonly on the side of the finger rather than in the center, and it may be thickened or malaligned. The condition can be unilateral or bilateral. Although initially described in Japan, the disease is found worldwide. A variety of bony changes of the phalanx under the affected nail have been reported and may be detected only by radiography.

Although the more severe cases are readily diagnosed, micronychia can be associated with other syndromes of absence of nails or dystrophic nails.

Leukonychia

The disorder has autosomal dominant inheritance. Leukonychia has been noted in several families in association with other features such as epithelial cysts and renal calculi.[28–31]

Leukonychia most commonly is an acquired disorder arising from a variety of causes. The hereditary leukonychias (Table 3–2) may manifest with a total, partial, or striate white color of the nail plate (Fig. 3–11). The first two of these conditions probably represent one entity, and both forms may be seen in the same patient. The nail changes may be present from birth or develop in childhood. The white color is very bright and is different from the color that results from a nail bed disorder. This can be confirmed by shaving off a piece of nail and observing that it is white. The white color results from retention of nuclei, which causes light scattering. The striate type may be single or multiple and may extend partially or completely across the nail. The condition is lifelong, but there may be periods when the nails look more normal.

Epidermolysis Bullosa

There are autosomal dominant and recessive forms of the scarring type, called *dystrophic* epidermolysis bul-

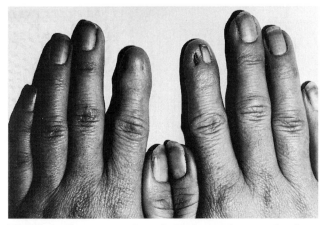

FIGURE 3–10 ■ Congenital onychodysplasia. Segments of nail are seen growing on the index finger.

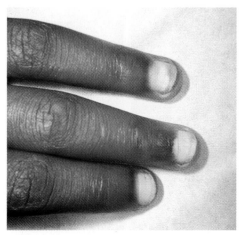

FIGURE 3–11 ■ Leukonychia. All the nail plates are bright white.

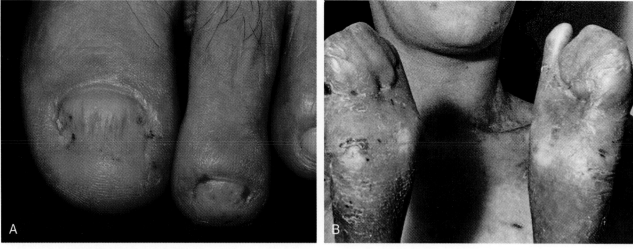

FIGURE 3–12 ■ Epidermolysis bullosa. Scarring of the nail bed in autosomal dominant dystrophic (*A*) and autosomal recessive dystrophic (*B*) types.

losa, and the latter tends to be more severe. These are caused by a mutation in the anchoring fibrils (collagen 7). Another subepidermal type, called *Herlitz' disease,* also produces loss of nails and results from mutation in laminin 5.

Epidermolysis bullosa consists of a group of disorders that manifest with blisters but may have a spectrum of other changes in the skin.[32–35] The blisters may occur in the epidermis or between the epidermis and dermis. In the latter group, scarring occurs and can result in permanent loss of the nail plate (Fig. 3–12) and hair. Scarring in the autosomal recessive form is usually more severe.

Keratinizing Disorders

A number of genetic disorders of keratinization are associated with nail changes; these are shown in Table 3–3 and Figures 3–13*A* and 3–14*A,B*). Pityriasis rubra pilaris, lamellar ichthyosis, and epidermolytic hyperkera-

TABLE 3–3 ■ Genetic Disorders of Keratinization with Nail Changes

Disorder	Nail Change	Inheritance
Pityriasis rubra pilaris	Dystrophic plate and subungual hyperkeratosis	AD
Lamellar ichthyosis	Dystrophic plate with grooves and subungual hyperkeratosis	AR Mutation of transglutaminase in some patients
Epidermolytic hyperkeratosis	Dystrophic plate and subungual hyperkeratosis	AD Mutation of K1 or K10
Porokeratosis	Ridging and splitting	AD
Linea nevus	Longitudinal ridges and depressions	Somatic mutation is likely
Palmoplantar keratoderma	Dystrophic plates and subungual hyperkeratosis	AD or AR depending on type; mutation of K1, K9, or loricrin depending on the disease

AD, autosomal dominant; AR, autosomal recessive; K, keratin.

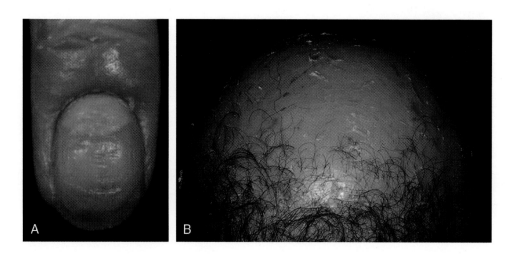

FIGURE 3–13 ■ Lamellar ichthyosis. *A,* The surface of the nail shows horizontal grooves and pits. *B,* Scarring of the scalp can be extensive.

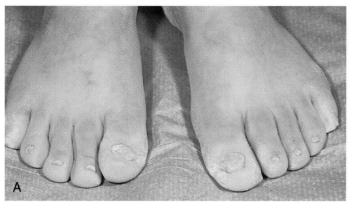
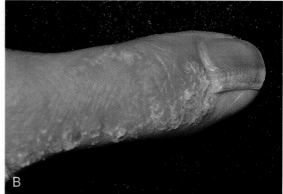

FIGURE 3–14 ■ Epidermolytic hyperkeratosis. There is subungal hyperkeratosis and marked dystrophy of the plates in the generalized form (A) and localized dystrophy in linear nevus that extends from the hand to the nail (B).

tosis produce a scaling disorder of the scalp that may cause scarring (see Fig. 3–13B).[36–39]

Nail-Patella Syndrome

The disease has an autosomal dominant inheritance and has been mapped to 9q34.1.[40, 41]

The nail-patella syndrome produces changes in the nails, bones, and kidneys. Nail changes are most pronounced in the thumbs and decrease toward the fifth finger (Fig. 3–15). The toenails usually are not affected. The nail may be absent or small and abnormal in size or shape. The lunula may have a **V** shape. The patella is hypoplastic or absent and may be subluxated (see Fig. 3–15C). Other bony changes are seen, but bilateral posterior iliac horns are characteristic. Glomerulonephritis is seen in about a third of the patients. Heterochromia of the iris and glaucoma occurs uncommonly.

Maternal Ingestion Causing Abnormal Nails

Hydantoin taken during pregnancy causes hypoplasia of nails and fingers[42] (Fig. 3–16). Other drugs that can cause small or dystrophic nails are listed in Table 3–4.

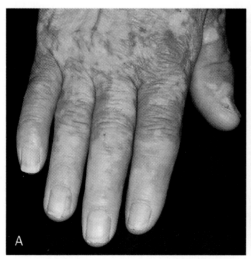
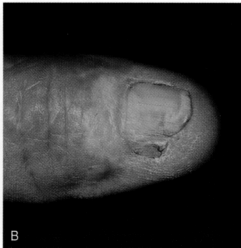
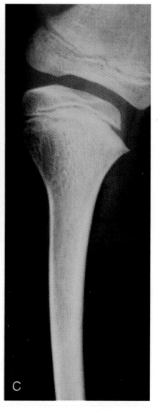

FIGURE 3–15 ■ Nail-patella syndrome. The thumbnail is small and dystrophic (A), and the other nail looks normal (B). The patella is absent on x-ray examination (C).

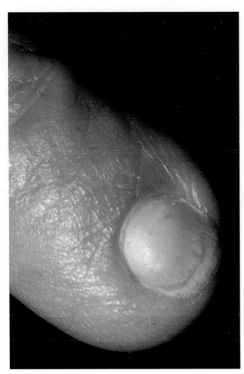

FIGURE 3–16 ■ Dilantin nail. The fifth hand nail is small.

Osler-Weber-Rendu Syndrome

The inheritance is autosomal dominant. The defect maps to chromosome 9q33–34.1 and is a mutation of the endoglin gene. However, genetic heterogeneity has been reported.[43–45]

The Osler-Weber-Rendu syndrome manifests in childhood as telangiectasia of the skin and mucous membranes, with nail bed involvement (Fig. 3–17). Telangiectasia may occur in internal organs, and bleeding is the major complication.

Essential telangiectasia can mimic the disorder, but it

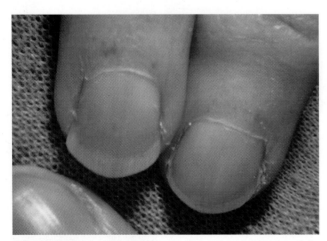

FIGURE 3–17 ■ Osler-Weber-Rendu syndrome. Telangiectasia of the finger and nail bed are seen.

TABLE 3-4 ■ Drugs and Chemicals That May Cause Defects If Ingested During Pregnancy

Trimethadione
Paramethadione
Valproic acid
Carbamazepine
Phenobarbitone
Warfarin
Alcohol
Polychlorinated biphenyl compounds

occurs in later childhood or early adult life. The presence of typical mucous membrane lesions of the Osler-Weber-Rendu syndrome usually allows the correct diagnosis to be established.

Periungual Fibroma

Tuberous sclerosis has autosomal dominant inheritance and is linked to chromosomes 9 (9q34) and 16 (16p13.3), indicating that the phenotype may be caused by mutations in different genes. The gene on chromosome 16 has been identified as *TSC2*, and the protein it expresses has been named tuberin.[46–48]

Periungual fibromas may represent an acquired fibrous tumor or a manifestation of tuberous sclerosis. The tumors associated with tuberous sclerosis (Koenen's tumors) are usually in the nail fold, first appear in the early teens, and increase with age (Fig. 3–18). They are multiple, small, round, smooth, skin-colored lesions that may press on the plate, causing a groove. They can at times destroy the plate by their size and number.

Histopathology in Koenen's tumors show increased collagen and blood vessels, with the former varying in

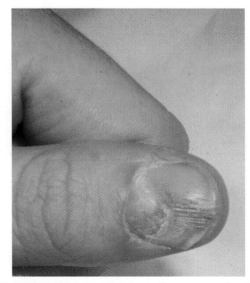

FIGURE 3–18 ■ Tuberous sclerosis. A fibroma protrudes from the nail fold.

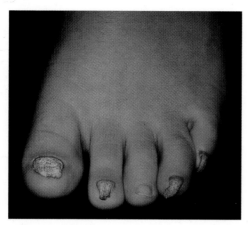

FIGURE 3–19 ■ Twenty-nail dystrophy. An isolated case of nail dystrophy with changes in all but one nail.

density and the latter in number.

The tumors can be excised, but this may result in significant defects of the nail plate.

Twenty-Nail Dystrophy

Inheritance of the disease is autosomal dominant.[49, 50]

Twenty-nail dystrophy occurs most commonly in children as an acquired disorder that may be idiopathic or a manifestation of alopecia areata, psoriasis, or lichen planus. In the hereditary type, changes are present at birth and increase in severity. The nails have longitudinal ridges and a rough surface, and they lack luster (Fig. 3–19).

Congenital Malalignment

Congenital malalignment of the nail is a developmental disorder, present from birth, in which the nail deviates

laterally.[51] With wearing of shoes and walking the nail becomes dystrophic, is raised at the free margin, has striations, and is discolored (Fig 3–20).

Problems with the nail can be avoided by a surgical procedure to realign the nail; this should be done early.

Periodic Shedding of the Nails

The inheritance is autosomal dominant.[52, 53]

There is periodic loss of nails without prior evidence of inflammation. The nails come loose, develop a dull color, and are shed spontaneously (Fig. 3–21). Spontaneous regrowth of the nail occurs. Both fingernails and toenails are affected.

Alopecia Congenita

Most cases are spontaneous occurrences, but autosomal dominant and recessive forms of inheritance have been described.[54–56]

Alopecia congenita is a heterogeneous group of diseases characterized by decreased number and size of hairs. In the most severe cases, the patients have few vellus-size hairs, but in some families the hair may attain a length of more than 1 cm (Fig. 3–22). Some areas, such as eyebrows and lashes, may appear normal. Other skin appendages, epidermis, and stratified epithelium appear normal.

Dermatopathology reveals a decreased number and size of hair follicles. Dystrophic follicles with abnormally keratinized hair shafts may be observed.

Atrichia with Papular Lesions

The inheritance in the classic cases has not been established, but autosomal recessive inheritance is suggested

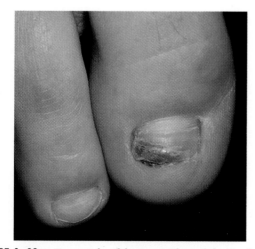

FIGURE 3–20 ■ Congenital malalignment. The nail deviates laterally, is raised at the free edge, is discolored, and has striations.

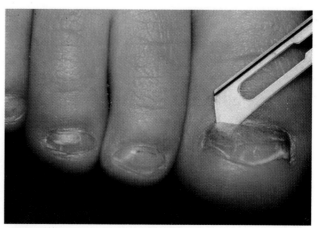

FIGURE 3–21 ■ Periodic shedding. The old nail (lifted up by the blade) is separating proximally from the new nail, which is pushing it out.

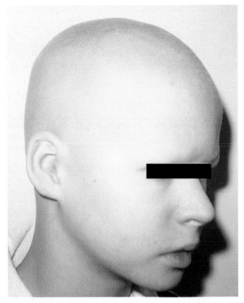

FIGURE 3-22 ■ Spontaneous occurrence of alopecia congenita. Only short vellus hair was present, except for the eyelashes.

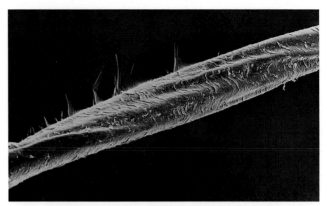

FIGURE 3-24 ■ Scanning electron microscopy of hair of Marie Unna hypotrichosis. The hair is very flat and has a damaged cuticle (magnification 200x).

in some pedigrees. Less severely affected families showed autosomal dominant inheritance.

Atrichia with papular lesion manifests as permanent alopecia after shedding of the fetal hair. Multiple papules are observed commonly on the face.[57, 58] This disease is discussed in more detail in Chapter 4.

Marie Unna Hypotrichosis

The inheritance is autosomal dominant.[59-61]

Marie Unna hypotrichosis produces a progressive scarring alopecia. The appearance of the scalp hair at different ages can vary considerably. Although the literature has described male patients as being more severely

affected, this is not true in all families. In patients followed by an author (HPB), the hair is very sparse during the first few years of life and then gradually increases in amount (Fig. 3-23). In older children and adults, the hair is characteristically coarse. With time there is a progressive loss of hair, with little if any evidence of perifollicular inflammation. Eyelashes and brows may be scanty from birth, and in adults the pubic, axillary, and body hair is sparse. The remainder of the skin usually is normal, although facial milia have been described.

The hairs as shown using light microscopy are flattened, twisted, and wider than normal (>100 μm) (Fig. 3-24). On scanning electron microscopy, the shafts have ridges and grooves, and the scales are chipped or lost. Dermatopathology shows fewer follicles than normal. In childhood the follicles may appear diminutive, with abortive attempts to form hair follicles manifested by hair cysts. Some anagen hairs demonstrate cellular degeneration of cortical epithelium and the outer root sheath. With progression of hair loss, granulomatous infiltrates around follicles and eventually scarring are seen.

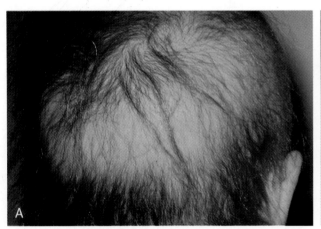
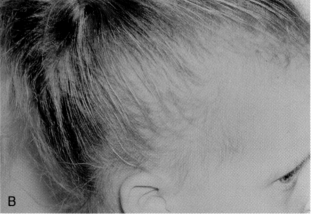

FIGURE 3-23 ■ Marie Unna hypotrichosis. The 1½-year-old child (A) shows very sparse hair, which increased in amount by age 3½ years (B).

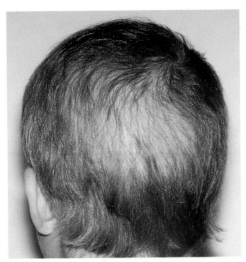

FIGURE 3–25 ■ Loose anagen hair syndrome. There is decreased density in the posterior scalp, and the hair is of uneven length.

Loose Anagen Hair

Most cases occur spontaneously, but dominant inheritance is well documented.[62–64]

Patients with the loose anagen hair syndrome present in childhood with scanty hairs of uneven lengths (Fig. 3–25). Localized areas of baldness may be apparent. Parents state that scalp hair is pulled out painlessly. Among affected individuals, females with light-colored hair predominate. In the teen years after puberty the scalp hair appears normal and can grow long. However, abnormal hairs can still be pulled from the hair without pain.

Light microscopy of hairs pulled from the head without pain have a characteristic appearance. The bulb end is misshapen, and the inner and outer root sheaths are

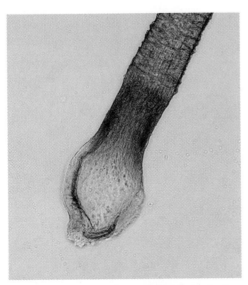

FIGURE 3–26 ■ Appearance of anagen hair from the loose anagen hair syndrome. The bulb is misshapen, and their inner and outer root sheaths are absent. Wrinkling of the cuticle can be seen.

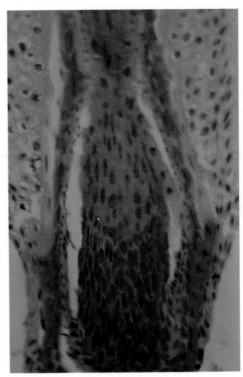

FIGURE 3–27 ■ Dermatopathology of follicle. Separation of the various layers is readily observed.

absent (Fig. 3–26). Characteristically, rippling of the cuticle is observed at the beginning of the hardened shaft. Dermatopathology of the scalp shows premature keratinization of the inner root sheath and areas of separation of the various layers of the follicles (Fig. 3–27). When the follicles are observed in cross-section, some have an abnormal shape.

Treatment early in life is to minimize pulling of the hair during normal grooming. After puberty, patients appear to have few problems with ordinary hair care.

Keratosis Follicularis Spinulosa Decalvans

Several large kindreds have been reported from the Netherlands with a sex-linked recessive form of inheritance in which males are more severely affected.[65–67] The disease is most severe early in life and subsides after puberty. In cases reported in the United States, both sexes are affected, the disease does not improve with puberty, and autosomal dominant inheritance is observed in some families.

Keratosis pilaris atrophicans includes a group of hereditary disorders characterized by an inflammatory follicular process that results in destruction and scarring. When the scalp is involved, the term *keratosis follicularis spinulosa decalvans* is used. Affected areas of the scalp are red, and the follicles are surmounted by a scale crust (Fig. 3–28). White, scarred areas of scalp skin represent the end stage of the disease. Follicular,

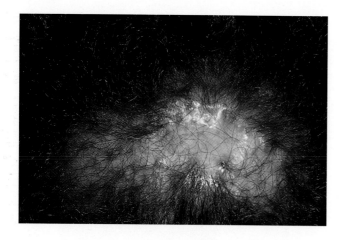

FIGURE 3–28 ■ Keratosis follicularis spinulosa decalvans. Inflammatory changes including redness and crusting are present at the periphery of the scarred scalp lesion.

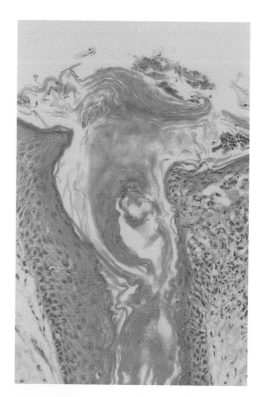

FIGURE 3–29 ■ Dermatopathology of the scalp. The ostium is distended by a keratotic plug.

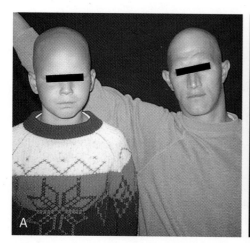

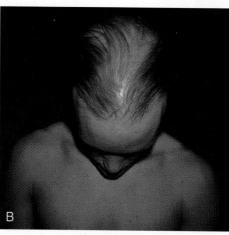

FIGURE 3–30 ■ Sparse hair in ectodermal dysplasia. A, Father and son with hidrotic ectodermal dysplasia. B, Anhidrotic ectodermal dysplasia.

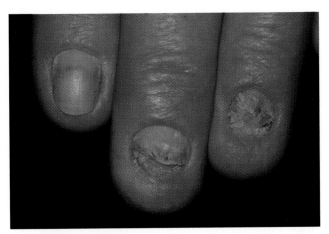

FIGURE 3–31 ■ Dystrophic nails in hidrotic ectodermal dysplasia.

red, papular lesions are usually present on the face, extremities, and trunk. In some families keratoderma of the palms and soles and corneal dystrophy have been reported.

Dermatopathology of early lesions shows the ostium distended by horny plugs and polymorphonuclear leukocytes in the perifollicular epidermis (Fig. 3–29). In older lesions a chronic inflammatory infiltrate and scarring surround the follicles, and even at a later stage, follicles are destroyed and replaced by horizontal scarring.

Intermittent bacterial infections occur and are treated by appropriate antibacterial drugs. Oral retinoid therapy results in some improvement, and etretinate may be the best choice.

Ectodermal Dysplasia

Hidrotic ectodermal dysplasia (HED) is inherited as an autosomal dominant disorder, and anhidrotic ectodermal dysplasia (AED) as an X-linked recessive disorder.[68–72]

The term *ectodermal dysplasia* has been used to define a number of hereditary disorders with abnormalities in several ectodermal tissues, including epidermis and its appendages. Until the genetic basis of the various types is determined, the clinical classification remains rather arbitrary and artificial. The two best known entities are HED and AED, which produce a decreased amount of scalp hair that may be fine and brittle (Fig. 3–30). Hair on other areas of body can be similarly affected. In HED, the nails are abnormal in shape, size, and color, and palmar hyperkeratosis is observed (Fig. 3–31). In AED, the sweat glands are drastically reduced in number, there are major defects or absence of teeth, and unusual facies are present (Fig. 3–32).

Light and scanning electron microscopy show numerous structural abnormalities of the shaft.

Monilethrix

Inheritance is autosomal dominant with variable expression. Clinical features include short, stubby hair associated with follicular hyperkeratosis and perifollicular erythema (Fig. 3–33). Hair fibers are characterized by uniform elliptical nodes and internodes. Linkage has been established to the keratin gene cluster on 12q11: q13.[73]

Premature Aging

Inheritance of the disorders of premature aging is autosomal recessive, except that dyskeratosis congenita also has X-linked recessive and dominant forms.[74–78]

In the premature aging disorders such as progeria, Werner's syndrome, Cockayne's syndrome, Rothmund-Thomson syndrome (Fig. 3–34A), and dyskeratosis con-

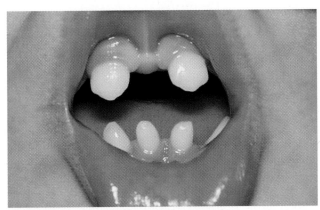

FIGURE 3–32 ■ Abnormal teeth in anhidrotic ectodermal dysplasia.

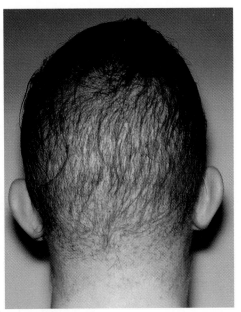

FIGURE 3–33 ■ Monilethrix. The patient has short, stubby hair associated with follicular hyperkeratosis and perifollicular erythema.

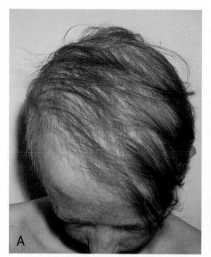
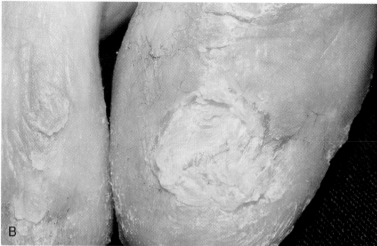

FIGURE 3–34 ■ Rothmund-Thomson syndrome. Decreased scalp hair (*A*) and dystrophic nails (*B*).

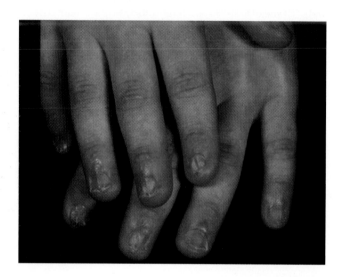

FIGURE 3–35 ■ Dyskeratosis congenita showing dystrophic nails.

FIGURE 3–36 ■ Acrodermatitis enteropathica. *A*, Dermatitis of the skin, paronychia with nail changes, and sparse hair. *B*, Closer view of nails.

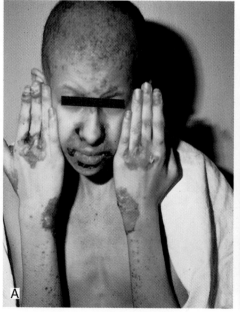
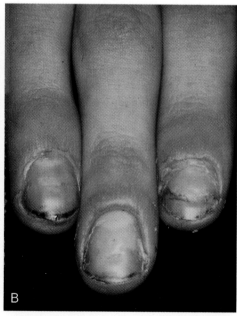

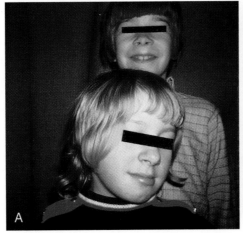
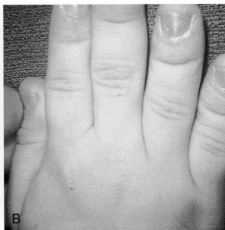

FIGURE 3-37 ■ *A.* Cartilage-hair hypoplasia. The patient, who is short in stature and has fine, sparse blond hair, is standing in front of an unaffected sibling who is 1½ years older. *B.* The nails are short and broad.

genita, thinning of the scalp hair is seen. The other features of these disorders are multiple and include cutaneous changes associated with photoaging or loss of subcutaneous fat. Dystrophic changes of the nails are also observed (Fig. 3–35; see Fig. 3–34*B*).

Metabolic Diseases

The metabolic diseases biotin-responsive multiple carboxylyase deficiency, 1,25-dihydroxy vitamin D unresponsiveness, and acrodermatitis enteropathica have been reported to have autosomal recessive inheritance.

There are two forms of hereditary multiple carboxylyase deficiency. The neonatal type may progress rapidly and is potentially fatal unless diagnosed early. The juvenile form manifests at a few months of age with periorificial dermatitis that persists in undiagnosed cases and may result in hair loss. The neonatal type is caused by holocarboxylase-synthetase deficiency and the other by biotinidase deficiency.[79-81]

Vitamin D–unresponsive rickets is a result of mutation in the vitamin D receptor gene and is associated with significant alopecia.[82]

Acrodermatitis enteropathica results from malabsorption of zinc and is associated with a dermatitis around mucocutaneous orifices, paronychia, nail dystrophy, and alopecia (Fig. 3–36). In all these diseases the patients exhibit decreased numbers of hairs, thinning of the shaft, and brittle hair, and the appearance depends on the severity of the condition.[83]

Treatment of the disorders is by replacement therapy, and early recognition is important.

Cartilage-Hair Hypoplasia

The inheritance is autosomal recessive.[84-87]

Cartilage-hair hypoplasia, manifested by short-limb dwarfism, produces fine, sparse, light-colored hair of scalp, lashes, brows, and body (Fig. 3–37A) in association with short, broad nails (Fig. 3–37B).

Focal Dermal Hypoplasia

Inheritance is X-linked dominant.[88-90]

Focal dermal hypoplasia (Goltz' syndrome) results in a variable expression of cutaneous lesions, including atrophic and hypertrophic scarring, hypopigmentation and hyperpigmentation, papillomas, and nodules. Involvement of other organs also occurs. Sparse hair or areas of absent hair may be observed, and the nails may be dystrophic or absent (Fig. 3–38).

Congenital Absence of Skin

Simple congenital absence of skin (aplasia cutis) is usually sporadic, but autosomal dominant inheritance has been reported. When it is associated with other findings, the inheritance depends on the primary disorder.[91-93]

Aplasia cutis of the scalp usually manifests as a single, 2- to 3-cm ulceration or a scarred bald area, usually near the vertex (Fig. 3–39). There may be defects of the underlying tissue extending to the meninges. There

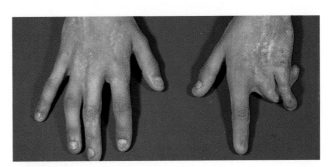

FIGURE 3-38 ■ Dystrophic nails in Goltz' syndrome.

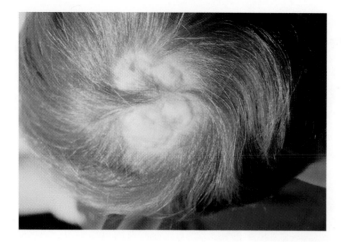

FIGURE 3-39 ■ Congenital absence of skin. The defect has healed with a scar.

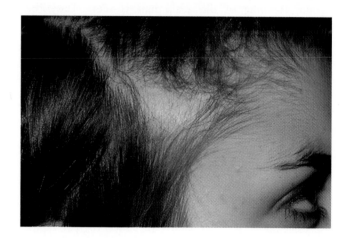

FIGURE 3-40 ■ Triangular alopecia at the frontal hair line.

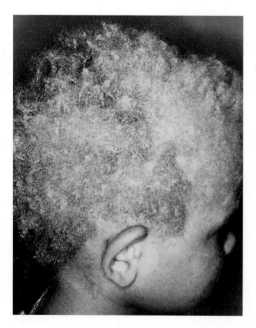

FIGURE 3-41 ■ Wooly hair. This Caucasian child has tightly coiled, light-colored hair.

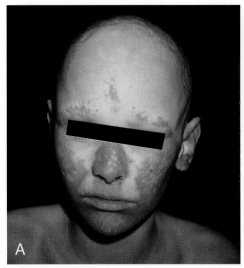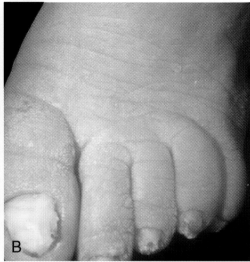

FIGURE 3–42 ▪ Keratitis, ichthyosis, and deafness (KID) syndrome. The patient has a generalized keratoderma and scarring alopecia of the scalp (*A*). Dystrophic nails are also observed (*B*).

are different genetic forms of the disease with other manifestations, including one associated with autosomal dominant dystrophic epidermolysis bullosa.

Dermatopathology of a healed lesion shows a thin epidermis, absent appendages, a dermal scar, and decreased or absent elastic fibers.

Small lesions are best treated by allowing them to heal spontaneously, using topical treatment that best controls infection.

Triangular Alopecia

There is no evidence for an inherited basis of this disease.

Triangular alopecia is a developmental defect that probably is present from birth but is not noted until later in life.[94] The base of the triangle is at the junctions of the frontal and temporal regions (Fig. 3–40). It is most commonly unilateral but can be bilateral.

Dermatopathology shows the presence of apparently normal vellus hairs.

Wooly Hair

Inheritance is autosomal dominant.[95, 96]

The scalp hair is tightly coiled and in some cases does not grow long because of breakage due to excessive grooming (Fig. 3–41). There is variability in hair color. Only the scalp hair is involved.

By light microscopy, the hair has an oval shape and shows repetitive coils that result from gradual twisting of the shaft. The hair shaft is flat at the turns. The hair tends to become less kinky and easier to manage in the adult years.

There is no specific treatment other than cosmetic straightening of the hair.

KID Syndrome

Most cases are sporadic, but autosomal dominant inheritance has been reported.[97–99]

The KID (*k*eratitis, *i*chthyosis, and *d*eafness) syndrome is a congenital disorder that is manifested as keratoderma, keratitis with blindness, and neurosensory deafness. Scarring alopecia (Fig. 3–42*A*) is a constant feature, as is dystrophy of the nails (Fig. 3–42*B*).

REFERENCES

1. Olsen EA: Disorders of Hair Growth. New York, McGraw-Hill, 1994.
2. Baran R, Dawber RPR: Diseases of the Nails and Their Management, 2nd ed. Oxford, Blackwell Scientific, 1994.
3. McKusick VA: Mendelian Inheritance in Man: Catalogs of Human Genes and Genetic Disorders, 11th ed (2 vols). Baltimore, Johns Hopkins University Press, 1994.
4. Rimoin DL, Connor JM, Pyeritz RE: Emory and Rimoin's Principles and Practice of Medical Genetics, 3rd ed. New York, Churchill-Livingstone, 1996.
5. Online Mendelian Inheritance in Man (OMIM). MIM {124200}. Baltimore, Johns Hopkins University. Available at: http://www3.ncbi.nim.nih.gov/omim/.
6. Kennedy JL, Berg D, Bassett AS, et al: Genetic linkage for Darier disease (keratosis follicularis). Am J Med Genet 55:307, 1995.
7. Rublevskaya I, Wakem P, Haake A, et al: Linkage mapping narrows the Darier's disease gene (DAR) region. J Invest Dermatol 108:645, 1997.
8. Online Mendelian Inheritance in Man (OMIM). MIM {167200, 167210, 184510}. Baltimore, Johns Hopkins University. Available at: http://www3.ncbi.nim.nih.gov/omim/.
9. Smith FJD, Corden LD, Rugg EL, et al: Missense mutations in keratin 17 cause either pachyonychia congenita type 2 or a phenotype resembling steatocystoma multiplex. J Invest Dermatol 108:220, 1997.
10. McLean WH, Rugg EL, Lunny DP, et al: Keratin 16 and keratin

17 mutations cause pachyonychia congenita. Nature Genet 9:273, 1995.

11. Bowden PE, Haley JL, Kansky A, et al: Mutation of a type II keratin gene (K6a) in pachyonychia congenita. Nature Genet 10: 363, 1995.

12. Novice FM, Collison DW, Burgdorf WHC, Esterly NB: Pachyonychia congenita. In: Handbook of Genetic Skin Disorders. Philadelphia, WB Saunders, 1994, p 427.

13. Online Mendelian Inheritance in Man (OMIM). MIM {206800}. Baltimore, Johns Hopkins University. Available at: http://www3.ncbi.nim.nih.gov/omim/.

14. Mahloudji M, Amidi M: Simple anonychia. Further evidence for autosomal recessive inheritance. J Med Genet 8:478–480, 1971.

15. Online Mendelian Inheritance in Man (OMIM). MIM {601675}. Baltimore, Johns Hopkins University. Available at: http://www3.ncbi.nim.nih.gov/omim/.

16. Baden HP, Jackson CE, Weiss L, et al: The physicochemical properties of hair in the BIDS syndrome (brittle hair, intellectual impairment, decreased fertility and short stature). Am J Hum Genet 28:514, 1976.

17. Weeda G, Eveno E, Donker I, et al: A mutation in the XPB/ERCC3 DNA repair transcription gene, associated with trichothiodystrophy. Am J Hum Genet 60:320, 1997.

18. Online Mendelian Inheritance in Man (OMIM). MIM {119900}. Baltimore, Johns Hopkins University. Available at: http://www3.ncbi.nim.nih.gov/omim/.

19. Curth HO, Firschein IL, Alphert M: Familial clubbed fingers. Arch Dermatol 83:829, 1961.

20. Fischer DS, Singer DH, Feldman SM: Clubbing: a review with emphasis on hereditary acropachy. Medicine (Baltimore) 43:459, 1964.

21. Basset H: Trois formes genotypiques d'ongles courts, le pouce en raquette, les doigts en raquette, les ongles courts simples. Bull Soc Fr Dermatol Syphil 69:15, 1962.

22. Online Mendelian Inheritance in Man (OMIM). MIM {149300}. Baltimore, Johns Hopkins University. Available at: http://www3.ncbi.nim.nih.gov/omim/.

23. Bumpers RD, Bishop ME: Familial koilonychia: a current case history. Arch Dermatol 116:845, 1980.

24. Kukuchi I, Ono T, Ogata K: Ectopic nail. Plast Reconstr Surg 61: 781–783, 1978.

25. Baran R, Stroud JD: Congenital onychodysplasia of the index fingers. Arch Dermatol 120:243–244, 1984.

26. Kitayama Y, Tsukada S: Congenital onychodysplasia. Arch Dermatol 119:8–12, 1983.

27. Millman AJ, Strier RP: Congenital onychodysplasia of the index fingers. J Am Acad Dermatol 7:57, 1982.

28. Online Mendelian Inheritance in Man (OMIM). MIM {151600}. Baltimore, Johns Hopkins University. Available at: http://www3.ncbi.nim.nih.gov/omim/.

29. Frydman M, Cohen HA: Leukonychia totalis in two sibs. Am J Med Genet 47:540, 1993.

30. Butterworth T: Leukonychia partialis. Cutis 29:363, 1982.

31. Bushkell LL, Gorlin RJ: Leukonychia totalis, multiple sebaceous cysts, and renal calculi. Arch Dermatol 111:899, 1975.

32. Online Mendelian Inheritance in Man (OMIM). MIM {131750, 226600}. Baltimore, Johns Hopkins University. Available at: http://www3.ncbi.nim.nih.gov/omim/.

33. Uitto J, Christiano AM: Molecular basis for the dystrophic forms of epidermolysis bullosa: mutations in the type VII collagen gene. Arch Dermatol Res 287:16–22, 1994.

34. Christiano AM, LaForgia S, Paller AS, et al: Prenatal diagnosis for recessive dystrophic epidermolysis bullosa in 10 families by mutation and haplotype analysis in the type VII collagen gene (COL7A1). Mol Med 2:59, 1996.

35. Christiano AM, Morricone A, Paradisi M, et al: A glycine-to-arginine substitution in the triple-helical domain of type VII collagen in a family with dominant dystrophic epidermolysis bullosa. J Invest Dermatol 104:438, 1995.

36. Online Mendelian Inheritance in Man (OMIM). MIM {242300, 113800}. Baltimore, Johns Hopkins University. Available at: http://www3.ncbi.nim.nih.gov/omim/.

37. Huber M, Rettler I, Bernasconi K, et al: Mutations of keratinocyte transglutaminase in lamellar ichthyosis. Science 267:525, 1995.

38. Bale SJ, Russell LJ, Lee ML, et al: Congenital recessive ichthyosis unlinked to loci for epidermal transglutaminases. J Invest Dermatol 107:808, 1996.

39. Rothnagell JA, Dominey AM, Dempsey LD, et al: Mutations in the rod domains of keratins 1 and 10 in epidermolytic hyperkeratosis. Science 257:1128, 1992.

40. Online Mendelian Inheritance in Man (OMIM). MIM {161200}. Baltimore, Johns Hopkins University. Available at: http://www3.ncbi.nim.nih.gov/omim/.

41. McIntosh I, Clough MV, Schaffer AA, et al: Fine mapping of the nail-patella syndrome locus at 9q34. Am J Hum Genet 60:133, 1997.

42. Johnson RB, Goldsmith LA: Dilantin digital defects. J Am Acad Dermatol 5:191, 1981.

43. Online Mendelian Inheritance in Man (OMIM). MIM {187300}. Baltimore, Johns Hopkins University. Available at: http://www3.ncbi.nim.nih.gov/omim/.

44. McAllister KA, Grogg KM, Johnson DW, et al: Endoglin, a TGF-beta binding protein of endothelial cells, is the gene for hereditary haemorrhagic telangiectasia type 1. Nat Genet 8:345, 1994.

45. Porteous MEM, Curtis A, Williams O, et al: Genetic heterogeneity in hereditary haemorrhagic telangiectasia. J Med Genet 31:925, 1994.

46. Online Mendelian Inheritance in Man (OMIM). MIM {191100, 191092}. (OMIM). MIM {242300, 113800}. Baltimore, Johns Hopkins University. Available at: http://www3.ncbi.nim.nih.gov/omim/.

47. Nellist M, Janssen B, Brook-Carter PT, et al: Identification and characterization of the tuberous sclerosis gene on chromosome 16. Cell 75:1305, 1993.

48. Green AJ, Johnson PH, Yates JRW: The tuberous sclerosis gene on chromosome 9q34 acts as a growth suppressor. Hum Mol Genet 3:1833, 1994.

49. Online Mendelian Inheritance in Man (OMIM). MIM {161050}. Baltimore, Johns Hopkins University. Available at: http://www3.ncbi.nim.nih.gov/omim/.

50. Pavone L, LiVolti S, Guarneri B, et al: Hereditary twenty-nail dystrophy in a Sicilian family. J Med Genet 19:337, 1982.

51. Baran R, Bureau H, Sayag J: Congenital malalignment of the big toe nail. Clin Exp Dermatol 4:359, 1979.

52. Martin SM, Rudolph AH: Familial dystrophic periodic shedding of the nails. Cutis 25:622, 1980.

53. Main R: Periodic shedding of the nails. Br J Dermatol 88:497, 1973.

54. Baden HP, Kubilus J: Analysis of hair from alopecia congenita. J Am Acad Dermatol 3:623, 1980.

55. Steijlen PM, Neumann HA, der Kinderen DJ, et al: Congenital atrichia, palmoplantar hyperkeratosis, mental retardation, and early loss of teeth in four siblings: a new syndrome? J Am Acad Dermatol 30:893, 1994.

56. Cantu JM, Sanchez-Corona J, Gonzalez-Mendoza A, et al: Autosomal recessive inheritance of atrichia congenita. Clin Genet 17:209, 1980.

57. Loewenthal LJA, Prakken JR: Atrichia with papular lesions. Dermatologica 122:85–89, 1961.

58. Kanzler MH, Rasmussen JE: Atrichia with papular lesions. Arch Dermatol 122:565, 1986.

59. Online Mendelian Inheritance in Man (OMIM). MIM {146550}. Baltimore, Johns Hopkins University. Available at: http://www3.ncbi.nim.nih.gov/omim/.

60. Solomon LM, Esterly NB, Medenica M: Hereditary trichodysplasia: Marie Unna's hypotrichosis. J Invest Dermatol 57:389, 1971.

61. Bentley-Phillips B, Grace HJ: Hereditary hypotrichosis: a previously undescribed syndrome. Br J Dermatol 101:331, 1979.

62. Online Mendelian Inheritance in Man (OMIM). MIM {600628}. Baltimore, Johns Hopkins University. Available at: http://www3.ncbi.nim.nih.gov/omim/.

63. Baden HP, Kvedar JC, Magro CM: Loose anagen hair as a cause of hereditary hair loss in children. Arch Dermatol 128:1349–1353, 1992.

64. Price VH, Bummer CL: Loose anagen syndrome. J Am Acad Dermatol 20:249–256, 1989.

65. Online Mendelian Inheritance in Man (OMIM). MIM {308800}. Baltimore, Johns Hopkins University. Available at: http://www3.ncbi.nim.nih.gov/omim/.

66. Baden HP, Byers HR: Clinical findings, cutaneous pathology and response to therapy in 21 patients with keratosis pilaris atrophicans. Arch Dermatol 130:469–475, 1994.

67. Oosterwijk JC, van der Wielen MJR, van de Vosse E, et al: Refinement of the localisation of the X linked keratosis follicularis spinulosa decalvans (KFSD) gene in Xp22.13-p22.2. J Med Genet 32:736, 1995.

68. Online Mendelian Inheritance in Man (OMIM). MIM {129500, 305100}. Baltimore, Johns Hopkins University. Available at: http://www3.ncbi.nim.nih.gov/omim/.

69. Clarke A, Burn J: Sweat testing to identify female carriers of X-linked hypohidrotic ectodermal dysplasia. J Med Genet 28:330, 1991.

70. Kere J, Srivastava AK, Montonen O, et al: X-linked anhidrotic (hypohidrotic) ectodermal dysplasia is caused by mutation in a novel transmembrane protein. Nat Genet 13:409, 1996.

71. Zonana J, Clarke A, Sarfarazi M, et al: X-linked hypohidrotic ectodermal dysplasia: localization with the region Xq11–21.1 by linkage analysis and implications for carrier detection and prenatal diagnosis. Am J Hum Genet 43:75, 1988.

72. Hayflick SJ, Taylor T, McKinnon W, et al: Clouston syndrome (hidrotic ectodermal dysplasia) is not linked to keratin gene clusters on chromosomes 12 and 17. J Invest Dermatol 107:11–14, 1996.

73. Stevens HP, Kelsell DP, Bryant SP, et al: Linkage of monilethrix to the trichocyte and epithelial keratin gene cluster on 12q11-q13. J Invest Dermatol 106:795–797, 1996.

74. Online Mendelian Inheritance in Man (OMIM). MIM {277700, 176670, 224230, 127550, 305000, 216500, 268400}. Baltimore, Johns Hopkins University. Available at: http://www3.ncbi.nim.nih.gov/omim/.

75. Drachtman RA, Alter BP: Dyskeratosis congenita: clinical and genetic heterogeneity. Report of a new case and review of the literature. Am J Pediatr Hematol Oncol 14:297, 1992.

76. Davidson HR, Connor JM: Dyskeratosis congenita. J Med Genet 25:843, 1988.

77. Knight SW, Vulliamy T, Forni GL, et al: Fine mapping of the dyskeratosis congenita locus in Xq28. J Med Genet 33:993, 1996.

78. Stefanini M, Fawcett H, Botta E, et al: Genetic analysis of twenty-two patients with Cockayne syndrome. Hum Genet 97:418, 1996.

79. Online Mendelian Inheritance in Man (OMIM). MIM {253270, 253260, 277440, 20110}. Baltimore, Johns Hopkins University. Available at: http://www3.ncbi.nim.nih.gov/omim/.

80. Suzuki Y, Aoki Y, Ishida Y: Isolation and characterization of mutations in the human holocarboxylase synthetase cDNA. Nat Genet 8:122, 1994.

81. Pomponio RJ, Norrgard KJ, Hymes J, et al: Arg538 to Cys mutation in a CpG dinucleotide of the human biotinidase gene is the second most common cause of profound biotinidase deficiency in symptomatic children. Hum Genet 99:506, 1997.

82. Malloy PJ, Eccleshall TR, Gross C, et al: Hereditary vitamin D resistant rickets caused by a novel mutation in the vitamin D receptor that results in decreased affinity for hormone and cellular hyporesponsiveness. J Clin Invest 99:297, 1997.

83. Moynahan EJ: Acrodermatitis enteropathica: a lethal inherited human zinc deficiency disorder. Lancet 2:399, 1974.

84. Online Mendelian Inheritance in Man (OMIM). MIM {250250}. Baltimore, Johns Hopkins University. Available at: http://www3.ncbi.nim.nih.gov/omim/.

85. Makitie O, Sulisalo T, de la Chapelle A, Kaitila I: Cartilage-hair hypoplasia. J Med Genet 32:39, 1995.

86. Sulisalo T, Sistonen P, Hastbacka J, et al: Cartilage-hair hypoplasia gene assigned to chromosome 9 by linkage analysis. Nat Genet 3:338, 1993.

87. van der Burgt I, Haraldsson A, Oosterwijk JC, et al: Cartilage hair hypoplasia, metaphyseal chondrodysplasia type McKusick: description of seven patients and review of the literature. Am J Med Genet 41:371, 1991.

88. Online Mendelian Inheritance in Man (OMIM). MIM {305600}. Baltimore, Johns Hopkins University. Available at: http://www3.ncbi.nim.nih.gov/omim/.

89. Goltz RW: Focal dermal hypoplasia: an update [editorial]. Arch Dermatol 128:1108, 1992.

90. Bellosta M, Trespiolli D, Ghiselli E, et al: Focal dermal hypoplasia: report of a family with 7 affected women in 3 generations. Eur J Dermatol 6:499, 1996.

91. Online Mendelian Inheritance in Man (OMIM). MIM {132000}. Baltimore, Johns Hopkins University. Available at: http://www3.ncbi.nim.nih.gov/omim/.

92. Zelickson B, Matsumura K, Kist D, et al: Bart's syndrome. Arch Dermatol 131:663, 1995.

93. Christiano AM, Bart BJ, Epstein EH, Uitto J: Genetic basis of Bart's syndrome: a glycine substitution mutation in the type VII collagen gene. J Invest Dermatol 106:778, 1996.

94. Garcia-Hernandez MJ, Rodriguez-Pichardo A, Camacho F: Congenital triangular alopecia (Brauer nevus). Pediatr Dermatol 12:301, 1995.

95. Anderson E: An American pedigree for woolly hair. J Hered 27:444, 1936.

96. Hutchinson PE, Cairns RJ, Wells RS: Wooly hair: clinical and general aspects. Trans St John's Hosp Derm Soc 60:160, 1974.

97. Online Mendelian Inheritance in Man (OMIM). MIM {148210}. Baltimore, Johns Hopkins University. Available at: http://www3.ncbi.nim.nih.gov/omim/.

98. Caceres-Rios H, Tamayo-Sanchez L, Duran-Mckinster C, de la Luz Orozco M, Ruiz-Maldonado R: Keratitis, ichthyosis, and deafness (KID syndrome): review of the literature and proposal of a new terminology. Pediatr Dermatol 13:105, 1996.

99. Wilson GN, Squires RH Jr, Weinberg AG: Keratitis, hepatitis, ichthyosis, and deafness: report and review of KID syndrome. Am J Med Genet 40:255, 1991.

c h a p t e r

4

Dermatological Diseases That Affect the Nail

ANTONELLA TOSTI

—

BIANCA MARIA PIRACCINI

Psoriasis

Nail involvement is observed in about 50% of adults and 10% of children with psoriasis. It is more common in patients with arthropathic psoriasis (70%). Psoriasis limited to the nails is not rare; in our experience, it affects about one third of patients who seek a nail consultation. In these patients a mild scalp involvement is often detected by clinical examination.

Repetitive trauma may favor the development of nail psoriasis through a Koebner phenomenon. Occupational trauma may therefore trigger or worsen fingernail psoriasis, and podiatric abnormalities may worsen toenail psoriasis.

CLINICAL FEATURES

Psoriasis produces several nail symptoms that may occur together or separately[1] (Fig. 4–1). Fingernail psoriasis usually manifests with multiple clinical signs; in order of frequency, they are pitting, reddish oily patches, onycholysis, subungual hyperkeratosis, and splinter hemorrhages. Toenail psoriasis usually is less polymorphic and manifests with subungual hyperkeratosis and diffuse yellow-brown discoloration of the nail plate (Fig. 4–2).

Pitting describes the presence of punctate depressions (pits) on the nail plate surface. Each pit results from a psoriatic focus in the proximal nail matrix, with persistence of clusters of loosely attached parakeratotic cells within the upper layers of the nail plate. Psoriasic pits are usually large, deep, and randomly scattered (Fig. 4–3). Pits are almost never observed in toenails.

Oily patches appear as yellowish or salmon-pink areas

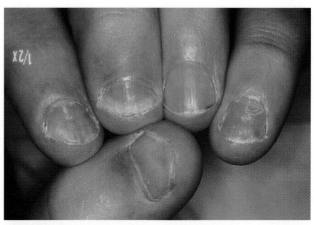

FIGURE 4–1 ■ Psoriasis. Several symptoms are randomly distributed in the different nails.

47

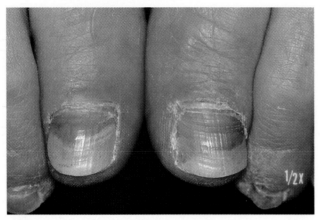

FIGURE 4–2 ■ Toenail psoriasis. Note prominent hyperkeratosis and onycholysis.

easily visible through the transparent nail plate. They result from a focal psoriatic involvement of the nail bed. Oily patches may be localized in the central portion of the nail or in the distal nail bed to surround an onycholytic area.

Onycholysis results from involvement of the nail bed and hyponychium. In psoriasis the onycholytic area typically is separated from the normal nail plate by an erythematous border.

Subungual hyperkeratosis results from the accumulation of parakeratotic cells under the distal portion of the nail plate. This produces a detachment of the nail plate from the nail bed. In fingernails, parakeratotic cells are usually shed and onycholysis is the prominent symptom. In the toenails, subungual hyperkeratosis usually is tightly adherent to the nail plate, which becomes hard, thick, and raised. Scales of subungual hyperkeratosis may have the typical whitish, silvery color of psoriatic scales or, more frequently, they may have a yellow, greasy appearance caused by the presence of a glycoproteic exudate between parakeratotic scales.

Splinter hemorrhages appear as longitudinal, linear, red-brown hemorrhages. They are most frequently seen in fingernails and usually are located in the distal portion of the nail plate. Splinter hemorrhages are a conse-

quence of psoriatic involvement of the nail bed capillary loops that run in a longitudinal direction along the nail bed dermal ridges.

Most frequently, patients with nail psoriasis present with a mild to moderate nail dystrophy that affects a few nails. The severity of the nail changes may vary considerably from nail to nail. Nail bed hyperkeratosis and onycholysis may considerably impair manual dexterity and foot biomechanics.

In a minority of patients, who usually are affected by severe skin or joint disease, psoriasis may cause severe nail changes owing to massive involvement of all of the nail unit. In these cases massive nail bed hyperkeratosis is associated with crumbling of the nail plate.

Typically, the disease has a variable course, with remissions and relapses that do not occur simultaneously in all nails.

PATHOLOGY

The pathological features of nail psoriasis are similar to those of skin psoriasis. However, hyperkeratosis usually is more marked, and spongiosis of the nail epithelia is a frequent finding.

DIAGNOSIS

The various signs of nail psoriasis may be present in one nail or may be randomly distributed in the different nails. The presence of multiple clinical signs makes the diagnosis easy.

The following nail findings are key to diagnosing psoriasis: onycholysis surrounded by an erythematous border; salmon patches of the nail bed; and irregular pitting associated with onycholysis, subungual hyperkeratosis, splinter hemorrhages, or some combination of these conditions.

In the absence of skin lesions or typical nail signs, the differential diagnosis of nail psoriasis includes contact dermatitis and onychomycosis. When psoriasis is limited to the toenails, differential diagnosis with onychomycosis may be impossible without a mycological study. However, fungal colonization of psoriatic nails is not uncommon.

TREATMENT

Nail psoriasis has an unpredictable course, but in most cases the disease is chronic and complete remissions are uncommon. Sunlight does not improve nail psoriasis, which may often worsen during summer.

Because topical drugs do not reach the nail matrix, treatment of nail matrix psoriasis requires systemic or intralesional drug administration. Systemic treatment with steroids, methotrexate, or cyclosporin A improves the nail but should be used only when nail psoriasis is associated with widespread disease or psoriatic arthritis. Intralesional steroid injections (triamcinolone acetonide, 5–10 mg/mL) at a dose of 0.2 to 0.5 mL per nail can be useful, even though the nail abnormalities usually relapse after discontinuation of therapy.

Psoriasis of the nail bed and hyponychium may bene-

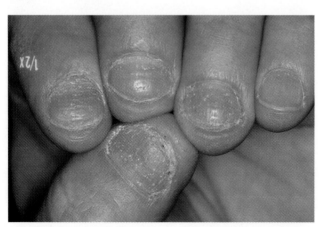

FIGURE 4–3 ■ Pitting caused by nail matrix psoriasis.

fit from treatment with topical steroids or calcipotriol (or both) after removal of the onycholytic nail plate.

Pustular Psoriasis

Pustular psoriasis can produce nail abnormalities. Prevalence, severity, and clinical presentation of nail changes are different in the various types of pustular psoriasis.[2]

In *acute palmoplantar pustular psoriasis* and *acute generalized pustular psoriasis,* nail abnormalities are uncommon but severe. Several or all nails are involved, with a large number of pustules affecting the entire nail unit. Definitive nail scarring is a common sequela.

In *Hallopeau's acrodermatitis continua,* nail abnormalities are found in the majority of patients. The condition usually is restricted to a single digit that shows recurrent painful pustular lesions in the periungual tissues and nail apparatus. The pustular eruption most commonly affects the nail bed. The affected nail may have a few pustular lesions that are visible through the nail plate (Fig. 4–4), or it may be severely dystrophic with nail bed hyperkeratosis and onycholysis (Fig. 4–5). Matrix involvement occasionally occurs and produces permanent scarring with partial or total loss of the nail plate. In long-standing lesions it is common to see a definitive atrophy of the nail apparatus and periungual soft tissues. Bone resorption is not rare.

In *chronic palmoplantar pustular psoriasis,* nail abnormalities are present in about one fifth of patients, with a clinical picture resembling that of nail psoriasis (Fig. 4–6) or of Hallopeau's acrodermatitis.

PATHOLOGY

The nail pathology shows spongiform pustules with parakeratosis.

DIAGNOSIS

In acute palmoplantar pustular psoriasis, acute generalized pustular psoriasis, and chronic palmoplantar pustu-

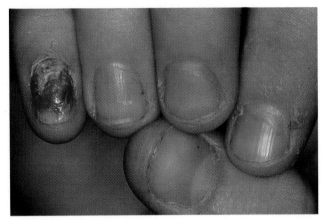

FIGURE 4–5 ■ Pustular psoriasis: typical involvement of a single nail in Hallopeau's acrodermatitis continua.

lar psoriasis, the diagnosis is suggested by the presence of typical skin lesions.

A diagnosis of Hallopeau's acrodermatitis should always be considered when the history reveals recurrent painful pustular eruption of the nail. Differential diagnosis when recurrent herpetic whitlow and bacterial infections are present usually is not difficult. In chronic cases, onychomycosis should be ruled out by cultures.

TREATMENT

Pustular psoriasis requires a systemic treatment. Etretinate (0.5–0.75 mg/kg) arrests the development of pustular lesions and avoids permanent scarring of the nail apparatus. Topical calcipotriol may be useful in some patients.

Lichen Planus

Specific nail involvement occurs in about 10% of patients with skin or oral lichen planus. Lichen planus limited to the nails is not uncommon.

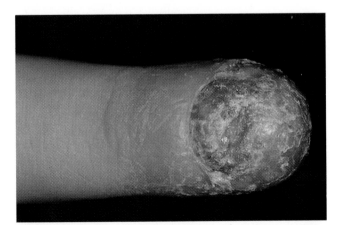

FIGURE 4–4 ■ Pustular psoriasis: diffuse pustular eruption in Hallopeau's acrodermatitis continua.

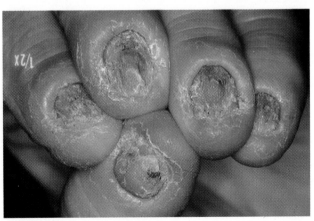

FIGURE 4–6 ■ Pustular psoriasis: severe nail changes in chronic palmoplantar pustular psoriasis.

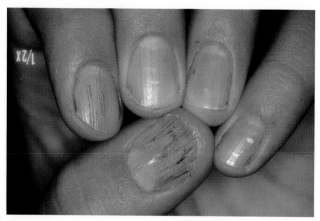

FIGURE 4-7 ■ Nail matrix lichen planus.

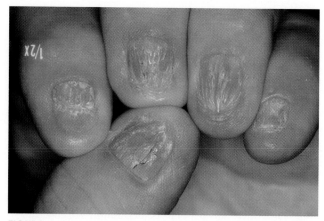

FIGURE 4-9 ■ Longstanding nail matrix lichen planus with diffuse nail pterygium.

CLINICAL FEATURES

The clinical manifestations of nail lichen planus depend on the localization of the disease in the nail apparatus and the duration and severity of the inflammatory changes.[3] Nail matrix lichen planus is a serious disease because it can definitively destroy the nails.

Most commonly, *nail matrix lichen planus* produces thinning, longitudinal ridging, and splitting of the nail plate (Fig. 4–7). Progression of the disease frequently results in permanent damage to the nail matrix with dorsal pterygium formation. In dorsal pterygium, the proximal nail fold epidermis adheres to the underlying nail bed epidermis, with the formation of a V-shaped extension of the skin of the proximal nail fold.

Nail bed lichen planus is less common and usually is associated with nail matrix involvement (Fig. 4–8). The affected nails show subungual hyperkeratosis and onycholysis.

In rare cases, nail lichen planus produces trachyonychia (20-nail dystrophy) or idiopathic atrophy of the nails.

PATHOLOGY

The pathological features of nail lichen planus are similar to those of skin lichen planus.

DIAGNOSIS

The diagnosis of nail lichen planus should be considered when nail thinning is associated with longitudinal ridging, splitting, and dorsal pterygium.

TREATMENT

Prompt treatment of nail lichen planus is mandatory, because the disease frequently results in a permanent destruction of the nail matrix with pterygium or onychoatrophy (Fig. 4–9). Permanent damage of at least one nail occurs in approximately 4% of patients.

Oral prednisone, 0.5 mg/kg every other day for 2 to 6 weeks, or intramuscular triamcinolone acetonide (Kenalog), 0.5 mg/kg every month for 2 to 3 months, usually produces recovery of the nail abnormalities. Intralesional injections of triamcinolone acetonide, 5 to 10 mg/mL, are a possible alternative when the disease is limited to a few nails. Mild relapses are frequently observed but usually are responsive to therapy.

Idiopathic Atrophy of the Nails

The term *idiopathic atrophy of the nails* describes a progressive and painless nail atrophy with scarring occurring during childhood.[4] Whether idiopathic atrophy of the nails should be considered a separate entity or a clinical variant of nail lichen planus is still controversial.

CLINICAL FEATURES

The nails show areas of complete absence of the nail plate with pterygium and nail bed scarring and areas of

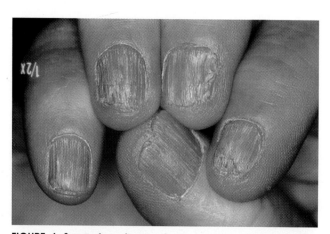

FIGURE 4-8 ■ Lichen planus with simultaneous involvement of the nail matrix and nail bed.

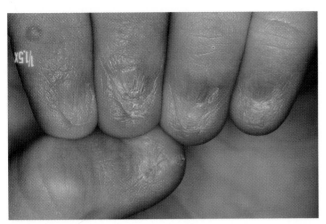

FIGURE 4–10 ■ Idiopathic atrophy of the nails producing pterygium of all nails.

severe thinning without obliteration of the proximal nail old (Fig. 4–10). When present, the hypoplastic nail plate is often yellow and detached from the nail bed.

PATHOLOGY

The nail pathology reveals nail matrix hypergranulosis with complete destruction of the keratogenous zone.

DIAGNOSIS

The diagnosis is suggested by the clinical history and the presence of severe nail atrophy both with and without pterygium.

TREATMENT

The condition is permanent.

Lichen Nitidus

Lichen nitidus is a rare, asymptomatic, chronic disorder that occasionally produces nail abnormalities.

CLINICAL FEATURES

Most commonly, the disease involves the proximal nail fold with multiple, pinhead-sized papules. These may be associated with nail pitting. In rare cases, nail lichen nitidus produces nail changes that resemble those of nail lichen planus, with thinning, longitudinal ridging, and splitting of the nail plate.

PATHOLOGY

The nail pathology reveals the presence of a lichenoid infiltrate with epithelioid and multinucleated giant cells.

DIAGNOSIS

The nail abnormalities are usually associated with typical skin lesions.

TREATMENT

Proximal nail fold involvement may be treated with topical steroids.

Lichen Striatus

When lichen striatus involves the fingers or the toes, nail involvement may occur as a consequence of inflammatory changes in the nail matrix. Usually a single nail is affected.[5]

CLINICAL FEATURES

Nail abnormalities closely resemble those of nail matrix lichen planus, with nail thinning associated with longitudinal ridging and splitting. Nail changes, however, are typically restricted to the medial or lateral portion of the nails (Fig. 4–11).

PATHOLOGY

The nail biopsy reveals lichen planus–like changes of the nail matrix.

DIAGNOSIS

The presence of linearly arranged papules along the affected extremity suggests the diagnosis.

In some cases lichen striatus is restricted to the nail. The diagnosis should be suspected when a child or a young patient has lichen planus–like abnormalities confined to the lateral or medial portion of a single nail.

TREATMENT

The nail lesions regress spontaneously in a few years.

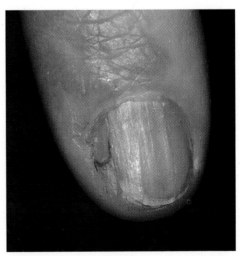

FIGURE 4–11 ■ Lichen striatus limited to the nail. Note lichenoid nail changes restricted to the medial portion of the nail plate.

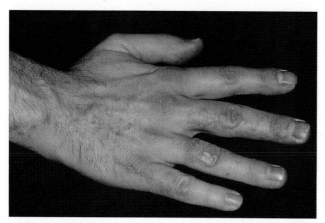

FIGURE 4–12 ■ Inflammatory linear verrucous epidermal nevus (ILVEN): psoriasiform nail changes.

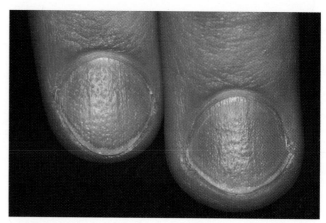

FIGURE 4–13 ■ Alopecia areata: geometric pitting.

Inflammatory Linear Verrucous Epidermal Nevus

Nail abnormalities in inflammatory linear verrucous epidermal nevus (ILVEN) are rare and are always associated with typical skin lesions of the affected digit.

CLINICAL FEATURES

Nail changes closely resemble those of psoriasis, with pitting, subungual hyperkeratosis, and onycholysis (Fig. 4–12).

DIAGNOSIS

The diagnosis is suggested by the presence of psoriasiform and verrucous skin lesions with a linear arrangement on the affected limb.

TREATMENT

Nail lesions are persistent and do not respond to treatment.

Alopecia Areata

Nail abnormalities occur in 46% of children[6] and 19% of adults with alopecia areata. Nail changes may precede or follow the diagnosis of alopecia areata; most commonly, however, nail changes and hair loss develop together, suggesting a common injury of both the hair and nail matrix.

CLINICAL FEATURES

Most frequently alopecia areata of the nails produces a regular and superficial pitting caused by focal involvement of the proximal nail matrix (Fig. 4–13). Pits may occasionally be associated with a mottled erythema of the lunulae that appears dishomogeneously red. Onycho-

madesis of all 20 nails may be seen during the acute onset of alopecia areata or alopecia universalis.

A peculiar form of punctate leukonychia characterized by white, pinpoint macules arranged in a repetitive fashion in longitudinal arrays is occasionally observed.

Trachyonychia (20-nail dystrophy) occurs in 12% of children and 3.3% of adults with severe alopecia areata (Fig. 4–14).

PATHOLOGY

The nail pathology shows a spongiotic inflammation of the nail apparatus.

DIAGNOSIS

The diagnosis of alopecia areata should always be considered in patients who have geometrical pitting or trachyonychia.

TREATMENT

Nail changes usually regress spontaneously and do not require treatment.

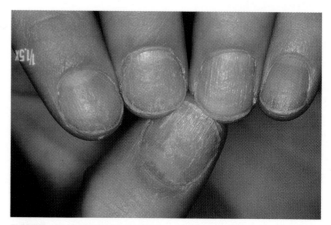

FIGURE 4–14 ■ Trachyonychia in a patient affected by alopecia areata.

Twenty-Nail Dystrophy (Trachyonychia)

The term *20-nail dystrophy*, or *trachyonychia*, describes a range of nail plate surface abnormalities that result in nail roughness.

Patients with trachyonychia can be divided into two main groups: patients with trachyonychia and a personal history or clinical evidence of alopecia areata, and patients with isolated nail involvement (idiopathic trachyonychia).

The frequency of idiopathic trachyonychia is unknown, but it is a rather rare nail disorder that is more commonly but not exclusively seen in children. Idiopathic trachyonychia may be a clinical manifestation of various nail diseases,[8] including lichen planus, psoriasis, eczema, and pemphigus vulgaris. It may also represent a clinical variety of alopecia areata limited to the nails.

CLINICAL FEATURES

Two varieties of trachyonychia were originally described by Baran and colleagues[7] in 1978: opaque trachyonychia and shiny trachyonychia. Either can occur in association with alopecia areata or idiopathically. Opaque trachyonychia is more common than shiny trachyonychia. In opaque trachyonychia, the nail plate surface shows severe longitudinal ridging and is covered by multiple, small, adherent scales. The nail is thin, opaque, and lusterless and gives the impression of having been sandpapered in a longitudinal direction (vertically striated sandpapered nails) (Fig. 4–15). The cuticle of the affected nails frequently is ragged, and a certain degree of koilonychia is often present.

In shiny trachyonychia, the nail plate surface abnormalities are less severe. Nail plate roughness is mild and is caused by a myriad of minuscule punctate depressions, that reflect the light.

In some patients, some nails have the sandpapered appearance and others have the shiny appearance.

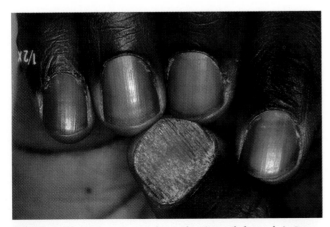

FIGURE 4–15 ■ Idiopathic trachyonychia (20-nail dystrophy). Severe nail roughness of one nail. The biopsy revealed spongiotic changes of the nail matrix epithelium.

The condition is symptomless, and patients complain only of brittleness and cosmetic considerations.

Although trachyonychia is better known as 20-nail dystrophy, the nail changes do not necessarily involve all 20 nails in every patient. Only fingernails or only toenails may be affected, and sometimes the onychodystrophy is limited to a few digits.

PATHOLOGY

Idiopathic trachyonychia is most commonly characterized by a spongiotic inflammation of the nail, but it can also be associated with the pathological features of lichen planus or psoriasis. Trachyonychia of alopecia areata is pathologically characterized by spongiotic changes.

DIAGNOSIS

Trachyonychia is a nail symptom that can be caused by several inflammatory diseases that disturb the nail matrix keratinization. There are no clinical criteria to distinguish spongiotic trachyonychia, the most common type, from trachyonychia caused by other inflammatory skin diseases.

TREATMENT

Trachyonychia is a benign condition that never produces nail scarring. This is true not only for trachyonychia associated with spongiotic changes, but also for trachyonychia caused by lichen planus or other dermatological diseases. Spongiotic trachyonychia regresses spontaneously in most patients.

Eczema

Involvement of the nails is commonly observed in atopic eczema and in irritant and allergic contact dermatitis. The proximal nail fold and hyponychium are most frequently affected.

CLINICAL FEATURES

Proximal nail fold involvement producing mild nail matrix damage is not uncommon in patients with hand eczema (Fig. 4–16). This results in nail plate surface abnormalities such as irregular pitting and Beau's lines. Onychomadesis may occur in severe cases (Fig. 4–17).

Chronic exposure to irritants or allergens may be responsible for the development of chronic paronychia, with loss of the cuticle together with erythema and swelling of the proximal nail fold.

Contact dermatitis of the hyponychium is usually chronic and associated with fingertip lesions (Figs. 4–18 and 4–19). The nails show subungual hyperkeratosis and onycholysis. Hyponychium contact dermatitis is most frequently occupational.

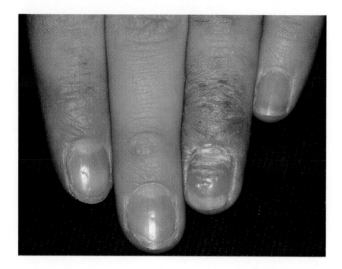

FIGURE 4-16 ■ Nail involvement in a patient affected by chronic contact dermatitis caused by nickel exposure.

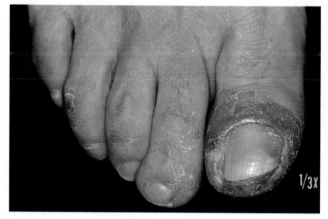

FIGURE 4-17 ■ Acute contact dermatitis caused by topical medicaments.

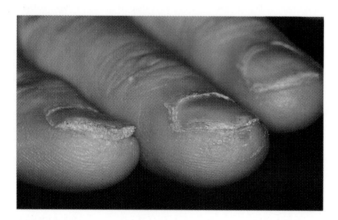

FIGURE 4-18 ■ Irritative contact dermatitis of the hyponychium.

FIGURE 4-19 ■ Allergic contact dermatitis of the hyponychium caused by acrylates.

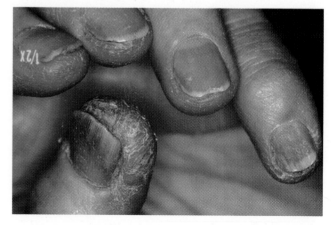

DIAGNOSIS

Patch testing is essential to discriminate between allergic and irritant reactions, the latter being more common.

TREATMENT

Avoidance of the causative factor is mandatory. Systemic or topical steroids are effective.

Pompholyx

Patients with palmoplantar hyperhidrosis may develop idiopathic onycholysis of several fingernails during summer.

CLINICAL FEATURES

Onycholysis usually develops simultaneously in all fingernails. The detachment regularly extends from one side of the nail to the other and shows a smooth proximal border. The nail bed is apparently normal. Nail abnormalities identical to those described for eczema may be associated.

DIAGNOSIS

Sudden development of onycholysis of all fingernails in summer should suggest the diagnosis.

Differential diagnosis includes idiopathic onycholysis and psoriasis.

Parakeratosis Pustulosa

This condition possibly represents a limited form of psoriasis. Parakeratosis pustulosa is a chronic condition that exclusively affects children, most commonly girls. It usually involves a single digit, most commonly the thumb or the index finger.[9]

CLINICAL FEATURES

In most cases the development of nail changes is preceded by fingertip erythema and scaling. However, this is not always true, and some patients may develop nail abnormalities in the absence of skin involvement.

The affected digit shows eczematous changes associated with mild distal subungual hyperkeratosis and onycholysis (Fig. 4–20). Nail abnormalities usually are more marked on one corner of the nail. Pitting of the nail plate may be present. The nail abnormalities closely resemble those seen in psoriasis.

DIAGNOSIS

Diagnosis of parakeratosis pustulosa should always be considered in a child with psoriasiform nail changes limited to a single digit.

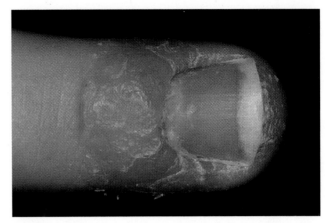

FIGURE 4–20 ■ Parakeratosis pustulosa: psoriasiform changes of the nail and periungual skin.

Patch tests can be useful to rule out contact dermatitis.

TREATMENT

The condition usually improves spontaneously when the child grows up. Some children, however, develop a typical nail psoriasis.

Pemphigus Vulgaris

In pemphigus vulgaris, acantholysis may occasionally involve the nail epithelia, especially the proximal nail fold.

CLINICAL FEATURES

Acantholysis restricted to the ventral portion of the proximal nail fold results in acute paronychia (Fig. 4–21). Patients complain of erythema, swelling, and pain of the paronychium. This usually is not associated with evidence of bullous lesions of the digits. Development of onychomadesis frequently follows the acute episode,

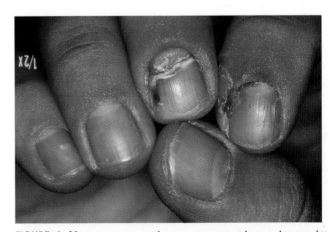

FIGURE 4–21 ■ Acute paronychia in a patient with pemphigus vulgaris.

and in some patients it may develop at each recurrence of the disease. Nail bed involvement is exceptional and may produce subungual hemorrhages and onycholysis.

PATHOLOGY

The pathology shows acantholysis with bulla formation.

DIAGNOSIS

The diagnosis of nail pemphigus may be difficult because the periungual inflammation is not specific and may suggest a bacterial infection or a herpetic whitlow. Direct immunofluorescence confirms the diagnosis.

TREATMENT

The nail lesions respond promptly to systemic steroids.

Bullous Pemphigoid

Nail involvement can occasionally be seen in patients with bullous pemphigoid or cicatricial pemphigoid.

CLINICAL FEATURES

Bullae affecting the proximal nail fold produce acute paronychia (Fig. 4–22). Nail matrix involvement may result in Beau's lines, onychomadesis or longitudinal splitting with pterygium. Nail atrophy has been reported in cicatricial pemphigoid.

PATHOLOGY

The pathology shows subepidermal splitting. Direct immunofluorescence is necessary for diagnosis.

DIAGNOSIS

Differential diagnosis with acquired epidermolysis bullosa requires immunoelectron microscopy or salt split-skin immunofluorescence.

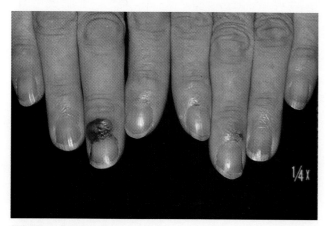

FIGURE 4–22 ■ Bullous pemphigoid involving the proximal nail fold.

Acquired Epidermolysis Bullosa

In acquired epidermolysis bullosa, erosions and blisters develop in the acral regions of the body, especially after trauma, and heal with scarring and milia formation. The nails may be affected.

CLINICAL FEATURES

Paronychia, onychomadesis, and nail scarring with pterygium may be seen.

TREATMENT

The disease scarcely responds to treatment. Avoidance of trauma is important to prevent bullae formation.

Erythema Multiforme

Although erythema multiforme commonly affects the digits, nail involvement is rare.

CLINICAL FEATURES

Typical papular or vesicular target lesions are commonly seen on the dorsal aspects of the digits and on the palms and soles. The nails may show paronychia or onychomadesis caused by the formation of blisters in the proximal nail fold and nail matrix. Nail scarring with severe pterygium may occasionally follow a severe episode of erythema multiforme major (Stevens-Johnson syndrome).

TREATMENT

Spontaneous recovery is usual, but nail pterygium may occur in severe cases.

Darier's Disease

Nail abnormalities are common in patients with Darier-White disease and may be helpful in the diagnosis of patients with minimal skin lesions.[10]

CLINICAL FEATURES

The clinical signs of Darier's disease are distinctive. The nail shows longitudinal, subungual, red and white streaks that typically are associated with a V-shaped notch in the nail plate free margin. This is caused by distal wedge-shaped subungual hyperkeratosis. Red streaks represent early lesions that in time develop into white streaks (Fig. 4–23).

Typical nail lesions frequently are associated with splinter hemorrhages and flat, keratotic papules on the

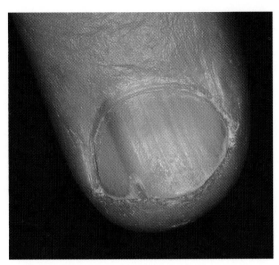

FIGURE 4–23 ■ Darier's disease.

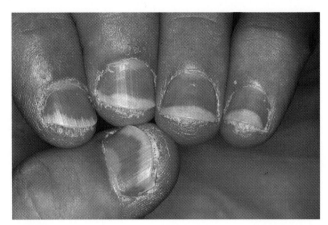

FIGURE 4–24 ■ Pityriasis rubra pilaris.

proximal nail fold. Severe splitting and massive thickening of the nail plate with nail bed hyperkeratosis may occasionally be observed.

PATHOLOGY

Pathological analysis of the white longitudinal streaks reveals the presence of numerous multinucleated onychocytes in the nail bed epithelium.

DIAGNOSIS

The longitudinal red and white streaks of Darier's disease are diagnostic.

TREATMENT

The nail lesions are usually persistent and not responsive to treatment with systemic retinoids.

Pityriasis Rubra Pilaris

Nail involvement is common in adult acute-onset type I pityriasis rubra pilaris and can occasionally be observed in other types of pityriasis rubra pilaris.

CLINICAL FEATURES

Fingernails are more severely affected, with yellow discoloration and thickening of the distal portion of the nail plate associated with subungual hyperkeratosis and splinter hemorrhages (Fig. 4–24).

DIAGNOSIS

Because skin and nail changes may be similar to those of psoriasis, a skin biopsy usually is necessary to confirm the diagnosis.

TREATMENT

Treatment with systemic retinoids improves the nail changes.

Palmoplantar Keratoderma

Patients with palmoplantar keratoderma may exhibit nail changes that are more commonly associated with diffuse palmoplantar keratoderma.

CLINICAL FEATURES

Psoriasiform changes with subungual hyperkeratosis, onycholysis, splinter hemorrhages, and irregular pitting are most commonly observed.

Onychogryphosis, nail thickening, longitudinal fissures, and onychomadesis can also occur.

PATHOLOGY

The nail pathology parallels that of the skin.

DIAGNOSIS

The diagnosis requires evaluation of the skin lesions and a pathological study.

TREATMENT

Although etretinate therapy usually produces a significant improvement of palmoplantar keratodermas, retinoids are in general of little value for the treatment of nail involvement.

Bazex Syndrome

Bazex syndrome, or acrokeratosis paraneoplastica of Bazex and Dupré, is a paraneoplastic disorder that oc-

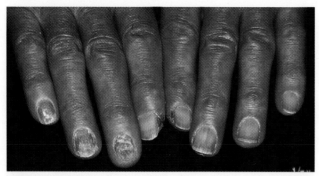

FIGURE 4–25 ■ Psoriasiform nail changes in a patient affected by Bazex syndrome.

curs in association with malignant tumors of the upper respiratory or digestive tracts.[11]

CLINICAL FEATURES

Skin lesions typically show an acral, symmetrical distribution with involvement of the hands, feet, nose, and ears. The periungual region shows psoriasiform changes with erythema and scaling. The nails may be markedly dystrophic, with subungual hyperkeratosis and onycholysis (Fig. 4–25).

DIAGNOSIS

Bazex syndrome may precede the symptoms of the associated malignancy by several months. This diagnosis should be considered in males with a psoriasiform erup-

tion that symmetrically involves the digits, the nose, and the ears.

TREATMENT

The skin lesions usually disappear when the tumor is removed and reappear with its recurrence. Topical steroids, systemic steroids, and etretinate may improve the eruption.

REFERENCES

1. Zaias N: Psoriasis of the nail: a clinical-pathological study. Arch Dermatol 99:567–579, 1969.
2. Burden AD, Kemmet D: The spectrum of nail involvement in palmoplantar pustulosis. Br J Dermatol 134:1079–1082, 1996.
3. Tosti A, Peluso AM, Fanti PA, et al: Nail lichen planus: clinical and pathologic study of 24 patients. J Am Acad Dermatol 28:724–730, 1993.
4. Tosti A, Piraccini BM, Fanti PA, et al: Idiopathic atrophy of the nails: clinical and pathological study of two cases. Dermatology 190:116–118, 1995.
5. Tosti A, Peluso AM, Misciali C, et al: Nail lichen striatus: clinical features and long-term follow-up of five cases. J Am Acad Dermatol 36:908–913, 1997.
6. Tosti A, Morelli R, Bardazzi F, et al: Prevalence of nail abnormalities in children with alopecia areata. Pediatr Dermatol 11:112–115, 1994.
7. Baran R, Dupré A, Christol B, et al: Vertical striated sand-papered twenty-nail dystropy. Ann Dermatol Venereol 105:387–392, 1978.
8. Tosti A, Piraccini BM: Trachyonychia or twenty-nail dystrophy. Curr Opin Dermatol 3:83–86, 1996.
9. Avci O, Günes AT: Parakeratosis pustulosa with dyskeratotic cells. Dermatology 189:413–414, 1994.
10. Zaias N, Ackerman AB: The nails in Darier-White disease. Arch Dermatol 107:193–199, 1973.
11. Bazex A, Griffiths A: Acrokeratosis paraneoplastica: a new cutaneous marker of malignancy. Br J Dermatol 102:301–306, 1980.

Nail Signs of Systemic Disease

MARK HOLZBERG

Because of specialized changes in the skin that occur in the nail, clues to systemic disease can be found by close examination of the proximal nail fold, the lunula, the nail bed, the hyponychium, and the nail plate. The skin and vasculature between the dorsal and ventral surfaces of the proximal nail fold thin to allow visualization of nail fold telangiectases in connective tissue diseases. The nail matrix may deposit nucleated cells into the nail plates of multiple nails in a characteristic pattern indicating transverse leukonychia, which is characteristic of Mees' lines in arsenic poisoning. The nail matrix may slow its growth, producing the transverse depression of Beau's lines, characteristic of a prior systemic illness. The nail plate may separate distally from the nail bed in the bilateral fourth fingernails, indicating Plummer's nails, characteristic of thyrotoxicosis. Alterations in nail bed color resulting from vascular alterations may indicate Lindsay's half-and-half nails of renal disease or Terry's nails of cirrhosis. This chapter examines nail changes associated with systemic disease in a stepwise approach, moving from the proximal nail fold to the lunula, nail bed, hyponychium, and nail plate.

Proximal Nail Fold

BYWATERS' LESIONS

Bywaters' lesions are small areas of palpable purpura in the proximal or lateral nail fold (or both). They classically are associated with rheumatoid vasculitis[1] (Fig. 5–1). Bywaters' lesions also have been associated with small-vessel vasculitis and Wegener's granulomatosis.

Small, red, tender nodules localized in the finger pulp or nail folds (or both) should also alert the clinician to Osler's nodes of subacute bacterial endocarditis.[2]

NAIL FOLD TELANGIECTASES

Nail fold telangiectases can be visualized in the proximal nail fold because capillary loops thin to a row of single loops at the distalmost portion of the fold, near the cuticle. Overt disruption of the capillaries can be seen without the aid of a magnifying device (Fig. 5–2), but the use of magnification with a dissecting microscope,

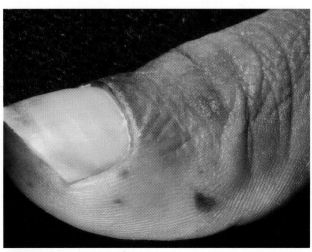

FIGURE 5–1 ■ Bywaters' lesions.

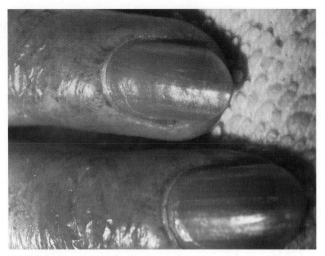

FIGURE 5-2 ■ Nail fold telangiectases.

ophthalmoscope, or stereoscope is necessary to appreciate specific telangiectatic patterns.[3]

Dilated capillaries with bordering avascular areas define the first fairly specific pattern. Distortion and budding of capillaries, enlargement of loops, and loss of capillaries are associated with dermatomyositis, scleroderma, and overlap diseases.[4, 5] Although scleroderma and dermatomyositis are frequently indistinguishable by capillary morphology, occasionally a bushy pattern is recognized; this has been seen more often with dermatomyositis.

Tortuous, meandering capillaries define the second, less-specific pattern. This pattern is associated with systemic lupus erythematosus and Raynaud's phenomenon.

Lunula (Matrix)

CHROMONYCHIA

Chromonychia, or color changes, in the proximal half-moon lunula may aid in the diagnosis of an underlying systemic illness. The lunula may be absent in patients with multiple myeloma, Raynaud's phenomenon, or acquired immunodeficiency syndrome (AIDS). A bluish discoloration of the lunula has been reported in Wilson's disease and with azidothymidine use.[6] In argyria, silver deposition in the lunula is thought to be photo-induced; it appears more commonly in the fingernails than in the toenails.[7] Blue lunulae have also been associated with quinacrine use; the antimalarial-melanin complex is reported to be deposited in the matrix and nail bed.[8]

Red lunulae are classically associated with cardiac failure and are thought to be produced by either an abnormal adhesion of the matrix to the nail plate or arteriolar blood flow changes.[2, 9] However, red lunulae also have been associated with alopecia areata, diabetes mellitus, polycythemia vera, carbon monoxide poisoning, and lymphogranuloma venereum.

Nail Bed

CHROMONYCHIA

Chromonychia can manifest as a diffuse, bluish discoloration of the nail bed, characteristically associated with ingestion of silver or antimalarial drugs. However, a small, painful, bluish macule in the nail bed should alert the clinician to the possibility of a glomus tumor. Pallor of the nail bed can be a sign of anemia. Cherry-red nail beds are a sign of carbon monoxide poisoning. Other specific color changes in the nail bed are described in the following sections.

SPLINTER HEMORRHAGES

Splinter hemorrhages are formed by extravasation of blood from longitudinally oriented nail bed vessels into adjacent longitudinally oriented troughs (Fig. 5-3).[8] Their appearance in multiple nails, especially if they are distributed closer to the lunulae, is frequently associated with systemic disease.[8]

Splinter hemorrhages are common. They are found in 10% to 20% of hospitalized patients. Although classically associated with subacute bacterial endocarditis, this association is probably overrated. In one large study of 574 consecutive hospitalized patients, none had subacute bacterial endocarditis.[10] Splinter hemorrhages are most frequently seen in trauma but have been associated with other systemic diseases (Table 5-1). The appearance of splinter hemorrhages in all nails simultaneously is reported as pathognomonic for trichinosis, and biopsy of the nail bed should demonstrate the responsible organism.[8]

TERRY'S NAIL

Terry's nail was described by Richard Terry in 1954 as a 1- to 2-mm, distal, pink nail bed band accentuated by

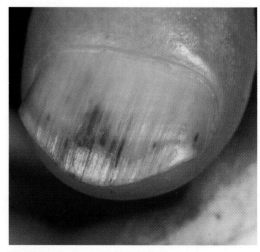

FIGURE 5-3 ■ Splinter hemorrhages.

TABLE 5–1 ■ Splinter Hemorrhages

1. Normal nails (10%–20% of normal population), light trauma
2. Cardiovascular
   a. Bacterial endocarditis
   b. Mitral stenosis
   c. Vascular/hematologic: vasculitis, scurvy, anemia, leukemia, Buerger's thromboangiitis obliterans, cryoglobulinemia, arterial emboli, hemachromatosis, hypertension, thrombocytopenia
3. Infection: trichinosis, fungus, rheumatic fever
4. Skin disease: psoriasis, pityriasis rubra pilaris, Darier's disease, lichen planus, subungual hyperkeratosis syndrome (idiopathic), eczema, exfoliative dermatitis, keratosis lichenoides chronica, mycosis fungoides, pemphigus
5. Rheumatologic: rheumatoid arthritis, Behçet's disease, Reiter's syndrome, dermatomyositis, Raynaud's disease, systemic lupus erythematosus, acrocyanosis, primary antiphospholipid antibody syndrome
6. Drug: tetracycline, psoralens, ketoconazole
7. Renal: chronic glomerulonephritis, dialysis
8. Hepatic: cirrhosis, hepatitis
9. Endocrinologic: diabetes, thyrotoxicosis, hypoparathyroidism
10. Miscellaneous: peptic ulcer, histiocytosis X, high altitudes, sarcoid, cystic fibrosis, general illness, irradiation, malignant neoplasms, Osler-Weber-Rendu syndrome

From Scher RK, Daniel CR: Nails: Therapy, Diagnosis, Surgery. Philadelphia, WB Saunders, 1990; Zaias N: The Nail in Health and Disease. New York, Spectrum, 1980; Pierre M (ed); The Nail. Edinburgh, Churchill Livingstone, 1981.

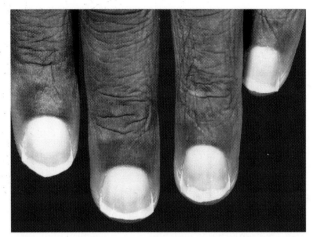

FIGURE 5–5 ■ Half-and-half (Lindsay's) nail.

congestion of the nail bed (Fig. 5–4).[11] He associated this change with cirrhosis but noted that other associations might exist. Holzberg and Walker modified Terry's original criteria to include any 0.5- to 3.0-mm wide, distal, brown-to-pink nail bed band with proximal pallor and found this change in approximately 25% of 512 consecutive hospitalized patients.[12] Affected patients more frequently had cirrhosis, chronic congestive heart failure, and adult-onset diabetes mellitus, especially if they were young. Pathological analysis in three patients showed that the clinical change was caused by distal nail bed telangiectases.

LINDSAY'S NAIL

Half-and-half nail (Lindsay's nail) was first described by Lindsay in 1967 as a nail exhibiting a red, pink, or brown transverse distal band occupying 20% to 60% of the total nail length, with proximal pallor[13] (Fig. 5–5). If the distal band was less than 20% of the total nail length, the patient was considered to have Terry's nail. Lindsay examined 1500 consecutive hospitalized patients and found the change in 1.7%; 84% of these patients had azotemia. No correlation between severity of the azotemia and distal band length was found. Stewart and Raffle studied similar patients with chronic renal failure and found distal brown arcs in 35%.[14] Histology showed melanin in the nail bed epidermis in two deceased patients. Both Terry's nail and Lindsay's nail are thought to be caused by a change in the onychodermal band, an anatomical entity in the distal nail bed with a distinct vascular supply.

MUEHRCKE'S LINES

Muehrcke's lines were described in 1956 as two transverse white bands of pallor representing an abnormality of the vascular nail bed[15] (Fig. 5–6). Pressure applied to the distal plate caused the bands to disappear, confirming a nail bed change. Muehrcke associated this change with hypoalbuminemia (<2.2 g per 100 mL). Muehrcke's lines are possibly caused by a localized edematous state in the nail bed that exerts pressure on

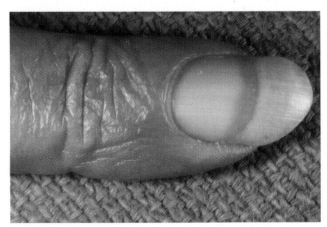

FIGURE 5–4 ■ Terry's nail.

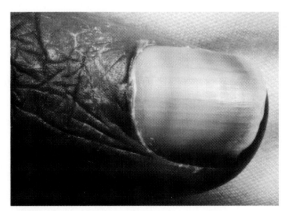

FIGURE 5–6 ■ Muehrcke's lines.

the underlying vasculature, decreasing the normal erythema seen through the nail plate. The nail change has been associated with nephrotic syndrome, glomerulonephritis, liver disease, malnutrition, and acrodermatitis enteropathica.[8] Some consider this sign interesting but nonspecific (M. Holzberg, unpublished observations).

QUENCKE'S PULSE

Quencke's pulse is an observable capillary pulse visualized in the nail bed or nail fold. It is associated with aortic insufficiency.

ONYCHOLYSIS

Onycholysis is defined as separation of the nail plate from the underlying nail bed causing a proximal extension of free air[2, 8, 16] (Fig. 5–7). Onycholysis is the third most common nail disorder seen in dermatology, after onychomycosis and warts. Although it is classically a sign of thyroid disease, the correlation of onycholysis with systemic disease is overrated, and it is more likely to be associated with common diverse local conditions such as trauma, local allergy, or irritant reactions.[8]

Both exogenous and endogenous factors cause onycholysis (Table 5–2). Exogenous factors predominate. Onycholysis is most frequently associated with occupations involving handling of water, chemicals, and irritants. Exposure "weakens" the attachment of the nail plate to the underlying nail bed. Systemic medications, with or without the influence of sunlight, also "weaken" this attachment. Tetracycline derivatives and psoralens

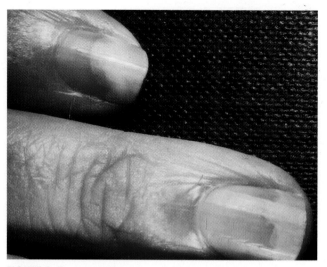

FIGURE 5–7 ■ Onycholysis.

predispose to a photo-induced onycholysis often associated with pain. Ultraviolet light combines with metabolites of the drug, releasing energy or changing cellular maturation, or both. The attachment of the nail plate to the underlying bed is broken, producing onycholysis. Administration of the medication at bedtime and use of sunscreen may be all that is needed if photo-induced onycholysis is suspected.

Endogenous systemic disease has also been responsible for onycholysis. Plummer's nail of hyperthyroidism most characteristically occurs in the fourth fingernail,

TABLE 5-2 ■ Onycholysis

Exogenous Causes

1. Nonmicrobial: trauma, maceration, chemicals, hot water with alkalis or detergents, sodium hypochlorite (exposure in swimming pool maintenance), solvents, burns, nail cosmetics, formaldehyde-containing nail hardeners, working with furs, thermal injury, and microwaves
   a. Occupations associated with onycholysis: housewives, washerwomen, domestics, laundry workers, dish and bottle washers, bartenders, typists, gardeners, farmers, cigar makers, leather and pelt workers, poultry pluckers, barbers and beauticians, brewers, miners, manual laborers, nut crackers, milkers, confectioners
2. Microbial: *Candida* species, dermatophytosis, *Pseudomonas aeruginosa*, *Corynebacterium minutissimum*, *Dermatophilus congolensis*
3. Drugs
   a. Photo-induced: benoxaprofen, chloramphenicol, chlorpromazine, chlortetracycline, demethylchlortetracycline (with pain), doxycycline (with pain), minocycline, oral contraceptives, psoralens, tetracycline (ultraviolet B), clorazepate dipotassium, spontaneous, fluoroquinolones, photochemotherapy in a patient with mycosis fungoides, trypaflavine, acriflavine hydrochloride, thiazides, systemic 5-fluorouracil, thorazine, practolol, captopril, quinine sulfate
   b. Non–photo-induced: bleomycin, doxorubicin, 5-fluorouracil (topical or systemic), retinoids, tetracycline, captopril, gold, mitozantrone, practolol, hydroxylamine, etoposide

Endogenous Causes

1. Dermatologic diseases: psoriasis, Reiter's disease, lichen planus, dermatitis, hyperhidrosis, porphyria cutanea tarda (photo-onycholysis), pemphigus vegetans, pemphigus foliaceus, lichen striatus, epidermolysis bullosa simplex, paronychial onycholysis, alopecia areata, multicentric reticulohistiocytosis
2. Neoplastic disorders: squamous cell carcinoma of the nail bed, mycosis fungoides, histiocytosis X, other neoplasms
3. Systemic diseases and states: impaired circulation, yellow nail syndrome, endocrine (hypothyroidism, thyrotoxicosis, diabetes mellitus), pregnancy, lupus, syphilis, iron deficiency anemia, shell nail syndrome, porphyria, pellagra, Cronkhite-Canada syndrome, human leukocyte antigen 27, tabes dorsalis, multicentric reticulohistiocytosis, amyloid and multiple myeloma, leprosy, Reiter's disease, scleroderma, carcinoma of the lung, histiocytosis X, neuritis

Idiopathic Acquired Onycholysis

Congenital or hereditary

Hereditary partial onycholysis, congenital onycholysis, pachyonychia congenita, congenital ectodermal defect, partial hereditary onycholysis, malalignment of the big toenail, hereditary ectodermal dysplasia, Darier's disease

From Scher RK, Daniel CR: Nails: Therapy, Diagnosis, Surgery. Philadelphia, WB Saunders, 1990; Pierre M (ed): The Nail. Edinburgh, Churchill Livingstone, 1981.

followed by the fifth fingernail. In Plummer's nail, the distal free edge of the nail plate is undulated and curves upward, producing onycholysis.[8] Impaired circulation from diabetes or iron deficiency is also reported to be associated with onycholysis.

ONYCHOMADESIS

Onychomadesis is the term used for complete onycholysis or spontaneous nail shedding. Neurovascular change most often causes this abrupt separation of the nail plate from the underlying matrix and bed. Exanthems (particularly measles and scarlet fever), hypocalcemia with arteriolar spasm, diabetes, and other vascular diseases have been reported as associated conditions. Onychomadesis has also been seen associated with athletics. Drug associations include etretinate, parathormone, carbamazepine, penicillin anaphylaxis, mercaptopurine, arsenic, lead poisoning, and quinacrine.

▌Hyponychium

PTERYGIUM INVERSUM UNGUIS

Pterygium inversum unguis is a persistent adherence of the distal portion of the nail bed or hyponychium to the ventral surface of the nail plate that obliterates the normal distal separation of the hyponychium from the plate.[8] Pain has been reported in 20% of patients with this condition, and all 10 fingernails are involved in 40%.[17] The condition is thought to be a consequence of abnormal circulation and microvascular ischemia, but genetic predisposition may also play a role.[17]

Pterygium inversum unguis may be inherited or acquired. Acquired vascular abnormalities, especially lupus erythematosus and scleroderma, are most commonly associated.[17] Other associated impaired circulatory conditions include acrosclerosis, causalgia of the median nerve, digital ischemia, Raynaud's phenomenon, diabetes, stroke, and leprosy. Nail contact allergy from formaldehyde-containing nail cosmetics has also produced similar nails.

▌Nail Plate

Changes in the nail plate can be reflected as a change in color (chromonychia) or a change in shape.

CHROMONYCHIA

Chromonychia can occur as a result of increased melanogenesis in the matrix (brown discoloration), imperfect keratinization (white discoloration), infection, or byproducts of metabolism or medications.[8] Pigmentation is more often associated with an internal than an external cause if the examiner is unable to scrape the color off the surface of the nail plate with a scalpel blade. Additionally, Zaias appropriately observed that nail discolor-

ation in which the proximal border mimics the shape of the lunula is more likely to result from an internal cause, whereas that in which the proximal border mimics the shape of the proximal nail fold is more likely a result of an external factor.[18]

Systemic illness can increase the production of melanin by matrix melanocytes, producing a brown, diffuse pigmentation of the nail plate. Brown-to-black, diffuse pigmentation of the nail plate is present in 52% of African-American patients with systemic lupus erythematosus.[19] Adrenal insufficiency and pituitary tumors may produce a diffuse brown discoloration of the nail plate caused by melanin production secondary to increased melanocyte-stimulating hormone.[18] Acanthosis nigricans, vitamin B_{12} deficiency, hemochromatosis, hyperbilirubinemia, hyperthyroidism, hypopituitarism, porphyria, and syphilis can all produce a similar dyschromia.

Brown-to-black discoloration of the nail plate has been associated with medications, including cancer chemotherapeutic agents (melphalan, hydroxyurea, doxorubicin [Adriamycin], busulfan, bleomycin), tetracycline derivatives, 8-methoxpsoralen, antimalarials, sulfonamides, phenothiazines, phenindione, mercury, gold, phenytoin, timolol, and azidothymidine.[6] Brown discoloration of the nail plate resulting from melanin deposition with azidothymidine use usually occurs 4 to 8 weeks after initiation of the medication but may occur as long as 1 year after initiation. Most affected patients have brown dyschromia on multiple nails that may be accompanied by mucosal pigmentation.[6]

These internal changes must be differentiated from externally applied local agents. Ink, photographic developer, shoe polish, nicotine (in cigarette smokers), henna, anthralin, and nail enamel can easily be scraped from the surface of a brown, diffusely discolored nail with a scalpel blade. Certain dematiaceous fungi can cause a diffuse brown-to-black discoloration in the nail (*Proteus mirabilis*, *Hormodendrum elatum*, *Alternaria grisea tenuis*, *Acrotherium niger*, *Botryodiplodia theobromae*, *Hendersonula toruloidea*), confirmed by culture or potassium hydroxide preparation.

The differential diagnosis of brown longitudinal bands is important because of the ramifications of an incorrect diagnosis of melanoma (Table 5–3). Certain features help the clinician to differentiate a systemic disease from an idiopathic change. First, longitudinal pigmented bands are more likely to be associated with systemic disease in lightly pigmented persons. Second, longitudinal pigmented bands associated with systemic changes usually occur in multiple nails, although African-American patients not infrequently manifest them idiopathically (Fig. 5–8).[8] The clinician should be suspicious of melanoma (Fig. 5–9) when the brown-pigmented nail plate band occurs as a single band in an older person, has an abrupt onset, has color variation or a blurred margin, suddenly darkens or widens proximally, or is accompanied by pigmentation of the nail fold (Hutchinson's sign).[20] Subungual melanoma usually is found on the thumb or second digit and may be associated with trauma.[20]

Pigmentation on a contiguous nail fold (Hutchinson's sign) may not be pathognomonic of melanoma. Pseudo-

TABLE 5-3 ■ Longitudinal Melanonychia

Single Bands		Multiple Bands	
Nonneoplastic	Neoplastic	Nonneoplastic	Neoplastic
Carpal tunnel syndrome, foreign body, hematoma, irradiation, postinflammatory pigmentation, trauma, nail biting, friction	Melanocytic: Acquired nevus, congenital nevus, lentigo (proliferation of normal or atypical melanocytes), postoperative, melanoma (in situ, metastatic, subungual) Nonmelanocytic: basal cell carcinoma, Bowen's disease, mucous cyst, fibroma, histiocytoma, verruca vulgaris	Dermatologic: Laugier-Hunziker syndrome, lichen planus, lichen striatus, prurigo vulgaris Drugs and ingestants: antimalarials, arsenic, bleomycin, busulfan, diquat, cyclophosphamide, daunorubicin, doxorubicin, fluoride, 5-fluorouracil, gold, hydroxyurea, ibuprofen, ketoconazole, melphalan, mepacrine, mercury, methotrexate, minocycline, nitrogen mustard, nitrosourea, phenytoin, phenothiazine, psoralen, sulfonamides, tetracycline, timolol, zidovudine Microbial: AIDS, *Acrothecium nigrum, Alternaria,* bacteria, *Blastomyces, Candida, Fusarium, Hendersonula toruloidea, Hormodendrum elatum, Pinta, Proteus mirabilis,* secondary syphilis, *Trichophyton sodanense, Trichophyton rubrum* Exogenous: irradiation (systemic) Racial variation: African-American, Hispanic, Indian, other dark-skinned races, Japanese Systemic disease: Addison's disease, adrenalectomy for Cushing's disease, hemosiderosis, hyperbilirubinemia, hyperthyroidism, malnutrition, Peutz-Jeghers syndrome, porphyria, pregnancy, vitamin D deficiency and megaloblastic anemia, AIDS without zidovudine	Breast cancer

From Baran R, Kechijian P: Longitudinal melanonychia (melanonychia striata): diagnosis and management. J Am Acad Dermatol 21:1165–1175, 1989.

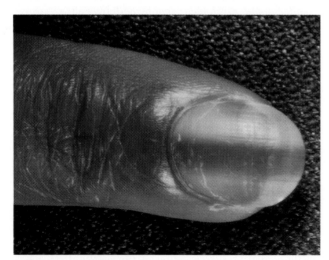

FIGURE 5–8 ■ Longitudinal melanonychia.

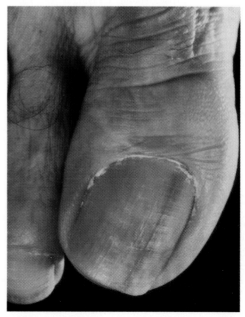

FIGURE 5–9 ■ Malignant melanoma.

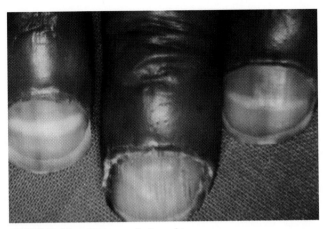

FIGURE 5-10 ■ Transverse leukonychia.

Hutchinson's sign is caused by the relative translucency of the cuticle and proximal nail fold, which allows the examiner to visualize pigment through them.[21] This sign has been associated with Laugier-Hunziker syndrome, use of minocycline, Peutz-Jeghers syndrome, trauma, biopsy, Bowen's disease, ethnic pigmentation, radiation therapy, malnutrition, AIDS, and congenital nevus.

If a treatment is recurrently started and stopped, transverse brown bands can occur in the nail plate. Transverse bands have been associated with radiotherapy, electron beam therapy, cancer chemotherapeutic agents, and azidothymidine.[6]

Blue discoloration of the nail plate is caused by copper in Wilson's disease and by silver deposition in argyria. Diffuse blue discoloration has been reported in bronchiectasis, with use of minocycline or azidothymidine, and idiopathically in "azure nails."

TRANSVERSE LEUKONYCHIA

Transverse leukonychia is a chromonychia characterized by transverse, opaque white bands that tend to occur in the same relative position in multiple nails (Fig. 5–10).[8] The bands' configuration mimics the contour of the lunula, and they grow out with the plate. Parakeratotic cells incorporated in the nail plate by a compromised matrix cause the condition. Measuring the distance of the line from the proximal nail fold can give an approximate time at which the insult occurred, because fingernails grow at a rate of about 0.10 to 0.15 mm/day. Many systemic illnesses and medications are associated with transverse leukonychia (Table 5–4). Mees' lines describe the association of transverse leukonychia with arsenic deposition in the plate as a manifestation of arsenic poisoning.[22]

YELLOW NAIL SYNDROME

Yellow nail syndrome is defined as the triad of yellow nails, lymphedema, and pulmonary complications.[23] The nails have a striking yellow color, increased transverse curvature, absent lunula and cuticle, a tendency to form a "hump," and a variable degree of onycholysis. Spontaneous clearing of nails has been described in association

TABLE 5-4 ■ Leukonychia

Transverse Leukonychia

1. Poisoning: arsenic (Mees' lines), thallium, carbon monoxide
2. Infection: leprosy, malaria, trichinosis, zoster, "infectious fevers"
3. Systemic disease: renal failure, after renal transplantation, myocardial infarction, cardiac insufficiency, Hodgkin's disease, deficiency states (acrodermatitis enteropathica, pellagra), pneumonia, expedition nails, sickle cell anemia, warm-reacting antibody immunohemolytic anemia, Addison's disease, other serious systemic diseases
4. Childbirth
5. Menstrual cycle
6. Drugs: chemotherapeutic drugs
7. Skin disease: psoriasis, exfoliative dermatitis
8. Trauma (occupational)

Diffuse Leukonychia

1. Congenital: leukonychia totalis, partial leukonychia, leukonychia associated with spoon nails and deafness, dominant knuckle pad/leukonychia/deafness, leukonychic koilonychia (also associated with deafness, leukonychia totalis/multiple sebaceous cysts/renal calculi, pili torti, and leukonychia)
2. Systemic disease: leprosy, hemochromatosis, hypocalcemia, acanthosis nigricans
3. Local agents: *Trichophyton rubrum*

Longitudinal Bands

1. Local agents: *Candida albicans*
2. Skin disease: Darier's disease (leukonychia striata longitudinalis), Hailey-Hailey disease
3. Drugs: quinacrine

Punctate Spots (Leukopathia punctata)

1. Congenital
2. Trauma and manicure
3. Local agents: contact with concentrated solvents, *Trichophyton mentagrophytes*, *Fusarium oxysporum*, *Aspergillus flavus*, *Cephalosporium*, cryotherapy
4. Systemic diseases: infectious diseases (typhus, scarlet fever, measles, acute rheumatic fever, diphtheria, syphilis), vascular diseases of varied origin (especially diabetes), poisoning (especially arsenic and lead), sympathetic symmetric punctate leukonychia
5. Skin diseases: psoriasis, dyshidrosis

From Baran R, Dawber RPR (eds): Diseases of the Nails and Their Management, 2nd ed. Oxford, Blackwell Scientific, 1994; Scher RK, Daniel CR: Nails: Therapy, Diagnosis, Surgery. Philadelphia, WB Saunders, 1990.

with no change in systemic disease, indicating that the nail change may be independent of systemic disease. Slow rate of growth or lipofuscin pigment may be the cause of the nail color. Growth rate is less than 0.2 mm/wk, and patients often remark that their nails have "stopped growing."[2]

The syndrome is associated with pulmonary disease, internal malignancy, infections, medications, immunological and hematological abnormalities, endocrine changes, and connective tissue disease (Table 5–5). Cancer patients appear to have associated lymphedema less frequently. Medical cure or removal of the cancer has been associated with resolution of the yellow nails.[24] The association of yellow nails and AIDS is controversial because patients did not exhibit the other characteristic nail changes of yellow nail syndrome.[2]

Thirteen cases of yellow nail syndrome were described by Samman and White in 1964, each of which

TABLE 5-5 ■ Yellow Nail Syndrome

1. Idiopathic
2. Edema; edema of the lower extremities, includes Milroy's disease, facial edema
3. Pulmonary/respiratory: pleural effusion, chronic bronchitis, sinusitis, bronchiectasis, chronic pulmonary infections, other upper and lower respiratory chronic disease, chronic pulmonic and hepatic tuberculosis, giant cell interstitial pneumonitis, asthma, chronic obstructive pulmonary disease, chronic nasal obstruction and rock-hard cerumen, pulmonary fibrosis
4. Internal malignancy: cancer of the larynx, lymphoma, sarcoma, adenocarcinoma of the endometrium, malignant melanoma, infiltrating ductal carcinoma of the breast, Hodgkin's disease, mycosis fungoides, carcinoma of the gallbladder
5. Infections: chronic sinusitis, chronic pulmonary infections, recurrent cellulitis, syphilis, acquired immunodeficiency disease
6. Drugs: D-penicillamine, bucillamine
7. Immunologic/hematologic: lymphopenia, hypogammaglobulinemia, complete absence of immunoglobulin A, low levels of immunoglobulin M, macroglobulinemia
8. Endocrine: thyroid disease (hypothyroidism, thyrotoxicosis, Hashimoto's thyroiditis), diabetes, breasts of unequal size
9. Connective tissue abnormalities: rheumatoid arthritis, high levels of rheumatoid factor, Raynaud's disease, systemic lupus erythematosus
10. Miscellaneous: mental retardation, nephrotic syndrome, hypoplastic kidney, myocardial disease

From Scher RK, Daniel CR: Nails: Therapy, Diagnosis, Surgery. Philadelphia, WB Saunders, 1990; Zaias N: The Nail in Health and Disease, New York, Spectrum, 1980.

was associated with some type of edema, often ankle edema but sometimes facial edema.[23] Patients had hypoplastic or smaller vessels detected by lymphangiography. Pleural effusion was later recognized as an additional sign of the syndrome.[2] It has been postulated that the pleural lymphatics are hypoplastic and are able to function normally until an extra load is placed on them (e.g., infection).[25] Histology shows dense fibrous tissue replacing stroma, with numerous ectatic, endothelium-lined vessels. Stromal sclerosis may lead to lymphatic obstruc-

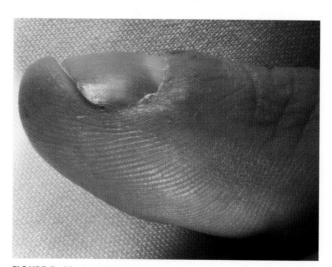

FIGURE 5-11 ■ Clubbing.

tion, explaining the clinical manifestations.[26] The age of onset of symptoms is variable and has been described from birth to the eighth decade of life. Women with the syndrome outnumber men. A family history is rare. Topical and oral vitamin E, intralesional and systemic corticosteroids, and parenteral zinc have all been used to treat yellow nails.

CLUBBING

Lovibond's angle, the angle between the proximal nail fold and the nail plate, is normally 160 degrees. *Clubbing* is defined as a Lovibond's angle of 180 degrees or more (Fig. 5–11). Clubbing is a long-recognized nail sign. Hippocrates described the association of clubbing and empyema in the 5th century B.C.[27] Synonyms for clubbing include Hippocratic nail, acropachy, dysacromelia, trommelschlagelfinger, distal hippocratism, drumstick fingers, parrot-beaked nails, serpent-headed nails, and watchglass nails.[8, 18]

Clubbed nails often develop a "spongy" feel as pressure is applied to the proximal nail fold, probably because of fibrovascular hyperplasia of the underlying soft tissue.[8] Mendlowitz found that the blood flow of the fingertip was abnormally high in all cases of simple clubbing that he studied, except in hereditary clubbing.[27] Blood flow changes may cause the distal matrix to occupy a relatively high position compared with the proximal matrix, causing clubbing.[28]

Clubbing can be inherited or acquired (Table 5–6). The inherited form may begin after puberty, may affect both fingernails and toenails,[8] may be associated with hyperkeratosis of the palms and soles, and may be associated with cortical hypertrophy of the long bones.[2] The most common association is thoracic disease; this is seen in 80% of cases of acquired clubbing, often with associated hypoxia.[28] Clubbing can be found in hypoxemic pulmonary and cardiovascular disease, especially congenital heart disease with cyanosis. Clubbing can be seen in gastrointestinal inflammatory bowel disease and cystic fibrosis. Clubbing is most frequently bilateral and often begins in the thumb and index finger.[8] It usually is painless, except for some forms of carcinoma of the lung, in which clubbing may cause severe pain and may develop abruptly.[2]

Hypertrophic osteoarthropathy[2, 8, 28] describes the association of clubbing of the fingers and toes, acromegalic hypertrophy of the upper and lower extremities, peripheral neurovascular disease, bone pain and pathology, joint pain and swelling, and muscle weakness.

Hypertrophic osteoarthropathy can be inherited (primary) or acquired (secondary). Pachydermoperiostosis (Touraine-Solente-Golé syndrome) is inherited in an autosomal dominant manner. Patients possess a connective tissue abnormality in which acidic mucopolysaccharides and some fibrillar material accumulate in the dermis. Increased levels of osteocalcin in serum indicate a higher osteoblastic activity. Pachydermoperiostosis is characterized by clubbing, enlargement of the hands, thickening of the legs and forearms, thickened facial features, and periosteal ossification. The pachydermal

TABLE 5-6 ■ Clubbing

Idiopathic

Hereditary and Congenital

1. Familial and genotypic pachydermoperiostosis
2. Racial forms (African-Americans, North Africans)
3. Citrullinemia
4. Hereditary: transmitted as simple autosomal dominant or as an autosomal dominant sex-linked trait with variable penetrance

Acquired Forms

1. Thoracic forms (80%)
   a. Bronchopulmonary disease, especially chronic and infective: bronchiectasis, abscess and cyst of the lung; tuberculosis, sarcoidosis, pulmonary fibrosis, emphysema, Ayerza's syndrome, chronic passive congestion, secondary amyloidosis, blastomycosis, acute pneumonia, pulmonary endarteritis
   b. Thoracic tumors: primary or metastatic bronchopulmonary cancers, pleural tumors, mediastinal tumors (infrequently: Hodgkin's disease, lymphoma, pseudotumor with esophageal dilatation), metastatic neoplasm (fibrosarcoma, giant cell tumor)
   c. Cardiovascular disease: congenital heart disease associated with cyanosis, acyanotic congenital heart disease, thoracic vascular malformations, subacute bacterial endocarditis, congestive heart failure, myxoma, Raynaud's syndrome, erythromelalgia, Maffucci's syndrome, chronic myelogenous leukemia, acyanotic congenital heart disease, heroin addiction
2. Gastrointestinal forms (<5%)
   a. Esophageal, colonic, and gastric cancers
   b. Diseases of the small intestine
   c. Colonic diseases with the following: amoebiasis and inflammatory states of the colon, ulcerative colitis, familial polyposis (Gardner's syndrome), ascariasis, whipworm infection, celiac disease, carcinoma, idiopathic steatorrhea, neoplasms, Crohn's disease
   d. Hepatic: active chronic hepatitis, primary or secondary cirrhosis, secondary amyloidosis, Hodgkin's disease, chronic obstructive jaundice
   e. Chronic use of senna (and long-term diarrhea)
   f. Cystic fibrosis
3. Endocrine origin: Diamond's syndrome (pretibial myxedema, exophthalmos finger clubbing), after thyroidectomy
4. Hematologic: primary or secondary polycythemia associated with hypoxia; poisoning by phosphorus, arsenic, alcohol, mercury or beryllium; hypervitaminosis A
5. Renal: chronic pyelonephritis
6. Unilateral or limited to only several digits: subluxation of the shoulder (paralysis of the brachial plexus), median neuritis, Pancoast-Tobias syndrome, brachial arteriovenous fistula, aneurysm of the aorta or the subclavian artery, erythromelalgia, sarcoid bone disease, tophaceous gout, local injury, whitlow, lymphangitis, subungual epidermoid inclusions
7. Neural: syringomyelia, peripheral neuritis
8. Transitory forms: physiologic in the newborn
9. Occupational acro-osteolysis: exposure to vinyl chloride
10. Miscellaneous: syphilis, Maffucci's syndrome, congenital dysplasia, angiectasis, chronic familial neutropenia, cretinism, leprosy, rheumatic fever, Raynaud's disease, acrocyanosis, chilblains, Kaposi's sarcoma, acrogeria, sarcoid, Osler-Weber-Rendu disease, laxative abuse, systemic lupus erythematosus, scleroderma (probably because of pulmonary manifestations)

From Stone OJ: Spoon nails and clubbing. Cutis 16:235–241, 1975.

change of the extremities and face, including furrowing and oiliness of the skin, is the most characteristic feature of this disorder.[2] It is familial in more than half of the cases.

The acquired secondary form is divided into two types.[2] First, hypertrophic pulmonary osteoarthropathy (Bamberger-Pierre-Marie syndrome) is characterized by hypertrophic osteoarthropathy confined to the lower extremities and is often caused by recurrent infections of the lower extremities after bypass grafting. The second type is most often associated with malignant tumors of the chest. When the syndrome has all six parts, a malignant thoracic tumor is seen in 90% of cases, and the tumor is usually bronchogenic squamous cell carcinoma. Associated joint pain and swelling is almost pathognomonic of malignant chest tumors. Hypertrophic osteoarthropathy occurs in 0.7% to 12% of patients with bronchogenic carcinoma.[2] Gynecomastia is a further indication of malignancy. Other associations include suppurative pulmonary lesions, rheumatic fever, rheumatoid arthritis, infective arthritis, thrombophlebitis, congestive heart failure, nutritional edema, peripheral neuropathy, acromegaly, and ulcerative colitis.[2]

KOILONYCHIA

Koilonychia is defined as spoon-shaped nail plates (Fig. 5-12). Koilonychia is thought to occur because of a relatively low distal matrix compared with the proximal matrix, which causes nail plate growth to occur in a downward direction as it grows toward the nail bed.[28] Koilonychia may be idiopathic, inherited, or acquired (Table 5-7). The idiopathic form has been noted more commonly in children than in adults.[8] Temporary koilonychia may be noted in some infants. It improves as the size and shape of the distal phalanx change. Persistent congenital and autosomal dominant forms are reported.[8] Koilonychia may be inherited as a part of several distinct syndromes. Acquired koilonychia, however, is the most common type. Koilonychia is most commonly acquired from trauma, dermatological disease (especially psoriasis and onychomycosis) and distal ischemia (especially Raynaud's phenomenon).[8] It has classically been a sign of iron deficiency anemia and can be seen in postgastrectomy patients and patients with Plummer-Vinson syndrome. In infants, there is a significant correlation between koilonychia and iron deficiency, and koilonychia

TABLE 5-7 ■ Koilonychia

Idiopathic

Hereditary and Congenital Forms

1. Fissured nails, sebocystomatosis
2. Monilethrix, keratodermal of the palms (mal de Meleda type), leukonychia
3. Nail-patella syndrome
4. Nezelof's syndrome
5. Focal dermal hypoplasia, Ellis–van Creveld syndrome
6. Steatocystoma multiplex
7. Temporary koilonychia
8. Leopard syndrome (leukokoilonychia)
9. Incontinentia pigmenti
10. Acrogeria
11. Ectodermal dysplasia with anhydrosis

Acquired Forms

1. Cardiovascular and hematologic
   a. Iron deficiency anemia (following gastrectomy, Plummer-Vinson syndrome)
   b. Iron malabsorption by the intestinal mucosa, cystine deficiency
   c. Hemoglobinopathy SG
   d. Polycythemia
   e. Hemochromatosis
   f. Banti's syndrome
   g. Coronary disease
   h. Polyglobias (erythropoietin-producing tumors)
2. Infections
   a. Syphilis
   b. Fungal disease
3. Endocrine
   a. Acromegaly
   b. Hypothyroidism
   c. Thyrotoxicosis
4. Traumatic and occupational
   a. Gasoline, various solvents, engine oils
   b. Acids, alkalis, thioglycolate (hairdressers)
   c. Housewives, chimney sweeps, rickshaw men (toenails)
   d. Nail biting
   e. Frostbite, thermal burns
5. Avitaminosis
   a. B_2, especially C, pellagra
   b. Cystine deficiency
   c. Malnutrition
6. Dermatoses
   a. Raynaud's disease, scleroderma
   b. Lichen planus
   c. Porphyria cutanea tarda
   d. Darier's disease
   e. Incontinentia pigmenti
   f. Alopecia areata
   g. Psoriasis
   h. Acanthosis nigricans
7. After kidney transplantation
8. Neurologic
   a. Carpal tunnel syndrome
9. Miscellaneous: primary amyloid

From Pierre M (ed): The Nail. Edinburgh: Churchill Livingstone, 1981.

may be noted before laboratory or clinical signs develop.[2]

HAPALONYCHIA

Hapalonychia (soft nail) has been associated with local occupational causes, skin diseases such as psoriasis and eczema, and systemic diseases. Systemic causes include hypochromic anemia, arsenic poisoning, infectious dis-

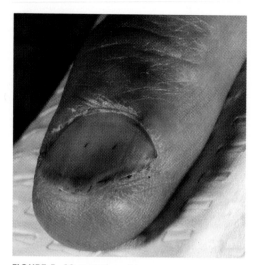

FIGURE 5–12 ■ Koilonychia.

eases, severe toxemia, rheumatoid arthritis, vitamin deficiency (A, B_6, C), osteoporosis, osteomalacia, myxedema, leprosy, hemiplegia, peripheral hypopituitarism, neuritis, Raynaud's disease, scleroderma, and multiple sclerosis.

BEAU'S LINES

Beau's lines were first described in 1846 as transverse grooves or depressions of the nail plate (Fig. 5–13) in patients with typhoid or other acute systemic disorders.[29] Beau's sign is one of the most common but least specific signs. Systemic disease is thought to cause a temporary cessation or decrease in nail plate deposition. The thumbnails and toenails are most frequently affected, and they are the most reliable indicators of previous disease.[2] The width of the furrow is an indicator of the duration of the disease. The distance of the line from the proximal nail fold can give an approximate time at which the insult occurred, because the fingernail grows at about 0.10 to 0.15 mm/day. If the entire activity of the matrix is inhibited for 1 to 2 weeks, a Beau's line will reach its maximum depth, causing a total division of the nail plate (onychomadesis).[2] Beau's lines are associated with both systemic disease and local factors

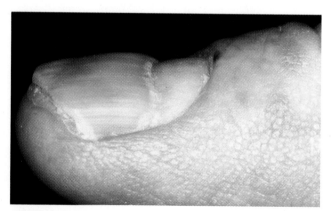

FIGURE 5–13 ■ Beau's line.

TABLE 5-8 ■ Beau's Lines

Systemic Disease

1. Febrile disease
2. Infectious disease: typhus, acute rheumatic fever, diphtheria, syphilis, parotitis, malaria, gonococcal arthritis, scarlet fever, epididymitis, erythema nodosum leprosum, mucocutaneous lymph node syndrome, AIDS
3. Nutritional disorders: protein deficiency, pellagra
4. Circulatory: myocardial infarction, peripheral vascular disease accompanied by arteriolar obliteration, Raynaud's disease, pulmonary embolism, prolonged tourniquet at surgery affecting all the digits on that limb
5. Dysmetabolic states: diabetes, hypothyroidism, hypocalcemia, hypoparathyroidism, Sheehan's syndrome (hypopituitarism)
6. Digestive diseases: diarrhea, chronic enterocolitis, subacute and chronic pancreatitis with malabsorption syndrome, sprue, severe gastritis, acrodermatitis enteropathica
7. Drugs: antimitotic drugs (dapsone, retinoids, carbamazepine, chemotherapeutic agents)
8. Surgical operations
9. Chronic alcoholism, arsenic toxicity
10. Strong psychic emotions (especially if prolonged), hysteria, after epileptic convulsions
11. Gynecologic: parturition, Sheehan's syndrome (hypopituitarism), dysmenorrhea
12. Congenital

Local

1. Chronic skin disease: paronychia, eczema, pustular psoriasis, pemphigus foliaceus
2. Trauma
3. Carpal tunnel syndrome

From Weismann K: J.H.S. Beau and his descriptions of transverse depressions on nails. Br J Dermatol 97:571–572, 1977; Pierre M (ed): The Nail. Edinburgh, Churchill Livingstone, 1981.

(Table 5–8). The condition is more often associated with a systemic disease when multiple nails are affected at the same relative position.

ONYCHORRHEXIS

The term *onychorrhexis* describes longitudinal ridges in the nail plate that are most often associated with old age (senile nail). The change can be inherited and the pattern has been described as specific enough to distinguish between identical twins and can be useful in forensic identification.[2] Onychorrhexis occurs with systemic disease, showing a strong correlation with rheumatoid arthritis. Sarcoidosis of the nail produces onychorrhexis, and often the diagnosis can be confirmed by nail fold biopsy.[30] Amyloidosis may manifest with onychorrhexis. Other systemic associations include iron deficiency anemia, peripheral circulatory disorders, multicentric reticulohistiocytosis, follicular mucinosis, genetic abnormalities, mycotic diseases, poisoning (especially arsenic), scleroderma, hypothyroidism, gout, Raynaud's phenomenon, hypoparathyroidism (hypocalcemia), amyloidosis, lupus, graft-versus-host disease, AIDS, and zinc deficiency. Associated medications include azidothymidine, lithium carbonate, penicillamine, and retinoids. Local factors such as skin diseases, localized radiotherapy, or trauma have been associated with longitudinal ridging. Onychorrhexis has been associated with leprosy, lichen planus, cicatricial pemphigoid, pemphigus foliaceus, lichen nitidus, and pityriasis rubra pilaris. A familial congenital form is associated with hereditary osteoungual dysplasia. This autosomal dominant inherited syndrome produces dyschromic, trachyonychic nails with longitudinal ridges.

TRACHYONYCHIA

Trachyonychia is the term used for rough nail plates with a characteristic gray opacity to the plate, brittle and split free ends, longitudinal ridging, and a rough sandpaperlike surface (Fig. 5–14).[31] Trachyonychia is associated with alopecia areata, lichen planus, psoriasis, ichthyosis vulgaris, and 20-nail dystrophy. Trachyonychia is a feature of 3.65% of patients with alopecia areata and 15.4% of those with alopecia universalis. Approximately one third of these patients exhibit spongiosis histologically in the nail fold, matrix, nail bed, or combinations of these. A lichenoid infiltrate may also be responsible for the clinical change. Miscellaneous conditions associated with trachyonychia include dark red lunulae and

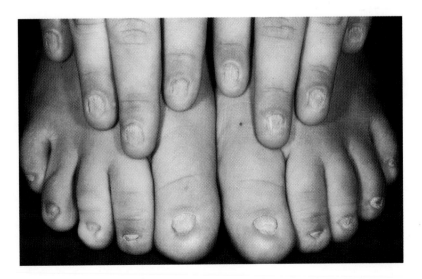

FIGURE 5-14 ■ Trachonychia.

knuckle pads, selective immunoglobulin A deficiency, ectodermal dysplasia, lithium, immune thrombocytopenic purpura, autoimmune hemolytic anemia, and mild depression of immunoglobulin levels. Twenty-nail dystrophy of childhood is an often self-limited trachyonychia originally described by Hazelrigg and colleagues in children with acquired trachyonychia of all 20 nails.[32]

REFERENCES

1. Bywaters EGL: Peripheral vascular obstruction in rheumatoid arthritis and its relationship to other vascular lesions. Ann Rheum Dis 16:84–103, 1957.
2. Baran R, Dawber RPR (eds): Diseases of the Nails and Their Management, 2nd ed. Oxford, Blackwell Scientific, 1994.
3. Minkin W, Rabhan NB: Office nail fold capillary microscopy using ophthalmoscope. J Am Acad Dermatol 7:190, 1982.
4. Maricq HR: Widefield capillary microscopy: technique and rating scale for abnormalities seen in scleroderma and related disorders. Arthritis Rheum 24:1159–1165, 1981.
5. Kenik JG, Maricq HR, Bole GG: Blind evaluation of the diagnostic specificity of nailfold capillary microscopy in the connective tissue diseases. Arthritis Rheum 24:885–891, 1981.
6. Greenberg RG, Berger TG: Nail and mucocutaneous hyperpigmentation with azidothymidine therapy. J Am Acad Dermatol 22:327–330, 1990.
7. Plewig G, Lincke H, Wolff HH: Silver-blue nails. Acta Derm Venereol 57:413–419, 1977.
8. Scher RK, Daniel CR: Nails: Therapy, Diagnosis, Surgery. Philadelphia, WB Saunders, 1990.
9. Wilkerson MF, Wilkin JK: Red lunulae revisited: clinical and histopathologic examination. J Am Acad Dermatol 20:453–457, 1989.
10. Kilpatrick ZM, Greenberg PA, Sanford JP: Splinter hemorrhages: their clinical significance. Arch Intern Med 115:730–735, 1965.
11. Terry R: White nails in hepatic cirrhosis. Lancet 1:757–759, 1954.
12. Holzberg M, Walker HK: Terry's nails: revised definition and new correlations. Lancet 1:896–899, 1984.
13. Lindsay PG: The half-and-half nail. Arch Intern Med 119:583–587, 1967.
14. Stewart WK, Raffle EJ: Brown nail bed arcs and chronic renal disease. Br Med J 1:784–786, 1972.
15. Muehrcke RC: The fingernails in chronic hypoalbuminemia. Br Med J 1:1327, 1956.
16. Kechijian P: Onycholysis of the fingernails: evaluation and management. J Am Acad Dermatol 12:552–560, 1985.
17. Caputo R, Cappio F, Rigoni C, et al: Pterygium inversum unguis: Report of 19 cases and review of the literature. Arch Dermatol 129:1307–1309, 1993.
18. Zaias N: The Nail in Health and Disease. New York, Spectrum, 1980.
19. Vaughn RY, Bailey JP Jr, Field RS, et al: Diffuse nail dyschromia in black patients with systemic lupus erythematosus. J Rheumatol 17:640–643, 1990.
20. Baran R, Kechijian P: Longitudinal melanonychia (melanonychia striata): diagnosis and management. J Am Acad Dermatol 21:1165–1175, 1989.
21. Baran R, Kechijian P: Hutchinson's sign: a reappraisal. J Am Acad Dermatol 34:87–90, 1996.
22. Marino MT: Mees' lines. Arch Dermatol 126:827–828, 1990.
23. Samman PD, White WF: The "yellow nail" syndrome. Br J Dermatol 76:153–157, 1964.
24. Guin JD, Elleman JH: Yellow nail syndrome. Arch Dermatol 115:734–735, 1979.
25. Gupta AK, Davies GM, Haberman HF: Yellow nail syndrome. Cutis 37:371–373, 1986.
26. DeCoste SD, Imber MJ, Baden HP: Yellow nail syndrome. J Am Acad Dermatol 22:608–611, 1990.
27. Mendlowitz M: Measurements of blood flow and blood pressure in clubbed fingers. J Clin Invest 20:113, 1941.
28. Stone OJ: Spoon nails and clubbing. Cutis 16:235–241, 1975.
29. Weismann K: J.H.S. Beau and his descriptions of transverse depressions on nails. Br J Dermatol 97:571–572, 1977.
30. Wakelin SH, James MP: Sarcoidosis: nail dystrophy without underlying bone changes. Cutis 55:344–346, 1995.
31. Tosti A, Fanti PA, Morelli R, Bardazzi F: Trachyonychia associated with alopecia areata: a clinical and pathologic study. J Am Acad Dermatol 25:266–270, 1991.
32. Hazelrigg DE, Duncan WC, Jarrat M: Twenty-nail dystrophy of childhood. Arch Dermatol 113:73–75, 1977.

Fungal Infections

PIET DE DONCKER

———

GERALD E. PIÉRARD

Accurate statistics on the causes of hair and nail fungal infections are limited by the fact that data are gathered systematically by only a minority of diagnostic centers. For this reason, the actual prevalence of tinea infections in various geographical locations worldwide cannot be accurately ascertained. The main fungi responsible for hair and nail diseases are dermatophytes, which include the genera *Trichophyton, Microsporum,* and *Epidermophyton.*[1] Dermatophytes can be categorized with the use of epidemiological criteria based on their natural habitat and host preference. Anthropophilic species infect humans almost exclusively. Zoophilic species infect animals, although human transmission may occur. Geophilic species are present in the soil and contaminate both humans and animals. Infections result from direct contact with the natural host. Indirect transmission is also common, through fomites and contaminated ground, particularly in public swimming pools and shower rooms. In addition to dermatophytes, yeasts and nondermatophytic molds cannot be overlooked as agents responsible for fungal infections.

Onychomycosis is an infection in which fungal organisms invade the nail unit, primarily the nail bed. This infection causes progressive changes in the color, texture, and structure of the nail.[2-4] Onychomycosis has an insidious onset and, if left untreated, progresses until it involves the entire nail plate. In contrast to some other diseases, onychomycosis rarely resolves spontaneously, nor does it respond to placebo therapy taken orally or applied topically.[5] Today this disease entity presents a clinical challenge marked by an increasing incidence over recent years.[6, 7]

Tinea capitis is a fungal infection of the scalp and hair caused by species of *Microsporum* and *Trichophyton.*[7] The disease takes on various clinical characteristics ac-cording to the causative organism. Anthropophilic fungi typically produce an inflammatory response that is less severe than that produced by the zoophilic and geophilic organisms. In general, children are more prone to tinea capitis than adults. However, adults may harbor anthropophilic dermatophytes without clinical signs. They are long-term carriers who intermittently shed viable propagules, possibly for decades.

Clinical Features

ONYCHOMYCOSIS

Prevalence

It is generally accepted that hair and nail fungal infections are influenced by age. Tinea capitis is more common in childhood. The reverse holds for toenail onychomycosis, which affects mainly adults in middle age and beyond.

Onychomycosis is the most common nail disorder, accounting for up to 50% of all nail problems.[2] The prevalence of onychomycosis ranges from 2% to 14% of the general population, but it is much higher among middle-aged persons.[8, 9] It has been estimated that as many as 15% to 20% of people between the ages of 40 and 60 years have the disease, whereas it is uncommon in children.[10, 11] In a study of North American children, the prevalence of onychomycosis was only 0.44%.[10] The reasons for the low prevalence of onychomycosis in children are not established, but several hypotheses exist, including differences in nail plate structure, less trauma, and faster linear nail growth in children.

Today, the consensus is that the prevalence of onychomycosis may be higher than previously estimated.

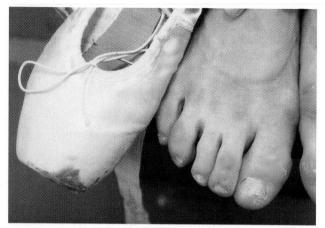

FIGURE 6–1 ■ Toenail onychomycosis in a ballet dancer.

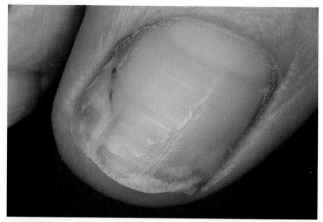

FIGURE 6–2 ■ Distal/lateral subungual onychomycosis caused by *Trichophyton rubrum.*

Onychomycosis is currently on the rise and undoubtedly constitutes one of the major causes of nail dystrophy.[12–14]

Onychomycosis affects a wide range of people, although there are groups at particular risk. For example, there is an expanding population of patients at risk from fungal infection because of immunosuppression as a result of human immunodeficiency virus (HIV) infection, long-term antibiotic treatment, or immunosuppressive therapies.[2, 15, 16]

An increased percentage of onychomycosis also is found in patients with clinically altered toenails. A study of patients with psoriasis demonstrated that the overall prevalence of pedal onychomycosis was 13%, but when the toenails were clinically abnormal the prevalence increased to 27%.[17]

Onychomycosis also has an employment-related component. Jobs that require continued standing, particularly when wearing ill-fitting shoes (Fig. 6–1), and occupations in which the hands are in contact with water and detergents for prolonged periods may increase the risk of onychomycosis. In one series, the prevalence of fungal infection of the nails was reported to be 27% among miners.

A very strong relation exists between onychomycosis and tinea pedis. The prevalence of onychomycosis and tinea pedis can vary from 34% to 96%.[18] This strongly suggests that onychomycosis is associated with tinea pedis, with *Trichophyton rubrum* as the major pathogen.

Various environmental factors such as hot and humid climates are known to predispose to the development of superficial fungal infections. A communal environment can clearly contribute to the higher prevalence of onychomycosis, for example in the Muslim community.[19] Furthermore, the increase in the prevalence of nail infection is believed to be secondary to socioeconomic, cultural, and occupational factors such as trauma, friction, occlusive footwear for sporting or professional activities, and the increasing use of enzymatic cleaning powders, which has made boiling of socks unnecessary. Patients are usually exposed by indirect contamination, such as walking barefoot in bathrooms, swimming pools, saunas, or showers. Therefore, this disease has come to

be regarded as an infection of "civilized countries." The increase in risk factors for onychomycosis parallels an increase in recreational activities and health-oriented behavior. In addition, the use of occlusive shoes may create an incubator-like repository for multiplication of offending fungi.

Classification

Classification by Portal of Entry

The site of invasion of the fungus determines the clinical form. The various types were originally described by Zaias.[20] In this chapter, we describe the clinical patterns associated with the portal of entry of fungi into the nail unit, as follows:

- Type 1: Entry via the distal or lateral nail bed, leading to *distal/lateral subungual onychomycosis (DLSO)*
- Type 2: Entry via the superficial dorsal nail plate, leading to *superficial white/black onychomycosis (SWO/SBO)*
- Type 3: Entry via eponychium/cuticle, leading to *proximal subungual onychomycosis (PSO)*

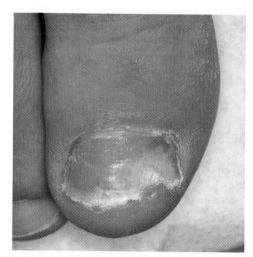

FIGURE 6–3 ■ Distal/lateral subungual onychomycosis caused by *Trichophyton rubrum.*

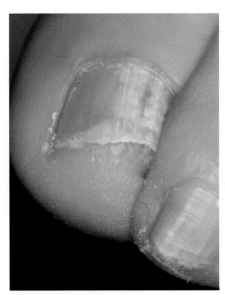

FIGURE 6-4 ■ Distal/lateral subungual onychomycosis caused by *Trichophyton rubrum.*

- Type 4: Entry directly inside the nail plate
- Type 5: Entry via the nail fold, leading to *paronychia onychomycosis*

TYPE 1: DISTAL/LATERAL SUBUNGUAL ONYCHOMYCOSIS. DLSO is the most common pattern of nail infection (Figs. 6–2 through 6–4). Fungi invade the distal nail bed near the ventral nail plate via the hyponychium or the lateral wall.[5, 8, 20] Although the fungal invasion originates at the nail bed (Fig. 6–5), it can secondarily involve the inner nail plate (Fig. 6–6).[21, 22] The primary site of infection is often the skin of the palms (Figs. 6–7 and 6–8) and soles. Dry-type or palmoplantar tinea pedis/manus with toenail infection (Fig. 6–9) or the involvement of one hand and both feet is a strong diagnostic feature for dermatophytosis caused by *T. rubrum.*[22] In the one hand–two feet syndrome, the hand in which tinea manus develops is often the one that is used to excoriate the soles of the feet or to pick the toenails.

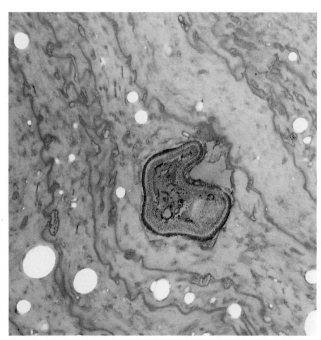

FIGURE 6-6 ■ Electron micrograph of a fungal invasion in the nail plate (via the nail bed), showing *Trichophyton rubrum* in the nail plate's onychocyte (big toenail of a 23-year-old patient). (Courtesy of Dr. J. André, Brussels, Belgium.)

Onychomycosis results in inflammation of the nail bed, a reaction comparable to subacute dermatitis. This in turn promotes hyperkeratosis of the nail bed epithelium and thickening, which may result in elevation of the nail plate (Figs. 6–10 and 6–11).

Onycholysis may occasionally follow, and in some cases the detached nail plate is partially destroyed (Fig. 6–12). Paronychia is also possible. The appearance of a gray to brownish color may be caused by bacterial invasion, and a green discoloration is suggestive of *Pseudomonas.*

Simultaneous presentation of different forms of onychomycosis (DLSO, PSO, SWO) can occur within the same patient (Fig. 6–13).

Finally, the nail plate can also be infected at its distal

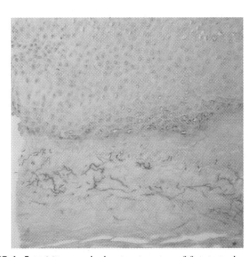

FIGURE 6-5 ■ Micrograph showing invasion of fungi via the nail bed (periodic acid–Schiff stain).

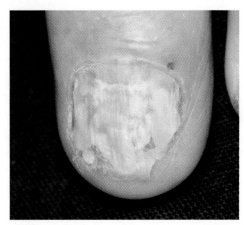

FIGURE 6-7 ■ Fingernail distal/lateral subungual onychomycosis caused by *Trichophyton rubrum.* (Courtesy of Dr. J. Del Rosso, Las Vegas, NV.)

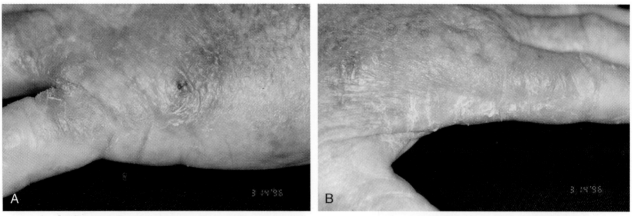

FIGURE 6–8 ■ *A*, Involvement of the hand (tinea manuum) of the same patient as in Figure 6–7. *B*, Closeup of the thumb side of the hand, simulating an eczema or dry skin. (Courtesy of Dr. Del Rosso, Las Vegas, NV.)

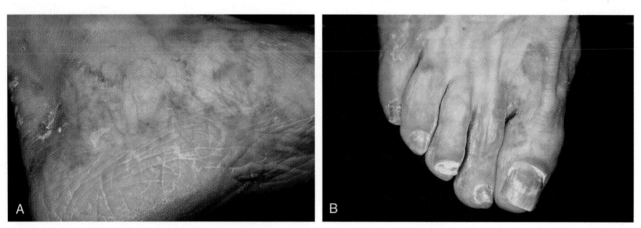

FIGURE 6–9 ■ *A* and *B*, Dry-type tinea pedis with toenail onychomycosis in the same patient as in Figure 6–7. (Courtesy of Dr. J. Del Rosso, Las Vegas, NV.)

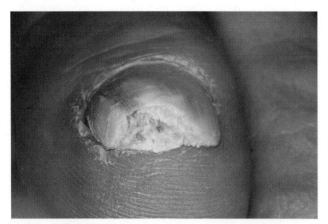

FIGURE 6–10 ■ Subungual hyperkeratosis of the nail bed resulting in lifting up of the nail plate.

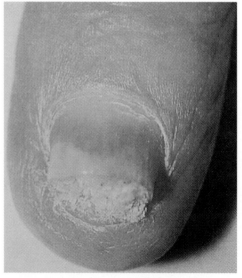

FIGURE 6–11 ■ Distal/lateral subungual onychomycosis: clinical presentation of the hyperkeratotic nail bed, evident after removal of the nail plate.

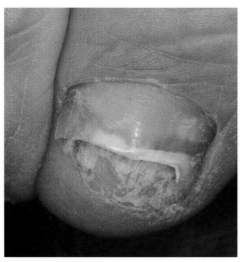

FIGURE 6-12 ■ Detached nail plate partially destroyed by onychomycosis.

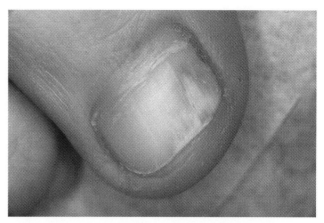

FIGURE 6-14 ■ Distal/lateral subungual onychomycosis caused by *Candida parapsilosis.*

end by *Candida* spp. (Fig. 6–14). The exact role of *Candida* as a causative agent in DLSO is still debated,[22] but it is certainly seen in immunocompromised patients (chronic mucocutaneous candidiasis, or CMCC) and with other immunodeficiencies. The infection may spread rapidly to all fingernails.[23] Gross hyperkeratosis can manifest as total nail plate involvement (see discussion of total dystrophic onychomycosis [TDO]). In other cases, *Candida* onychomycosis manifests with minimal thickening of the nail plate.[22] *Candida albicans* may also occur as a secondary pathogen in nails previously damaged by local or systemic factors (e.g., trauma, chronic paronychial infection, other skin diseases).

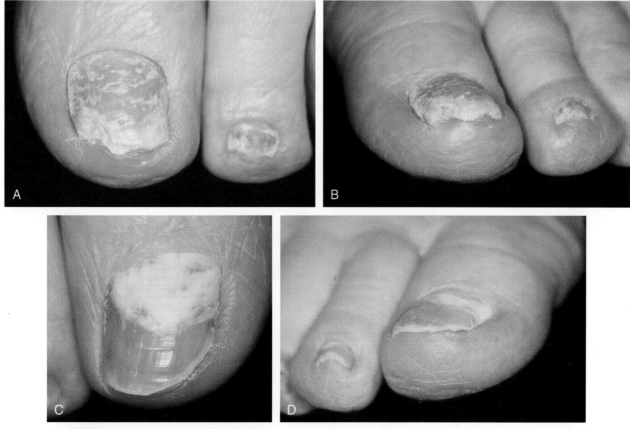

FIGURE 6-13 ■ Fifty-three-year-old woman with rheumatoid arthritis taking oral low-dose prednisone and oral methotrexate with a 12-month history of distal/lateral subungual onychomycosis on the left foot (*A* and *B*) and proximal white subungual onychomycosis on the right foot (*C* and *D*). The proximal nail shows an area of leukonychia. (Courtesy of Dr. J. Del Rosso, Las Vegas, NV.)

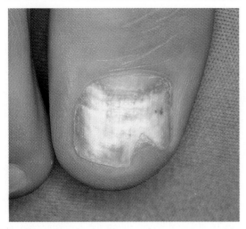

FIGURE 6–15 ■ Superficial white onychomycosis caused by *Tricho-phyton mentagrophytes.*

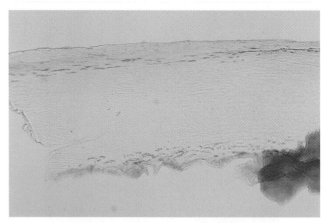

FIGURE 6–17 ■ Histological section of an onychomycosis with involvement of the surface and deep portion of the nail plate (periodic acid–Schiff stain).

TYPE 2: SUPERFICIAL WHITE/BLACK ONYCHOMY-COSIS. SWO is characterized by fungal invasion via the superficial nail surface, caused primarily by molds or dermatophytes (Fig. 6–15).[20, 22–26] This form affects the toenails, particularly the big toenail, more often than fingernails.

The first signs of SWO are discrete, soft, dry, white, opaque, well-defined spots on the nail surface, which result from invasion of the dorsal or superficial aspect of the nail plate. The spotty discoloration can coalesce to form a larger white plaque that can easily be scraped away. The nail surface begins to disintegrate, becoming crumbly and rough. However, the nail plate is not thickened, as in DLSO, and it continues to adhere to the nail bed.

SWO is frequently associated with tinea pedis interdigitalis (Fig. 6–16) and is diagnostic for dermatophytosis caused by *Trichophyton mentagrophytes* var. *interdigitale*, although this association is less frequent than that of *T. rubrum* dermatophytosis with DLSO.

When the superficial nail plate is invaded by *T. rubrum* var. *nigricans* or the mold *Scytalidium dimidiatum*, the dark discoloration contrasts with the SWO; this is termed SBO.

In some cases, the fungus also penetrates deeper into the nail plate and forms a second level of invasion, which may not be perceptible by clinical inspection alone (Fig. 6–17).[24]

TYPE 3: PROXIMAL SUBUNGUAL ONYCHOMYCOSIS. PSO is rare in immunocompetent persons but is increasingly being recognized with the rising number of immunocompromised patients (see Fig. 6–13). A subtype of PSO, called proximal white subungual onychomycosis, is commonly seen in patients with the acquired immunodeficiency syndrome (AIDS). This type of infection may be indicative for AIDS and is generally caused by *T. rubrum*[2, 27, 28] (Fig. 6–18). Unlike onychomycoses in the immunocompetent patient, this disorder can spread rapidly to all fingernails and toenails.

PSO usually results from a fungal infection of the skin surrounding the proximal nail fold that invades the lower nail plate via the eponychium and cuticle (hence, its proximal location); the superficial surface of the nail

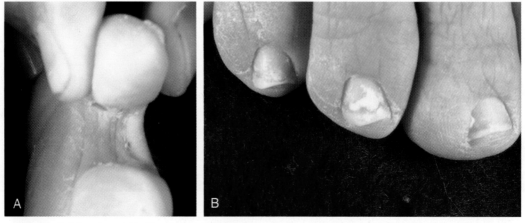

FIGURE 6–16 ■ *A* and *B*, Tinea pedis (athlete's foot) in a patient with superficial white onychomycosis. (Courtesy of Dr. A. Gupta, Toronto, Ontario, Canada.)

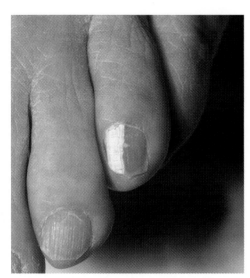

FIGURE 6–18 ■ Proximal subungual onychomycosis in an AIDS patient (caused by *Trichophyton rubrum*). (Courtesy of Dr. R. Scher, New York, NY.)

plate remains smooth and intact. Hyperkeratotic debris may accumulate under the nail plate. Clinically, it appears as irregular white spots or bands that grow distally from under the cuticle along the ventral aspect of the nail plate or along the nail bed. The distal end of the nail may continue to appear normal, and the infection usually is limited to the ventral surface of the proximal nail plate.

TYPE 4: INVASION INSIDE THE NAIL PLATE ONLY. In this type, fungi are seen only within the nail plate.[24] In contrast to the nail bed and other parts of the nail unit, immunological effectors are not present in the nail plate to eradicate the fungus. Therefore, fungi that flourish inside the nail plate may be different from those invading the nail bed. It is not known whether this type of onychomycosis represents an early fungal infection or whether it represents evolution of a particular type of onychomycosis in which the entry site is cleared either spontaneously or after insufficient treatment. This type of onychomycosis may be overlooked at the clinical examination. It may be a frequent cause of recurrent onychomycosis. This form was called "endonyx onychomycosis" in a single case caused by *Trichophyton soudanense*,[25] which may manifest as white discoloration of the nail plate without hyperkeratosis or onycholysis. Like DLSO and SWO, association with tinea pedis is possible.

TYPE 5: PARONYCHIA ONYCHOMYCOSIS. Candida paronychia corresponds to invasion of the proximal and lateral folds by *Candida*.[5, 8, 13, 23, 26] The affected digits have a bulbous appearance, with an edematous, reddened pad around the nail that causes an inflamed, swollen, and painful nail fold (Fig. 6–19). Pus may be expressed by applying pressure on the cuticle that has

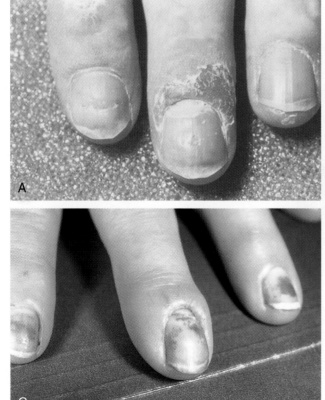

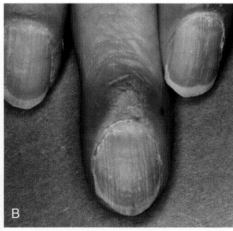

FIGURE 6–19 ■ *A* through *C*, Paronychia caused by *Candida albicans*. Note the presence of an inflammatory swollen pad, which can be painful.

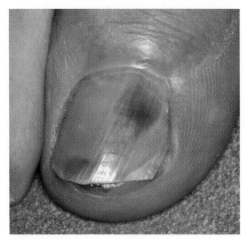

FIGURE 6-20 ■ Presence of a longitudinal band of fungal melanonychia.

separated from the nail plate. A dark, yellowish to black-brown zone can also be observed along the lateral border of the nail.

Whether *Candida* is the primary pathogen or is secondarily involved, acting as a colonizer in chronic paronychia and onycholysis, is a long-standing controversy in this type of onychomycosis.[29]

Classification by Evolution

The evolution of a fungal invasion in the nail provides another way to distinguish the various clinical appearances of fungal infection. There are three types: linear evolution (streak, longitudinal fungal melanonychia), macular spreading evolution, and total dystrophic evolution (TDO).

LINEAR EVOLUTION. The clinical appearance is caused by nail invasion in a longitudinal, narrow band that follows the ridges of the nail bed. In some patients, a brownish-black longitudinal band (Fig. 6–20) is caused by the direct production of melanin-related pigment by the fungus.[22, 25] More rarely, fungi produce tunnels that

contain air and are surrounded by a thickened wall (onychomycetoma). These appear as opaque white streaks in the nail plate (Fig. 6–21), a clinical feature not infrequently seen in dermatophyte and mold infections.[23]

MACULAR SPREADING EVOLUTION. This term denotes invasion of the nail plate in a three-dimensional volume. It induces a widespread heterochromic onychomycosis associated with focal onycholysis.

TOTAL DYSTROPHIC EVOLUTION. Although each pattern of nail infection is associated with a different clinical presentation, they all may eventually result in TDO, which involves the entire nail plate (Fig. 6–22).[5, 13, 22–26] More than one clinical type of onychomycosis may be associated with a single affected nail, and different types of onychomycosis may be present on separate nails in the same patient (Fig. 6–23). In TDO, the nail becomes thickened (claw-like) and crumbles away. The infection is characterized by complete loss of the nail structure, which may be replaced by a coarse-appearing keratotic mass. The toenails, in particular, may develop this pattern of onychomycosis.

Primary TDO is observed in patients with CMCC or other immunodeficiencies and may involve the entire nail plate and all the nails (Fig. 6–24).

TINEA CAPITIS

There are two main types of hair invasion by dermatophytes, namely the ectothrix and the endothrix patterns (Table 6–1).[1, 7, 30] The ectothrix type is characterized by the presence of arthroconidia coating the surface of the hair shaft that may contain hyphae (Fig. 6–25). In the endothrix type, arthroconidia are produced inside the hair shaft. In a much rarer type of tinea capitis corresponding to favus, hyphae without arthrospores are present throughout the hair length.

The prevalence of certain causative organisms of tinea capitis has, if anything, decreased in recent years, and other fungi are emerging or gaining in importance in some communities. The number of known cases of tinea capitis is probably vastly exceeded by those that go undiagnosed. Many physicians fail to diagnose the condition because they lack the necessary aids (e.g., Wood's

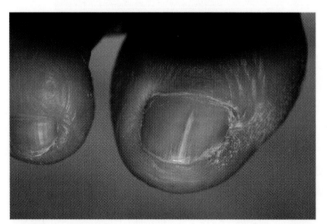

FIGURE 6-21 ■ Yellow streak. (Courtesy of Dr. H. Degreef, Leuven, Belgium.)

TABLE 6-1 ■ Dermatophytes in Tinea Capitis

Ectothrix Types	Endothrix Types
Microsporum audouinii	Trichophyton gourvilli
Microsporum canis	Trichophyton soudanense
Microsporum fulvum	Trichophyton tonsurans
Microsporum gypseum	Trichophyton violaceum
Microsporum ferrugineum	Trichophyton yaoundei
Trichophyton mentagrophytes	
Trichophyton megninii	
Trichophyton ochraceum (Trichophyton verrucosum)	
Trichophyton rubrum	

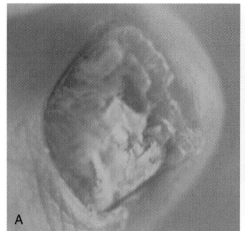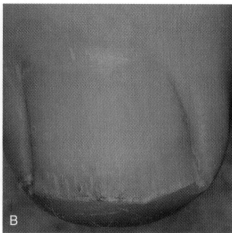

FIGURE 6-22 ■ *A* and *B*, Total dystrophic onychomycosis caused by *Trichophyton rubrum* and cured with itraconazole.

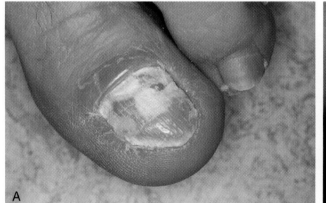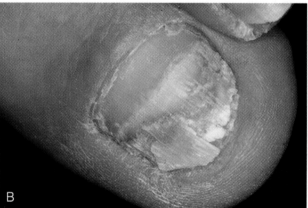

FIGURE 6-23 ■ *A*, Total dystrophic onychomycosis (caused by a dermatophyte and a nondermatophytic mold), showing different sites of invasion—lateral, proximal, superficial, and distal (removed)—in one toenail with the presence of a periungual inflammation. *B*, In this patient, oral itraconazole and terbinafine failed, but clear amelioration occurred after 3 to 4 months of topical therapy.

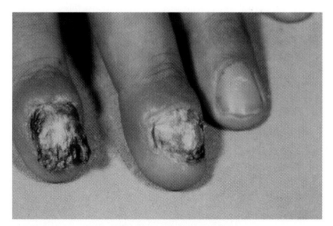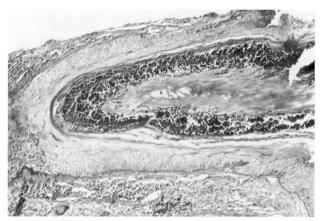

FIGURE 6-24 ■ Primary total dystrophic onychomycosis in a patient with chronic mucocutaneous candidiasis. (Courtesy of Dr. R. Willemsen, Brussels, Belgium.)

FIGURE 6-25 ■ Histological section of an ectothrix tinea capitis with multiple arthroconidia surrounding the hair shaft.

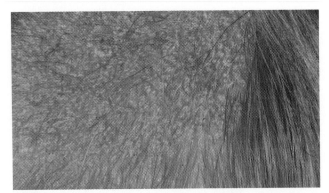

FIGURE 6–26 ■ Ectothrix tinea capitis (caused by *Microsporum canis*).

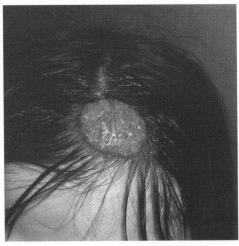

FIGURE 6–28 ■ Kerion Celsi (caused by *Trichophyton mentagrophytes*).

light) or the ability to carry out a mycological examination to confirm the diagnosis. In some instances the clinical presentation is subtle; for example, it may be suggestive of seborrheic dermatitis of the scalp.

Ectothrix Type

In many countries ectothrix infections are the most common cause of tinea capitis (see Table 6–1).[31] Historically, the anthropophilic *Microsporum audouinii* was the most predominant species in temperate countries. It is highly contagious and may represent a notifiable disease. Because the infection can be endemic, causing epidemics in schools and orphanages, it was dreaded in such public institutions.

Nowadays, the most common agent of ectothrix tinea, particularly in Europe, is *Microsporum canis* (Fig. 6–26). It is transmitted by infected animals and pets such as cats, particularly kittens (Fig. 6–27). Microsporosis tends to affect people within a close circle, often children of the same family. Transmission from person to person is the exception.

The signs of *M. canis* infection consist of broken hairs and fine, powdery dandruff in rounded, circumscribed areas of the scalp. The fact that the broken-off hairs tend to be of equal length has prompted comparison with a newly-cut lawn. The stumps of hair are dusted

with fine scales. Inflammation of the scalp is mild to moderate. The lesions may be pruritic, spreading peripherally to form patches. The infection tends to be self-limited. In addition to the scalp, *M. canis* infection tends to affect the face, arms, neck, and chest in children and chiefly the arms and trunk in adults. Small inflammatory papules tend to develop in the early stages of the disease. They later extend to the periphery while remaining sharply marginated.

Microsporum gypseum is rare in most parts of the world except South America. It is also transmitted by young animals, more often puppies than kittens. It has not infrequently been isolated from garden soil. The tinea is characterized by marked inflammation, indicative of a substantial defense reaction of the host, which explains the high rate of spontaneous remission.

Infections of the scalp by *T. mentagrophytes* and *Trichophyton ochraceum* (*Trichophyton verrucosum*) are characterized by deep and severe inflammatory reactions known as kerions (Fig. 6–28).[1, 30] The pustular folliculitis of adjacent hair follicles creates rounded, circumscribed, boggy areas with abscesses, pus, and crusting.

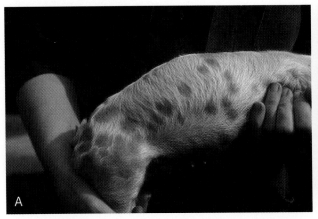
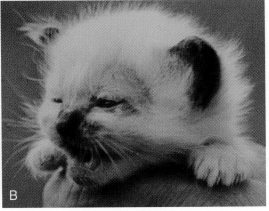

FIGURE 6–27 ■ *A*, A pig with *Microsporum canis* infection. *B*, A young cat with a lesion above the eye.

Kerions were formerly much more common than they are today. The chief sources of infection are calves and young cattle. The coats of infected animals show lesions of different sizes that appear bald but actually are covered with scales, crusts, and stumps of hairs. Contact with farm animals is restricted to relatively few people, but those exposed to these fungi, especially (but by no means exclusively) children, may develop deep trichophytosis. It typically attacks the scalp in children and the beard region in men, but other hairy regions may also be affected. In adults, trichophytosis of the scalp is more common than infections with *Microsporum* species.

Endothrix Type

Endothrix tinea is generally caused by *Trichophyton* species (see Table 6–1).[1, 7, 30, 32] The predominant agent in North America is now *Trichophyton tonsurans* (Fig. 6–29). In other countries, particularly in tropical and subtropical regions, species such as *Trichophyton violaceum* are prevalent. These infections are spread from person to person. Adult scalps do not have as much immunity to *Trichophyton* infections as to *Microsporum* infections. When the disease is acquired in childhood, it tends to persist through puberty and is more resistant to treatment. *T. violaceum* and *T. tonsurans* may be associated with tinea capitis that is particularly refractive to treatment.

These endothrix dermatophytes produce "black dot" ringworm, in which the infected hairs, which are invaded almost entirely within the shaft, break off at the surface and leave stumps that look like black dots in the follicles. Detection of the disease may be difficult, because it may be confused with dandruff or psoriasis. The lesions are small and chronic, with only a few hairs being infected.

Favus

Favus is a chronic scalp infection caused by *Trichophyton schoenleinii*[30] (Fig. 6–30). The initial lesion may manifest as yellow patches that develop into large, ele-

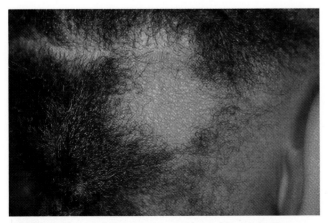

FIGURE 6–29 ■ Endothrix tinea capitis (caused by *Trichophyton tonsurans*). (Courtesy of Dr. A. Gupta, Toronto, Ontario, Canada.)

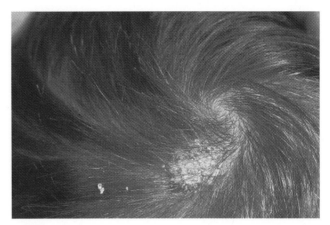

FIGURE 6–30 ■ Favus. (Courtesy of Dr. P. Dockx, Antwerp, Belgium.)

vated, cup-shaped crusts called *scutula*. Such a structure consists of mats of hyphae spreading from the ostia of the follicles. They range in diameter from a few millimeters to a centimeter. Scutula may eventually cover the scalp. A mousy odor is associated with the process. The hairs do not break off.

Children are most often affected, although the disease may progress into adult life, resulting in permanent postinflammatory cicatricial alopecia. In rare cases, the condition may spread to other parts of the skin as well as the nails. By contrast with favus of the scalp, the skin also shows inflammation with scaling and crust formation but no cicatricial atrophy.

Pathology

ONYCHOMYCOSIS

Onychomycosis is caused by a variety of organisms that affect either healthy or abnormal-appearing nail structures.[5, 6, 33] The prevalence of onychomycosis varies from country to country. Usually, dermatophytes are the most common causative agent of fungal nail infections, accounting for about 90% of the cases of onychomycosis.[34] Yeasts and nondermatophyte molds are also capable of causing the disease.

Infection by yeasts seems to be almost exclusively observed in fingernails. In general it spreads from infection of the surrounding periungual skin (paronychia) and invades the nail keratin secondarily. Direct nail invasion by *C. albicans* is limited to CMCC.[22, 23]

Molds are responsible for 1.5% to 6% of onychomycosis. This figure increases to more than 10% if only abnormal toenails are taken into account, particularly the great toe in elderly persons. Molds are usually considered contaminants or facultative pathogens, but they have been isolated from infected nails and in some patients should be considered a primary pathogen.

Onychomycosis Caused by Dermatophytes

This condition affects both sexes equally. This type of infection predominantly infects the feet (>75%), usually

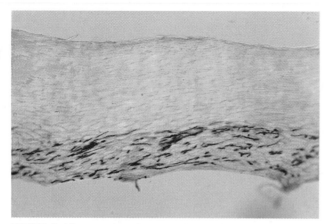

FIGURE 6–31 ■ Histological section of the nail plate showing a deep infiltration by dermatophytes (periodic acid–Schiff stain).

the big toenail.[2–5, 8, 13, 14] Fingernail fungal infection is rare in the absence of toenail involvement or tinea pedis.[35] Fungal nail infection is accompanied in more than 75% of the patients by infection of the skin (especially the feet).[18, 22]

As far as the dermatophytes are concerned, *T. rubrum* is the most common organism isolated from nails (Fig. 6–31). It often causes gross nail-plate destruction. *T. mentagrophytes* var. *interdigitale* is the second most common cause, but it is associated predominantly with SWO. Other dermatophytes are less commonly implicated.

Dermatophyte infection is also common in patients with HIV infection or AIDS.[9, 15, 16, 27, 28] The causative organisms and clinical presentation of onychomycosis are usually similar in patients with and without HIV infection, but there are some important differences. The proximal or diffuse leukonychia type has been found to be relatively common in people with AIDS but unusual in the general population. In immunocompromised persons, this type of onychomycosis usually is caused by *T. rubrum*. Unlike classic onychomycosis, the disorder can spread rapidly to all fingernails and toenails.

Finally, in some families *T. rubrum* nail infections seem to be transmitted to other family members. This appears to relate to hereditary susceptibility (autosomal dominant) rather than actual contagiousness.[36]

Onychomycosis Caused by Yeasts

This condition affects women two to three times more often than men. *Candida* infections usually involve the fingernails. There are two patterns of infection, depending on whether periungual tissues or the nail plate are affected.[8, 9, 13, 23] In the first pattern, the nail fold is the main site of infection causing paronychia. The second pattern results from colonization and infection of the skin beneath the nail, where the nail splits off the nail bed.

The species that cause paronychia are mainly *C. albicans* and less commonly *Candida tropicalis*, *Candida guilliermondii*, and other *Candida* species.[37] Proximal

nail invasion may develop secondarily to *Candida* paronychia. These infections are thought by some to represent secondary colonization because they secondarily affect the nail folds, eponychium, hyponychium, or nail bed after trauma, moisture, or contact irritants have first altered the structure of the nail unit. Furthermore, topical or systemic antimycotics do not always cure the condition in patients with nail abnormalities. In such cases, topical treatment with steroids and antibiotics can be effective.

Direct nail invasion by *C. albicans* suggests an underlying immunological cause (e.g., CMCC) in immunocompromised patients and patients with peripheral vascular disease.[29] This invasion may produce thickening and destruction of the nail. In immunocompetent patients, *Candida* pseudofilaments have been detected by histology, immunohistochemistry, and dual-flow cytometry[21] (Fig. 6–32). The morphological aspects are identical to those of systemic candidiasis that has invaded any other tissue, confirming the existence of primary infections of the nail by some *Candida* spp.

Maceration, occlusion, regular contact with water or with sugar-containing materials, and trauma (physical or chemical) are predisposing factors; systemic factors such as diabetes, compromised immune function, malnutrition, malabsorption syndrome, and iatrogenic factors (corticosteroids, antimitotics, antibiotics) are also important considerations.

Onychomycosis Caused by Molds

Molds most frequently invade altered keratin, particularly that of the big toe. Molds such as *Scopulariopsis brevicaulis*, *Scytalidium hyalinum*, *S. dimidiatum*, *Fusarium*, *Acremonium*, *Pyrenochaeta*, *Alternaria tenuis*, *Cephalosporium*, and various *Aspergillus* spp. have been reported to cause onychomycosis.[5, 8, 13, 23, 33]

Infections by *S. brevicaulis* are usually confined to the big toenail (Fig. 6–33), although the interdigital spaces may be involved. The fungal pathogens *S. dimidiatum* and *S. hyalinum* are usually seen in the tropics but also in immigrants from tropical countries. There is evidence that in some tropical areas these fungi are very common

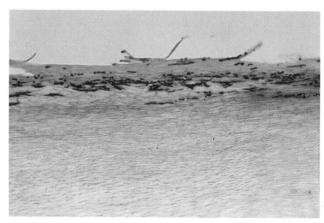

FIGURE 6–32 ■ Onychomycosis caused by *Candida albicans*. Pseudofilaments are observed in the nail plate (periodic acid–Schiff stain).

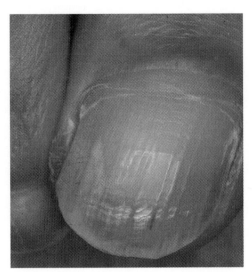

FIGURE 6–33 ■ Onychomycosis caused by *Scopulariopsis brevicaulis.*

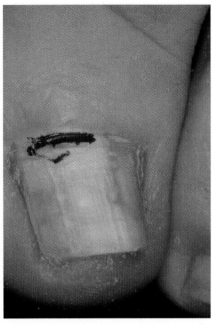

FIGURE 6–35 ■ Onychomycosis caused by *Fusarium oxysporum.* (Courtesy of Dr. R. Baran, Cannes, France.)

causes of onychomycosis and of extensive plantar infections mimicking dry-type infections caused by dermatophytes.[38]

In addition to these organisms, a number of molds not normally considered pathogenic are sometimes isolated from dystrophic nails, particularly in elderly patients.[39] These infections can be attributed to local environmental conditions, peripheral circulatory disturbance, specific anatomical conditions (e.g., overlapping toes, onychogryphosis), or certain occupations (e.g., coal mining). Often the big toenail is infected. The usual clinical pattern of nail involvement closely resembles DLSO, but the nail can show changes of onychogryphosis as well. Other molds isolated from infected nails include *Aspergillus* species (Fig. 6–34) such as *Aspergillus sy-*

dowii, Aspergillus terreus, Aspergillus versicolor; Acremonium spp., *Penicillium* spp.; and *Pyrenochaeta unguishominis.*

In some cases it is difficult to prove that these fungi genuinely contribute to the destruction of the nail, but in others the connection is made clear by various diagnostic techniques.[21] The findings indicate that these fungal organisms are actively growing in the nail. It has also been reported that *Acremonium* and *Fusarium* species can cause SWO (Fig. 6–35).[40] Besides being a well-recognized cause of onychomycosis, the latter species have been reported to disseminate in the immunocompromised patient, with a potentially fatal outcome.[35]

TINEA CAPITIS

Infection of the hair shafts distinguishes tinea capitis from infection on glabrous skin. Infected hairs are broken in ectothrix and endothrix tinea but are preserved in their full length in favus.[1, 7, 30, 41]

In ectothrix infection, hyphae invade the hair shaft at midfollicle (Fig. 6–36). In the upper location they emerge from the shaft and coat the hair surface with arthroconidia. Both the size and pattern of distribution of the arthroconidia are distinctive according to the fungal species. *M. canis* and *M. audouinii* form small arthroconidia, 1 to 3 μm in diameter, packed in a dense mosaic sheath around the hair. The arthroconidia of *M. gypseum* and *Microsporum fulvum* are 3 to 4 mm thick, few in number, and scattered. *T. mentagrophytes* produces small arthroconidia, about 2 μm in diameter, forming rare chains on the surface of the hair shaft. *T. ochraceum* forms larger arthroconidia, 6 to 11 μm thick, and manifests as large peripilar chains.

Endothrix infection by various *Trichophyton* species is

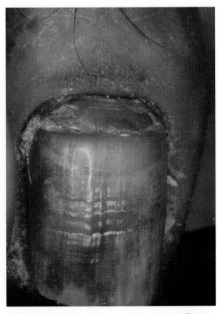

FIGURE 6–34 ■ Onychomycosis caused by *Aspergillus* spp. (Courtesy of Dr. J. DeCroix, Wilrijk, Belgium.)

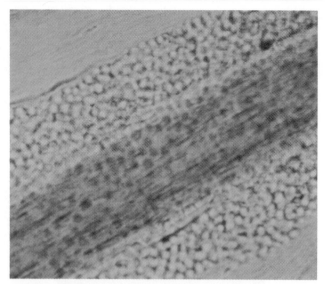

FIGURE 6-36 ■ Ectothrix type of tinea capitis with multiple arthroconidia surrounding the hair shaft.

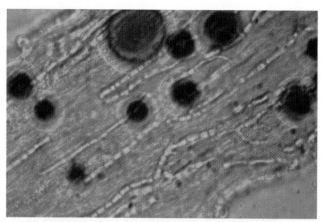

FIGURE 6-38 ■ Microscopic presentation of favus. Note the formation of air bubbles in the tunnels caused by *Trichophyton schoenleinii*.

characterized by the presence of chains of arthroconidia, 3 to 4 μm in diameter, inside the hair shaft (Fig. 6–37).

The unbroken favic hair contains many rounded arthroconidia and short, thick fragments of mycelium (Fig. 6–38). Air bubbles and empty tunnels are also present.

Diagnosis

COLLECTION OF MATERIAL FOR MICROSCOPY AND CULTURE

It is extremely important to obtain mycological confirmation of onychomycosis before beginning administration of an oral antifungal agent.[23] Various nail disorders may simulate onychomycosis, and fungi belonging to different genera may be responsible for the same clinical picture.[20–25] Therefore, the diagnosis must be confirmed before treatment can be given.[42, 43]

If a patient fails to respond to a treatment course

with an antifungal agent, mycological confirmation of the diagnosis will help in the subsequent management. The mycological confirmation of the diagnosis includes direct microscopy of nail material in potassium hydroxide (Fig. 6–39) and culture on Sabouraud agar (with or without cycloheximide).[5, 9] In addition, the laboratory outcome depends on observing the following: no antifungal treatment in the preceding weeks; prior cleaning of the nail with ethanol; sample taken from within the lesion; and separate collection of fingernails and toenails.

When examining nails, attention should be paid to whether the actual nail, the nail bed, hyponychium, or the nail folds are affected. For best results, it is essential to sample the portion of nail most likely to be infected. Sampling can be done by clipping, curetting, scraping by scalpel, punch, or dental drill. This entails reaching the site of the pathological process that contains the maximal yield of viable fungal filaments—the junction between infected and normal-appearing nail. If the nail fold is affected, the diseased tissue can easily be reached with the use of a bent inoculation loop. Surgically avulsed nail specimens should be carefully cleaned

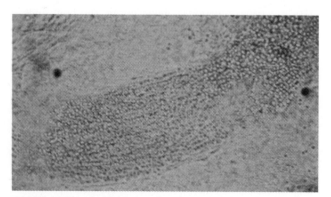

FIGURE 6-37 ■ Endothrix type of tinea capitis with a large quantity of spores in the hair.

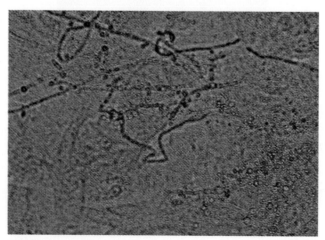

FIGURE 6-39 ■ Potassium hydroxide preparation of a nail sample: mycelium with arthrospores (dermatophyte).

and processed so that smaller pieces are used for light microscopy and culture. In certain instances, a nail biopsy may be helpful. The specimen can be stained with periodic acid–Schiff stain to outline fungal filaments.

If specimens are collected from the scalp or other hair-covered regions, it is advisable not to simply epilate or cut hairs from the suspect region but to collect stumps of hair, which are most likely to yield positive results.[7, 30] Extra care is needed in severely contaminated areas so as not to prejudice growth in culture. This applies equally to the examination of animal hair.

EXAMINATION OF THE SCALP UNDER WOOD'S LIGHT

The examination of ectothrix tinea under Wood's light at 365 nm reveals a bright green fluorescence in cases of infection by *M. canis, M. audouinii,* and *Microsporum ferrugineum.* Other ectothrix pathogens and the endothrix species exhibit no fluorescence. However, a nonspecific fluorescence may emanate from the residue of fluorescing material contained in shampoos or other preparations. A dull green fluorescence is typically seen in favus.

MICROSCOPY AND CULTURE IN TINEA CAPITIS

On potassium hydroxide mount, the size and distribution of arthroconidia are evaluated both inside and outside the hair shaft (see Pathology). Neither the clinical presentation nor direct examination enables species identification. Fungal culture is essential for accurate speciation. Details of the diverse test media and aspects of fungal growth are beyond the scope of this article, and the reader is referred to mycology textbooks.

OTHER LABORATORY TECHNIQUES FOR DIAGNOSIS OF ONYCHOMYCOSIS

The classic techniques (direct examination, culture, and light microscopy) in many cases produce a correct diagnosis but are often insufficient to detect mixed infections or to rule out the pathogenic role of certain nondermatophyte fungi. The systematic application of more recently described techniques (e.g., immunohistochemistry, flow cytometry) may be an effective means of identifying dermatophytes, yeasts, and molds.[21, 24, 42, 44] In addition, these techniques may provide evidence of the invasiveness of the different fungal organisms and help determine the extent of mixed infections.

Differential Diagnosis

NAIL INFECTIONS

Diagnosis of onychomycosis can be difficult. It is generally accepted that clinical examination alone is inadequate, because it may be difficult to distinguish onychomycosis from other nail diseases. A differential diagnosis of onychomycosis should rule out nail disease caused by age, psoriasis, Reiter's syndrome, Darier's disease, lichen planus, circulatory insufficiency, pachyonychia congenita, Norwegian scabies, chronic eczematous dermatitis of the distal phalanx, and various bacterial agents.[5, 8, 13, 14, 22, 23] Most of these disorders can be distinguished from onychomycosis by the history or the presence of characteristic skin lesions.

The clinical presentation of concurrent pathologies in one nail does not make the diagnosis of onychomycosis easier (Fig. 6–40). Differentiation of dermatophyte invasion of psoriatic nails and onychomycosis from psoriasis presents a challenge for correct diagnosis and adequate treatment.[17]

The clinical signs most commonly observed to make a differential diagnosis are paronychia, pachyonychia (subungual hyperkeratosis), onycholysis, dyschromia, onychogryphosis, modifications of the nail surface, and presence of cutaneous fungal skin infection at other anatomical sites.

TINEA CAPITIS AND FAVUS

To make the diagnosis of tinea capitis or favus, it is necessary to rule out alopecia areata, impetigo, psoriasis,

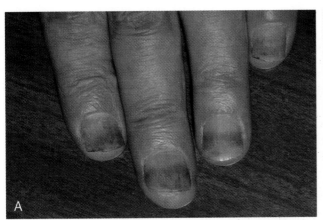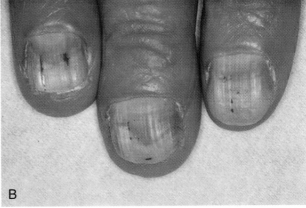

FIGURE 6–40 ■ *A* and *B*, Psoriasis of the nails with coexistence of a dermatophyte infection.

TABLE 6–2 ■ Management Guidelines in the Treatment of Onychomycosis

Type of Infection	Mild Type (<50% Distal Involvement)	All Types (Mild to Extensive Onychomycosis)
Dermophytes only	Topical imidazoles nail lacquers: miconazole° twice weekly tioconazole° with undecylenic acid bid bifonazole + 40% urea° for 11–12 days followed by bifonazole cream° od 5% amorolfine nail lacquer° once weekly	Terbinafine: continuous 250 mg/day for 12 wk (6 wk fingernails) Itraconazole: continuous 200 mg/day for 12 wk (6 wk fingernails) or pulse 400 mg/day for 1 wk/mo (3 pulses toenails, 2 pulses fingernails) Fluconazole: pulse 300 mg once weekly for 6 mo (3 mo fingernails) or pulse 150 mg once weekly for 9–12 mo (6 mo fingernails)
	8% ciclopirox nail lacquer° od	± topical add-on or combination with topical antifungals
		± nail debridement chemical: 40% urea 15% salicylic acid mechanical: fraizing, filing, surgical
Nondermophytes only	Same as for dermatophytes	Itraconazole: pulse 400 mg/day for 1 wk/mo (3–4 pulses) Terbinafine: continuous 250–500 mg/day for 3–6 mo
		± topical add-on or combination with topical antifungals

Chronic Paronychia/*Candida* Nail Infection (Mild to Severe)

Itraconazole: continuous 200 mg/day for 12 wk (6 wk fingernails) or pulse 400 mg/day for 1 wk/mo for 2–3 mo
Ketoconazole: continuous 200 mg/day 3 mo
Fluconazole: 150 mg once weekly for 3–6 mo
Terbinafine: Continuous 500 mg/day for 3–6 mo for *Candida parapsilosis*, less effective in *Candida albicans*

Distal Type (<50% Involvement)

Topical imidazoles nail lacquers (as above)
5% amorolfine once weekly

Paronychia (Localized)

Topical imidazole creams/ointments
± topical corticosteroids (inflamation)
± antiseptic bathing

Type of Infection		
Candida only or mixed infection including *Candida*		

° Not available in the United States.

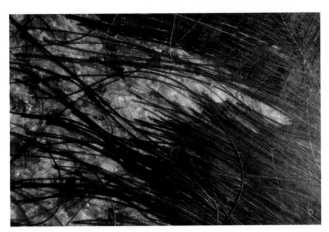

FIGURE 6–41 ■ Seborrheic dermatitis of the scalp with a squamous aspect and alopecia without broken hairs.

seborrheic dermatitis (Fig. 6–41), dandruff, folliculitis, trichotillomania, lupus erythematosus, lichen planus, scleroderma, and secondary syphilis.[1, 7, 30]

Management and Treatment

ONYCHOMYCOSIS

Management guidelines for the treatment of onychomycosis are outlined in Table 6–2. A number of topical therapies, including nail lacquers and creams, have been described.[2, 3, 5, 9, 22, 23, 45] Examples are organic acids, ciclopirox (olamine), sodium pyrithione, amorolfine, imidazoles (bifonazole-urea), allylamines, and propylene glycol–urea–lactic acid. The lacquers and creams are applied directly to the nail, with variable results. However, they should not be expected to be beneficial when there is moderate to severe proximal nail plate and nail bed involvement. The limited success of topical agents in curing onychomycosis, particularly the toenails, may be explained by insufficient penetration into and permeation through the nail unit or by the duration of treatment needed for complete cure. Patient compliance is clearly affected by long treatment durations with topical agents.

SWO, usually caused by *T. mentagrophytes*, is one clinical form of onychomycosis that responds well to topical therapy, especially if it is combined with superficial scraping or debridement of the surface of the nail plate.

Surgical avulsion of all diseased parts of the nail, when combined with topical antifungal therapy, may shorten the duration of treatment, but relapse is common, and treatment may need to be continued for several months. Mechanical reduction of the infected nail plate can be done by physical debridement or by chemical removal using a keratolytic agent such as 40% urea/15% salicylic acid applied under occlusion.[22, 46]

In the past, griseofulvin and ketoconazole were the main oral antifungal agents used to treat onychomycosis.

However, the requirement for long-term administration, low cure rates (especially with toenail infections), high relapse rates, and poor patient compliance made these traditional agents less attractive than the newer antifungals for the treatment of onychomycosis.[23, 45, 47] Ketoconazole may still be considered for *Candida* onychomycosis, including CMCC.[48]

Oral therapy with itraconazole (200 mg daily) or terbinafine (250 mg daily) has shown efficacy with reduced periods of treatment—6 weeks for fingernails and 12 weeks for toenails.[9, 22, 23, 45] These agents are currently the drugs of choice for this disease. Cure rates of terbinafine in onychomycosis caused by dermatophytes range between 75% and 80%. Its efficacy in fingernail onychomycosis caused by *C. albicans* is not established.

The development of intermittent itraconazole therapy, using 400 mg/day for 1 week each month, meant a further breakthrough for the treatment of this chronic disorder.[49] Cure rates are reported to be 70% to 80% with three pulses for toenail infections and 80% to 90% with two pulses for fingernail infections.[45] Cure rates with a 1-week regimen are as effective as the longer, continuous treatment regimens (100 to 200 mg itraconazole daily or 250 mg terbinafine daily).

A once-weekly 150 to 300 mg fluconazole regimen has also shown efficacy, although the optimal treatment regimen is not yet settled.[9, 45]

In an attempt to increase cure and avoid relapses, adjunctive therapies have been proposed for the treatment of onychomycosis with oral antifungals. Not all of these combinations have been proved statistically to be more beneficial than oral monotherapy, but some are certainly helpful. Nail avulsion (mechanical abrasion of the nail or chemical maceration with urea 40% or potassium iodide 50%) and topical antifungals in appropriate formulation represent adjunctive therapies that may be beneficial in cases that are difficult to treat.

For successful management of *Candida* paronychia, topical and/or antifungal treatment should be supplemented with patient education to enhance a successful outcome. The patient should be encouraged to eliminate predisposing factors; avoid exposure to contact irritants, water, and sugars; wear gloves; avoid trauma; and keep the nails as short as possible.

TINEA CAPITIS

Oral therapy is mandatory for tinea capitis.[7, 30] Topical monotherapy is likely to fail, but it may help minimize spread of infection to other family members or school friends. In this respect, shampoos containing imidazoles have been shown to be helpful.

One of the most difficult-to-treat types of tinea capitis is that caused by *M. canis*. Griseofulvin is still recognized as the gold standard for this type of infection,[50] although itraconazole is equally as effective. With terbinafine and fluconazole, *M. canis* infections causing tinea capitis seem more difficult to eradicate than those caused by *Trichophyton* spp. and may require longer treatment. In tinea capitis caused by *Trichophyton* spp., a short course of therapy with terbinafine or itraconazole may be effective.[51, 52] In children, a liquid is the ideal galenic formulation available for griseofulvin, ketoconazole, itraconazole, and fluconazole in many countries. Adjunctive therapy may consist of a shampoo containing an antifungal, corticosteroids, and oral antibiotics.

The recommended dosage for children is 15 to 20 mg/kg/day of micronized griseofulvin (9.9 to 13.2 mg/kg/day of ultramicronized griseofulvin) given for 6 to 8 weeks. Ketoconazole should be administered at a dosage of 20 mg three times daily for a median of 8 weeks if the child weighs less than 15 kg, or 100 mg once daily for a weight of 15 to 30 kg; for heavier children, the dosage should be the same as for adults. The fluconazole dosage instructions are 200 mg once weekly if the child weighs 20 to 40 kg, and 300 mg once weekly or 100 to 200 mg on alternate days if the weight is more than 40 kg. Treatment should be sustained until cure is obtained. The recommended dosage for itraconazole is 5 mg/kg/day. If the body weight is between 20 and 40 kg, 100 mg itraconazole can be administered, and if it is greater than 40 kg, 200 mg itraconazole daily can be used. Although most experience has been obtained with the use of a continuous treatment regimen for 6 weeks, studies exploring a 1-week pulse regimen given for two to three consecutive months suggest that short-duration pulse therapy may be effective in tinea capitis. The dosage for terbinafine is 62.5 mg/day if the body weight is less than 20 kg, 125 mg/day if between 20 and 40 kg, and 250 mg/day if greater than 40 kg. A 2-week treatment regimen may be sufficient for tinea capitis caused by *Trichophyton* spp., whereas treatment duration should be prolonged in the case of *M. canis*.

Prophylactic hygienic measures should be carried out in infected patients and their relatives.[7] They should wash the scalp regularly with shampoos containing antifungal agents and avoid sharing combs, brushes, and headgear such as caps.

SYSTEMIC TREATMENTS

The oral administration of antifungals has certain advantages over topical therapy in difficult-to-treat lesions. Oral antifungals are generally required for the treatment of chronic widespread or extensive skin infections and for hair or nail involvement (see Table 6–2). They are also used in patients for whom topical therapy has failed, patients with granulomatous lesions, and in patients who are immunosuppressed by disease or drugs.

Today, griseofulvin and ketoconazole are losing ground in the treatment of dermatomycoses because of their relatively long duration of treatment, the low cure rate, and uncertainty about the safety profile.[53, 54] The advent of new and more effective oral therapies has marked a turning point in the treatment of cutaneous fungal infections, especially for pedal onychomycosis. For terbinafine and itraconazole, wide and overlapping responses have been reported in studies of dermatophyte onychomycosis. The choice of an antifungal agent

in the future will depend not only on efficacy, safety, and cost but also on factors such as concomitant medication and disease, patient compliance, and the complexity and conformity level of a drug regimen.[45, 53]

The antifungal agents show diversity in their pharmacokinetic profiles, mechanisms of action, and toxicities. They may cause minor to moderate side effects. In addition, some antifungals (e.g., ketoconazole, itraconazole, fluconazole) can cause drug-drug interactions that may be difficult to recognize. The clinical significance of these interactions may not always be evident. A number of drugs need to be used cautiously in conjunction with these antifungal agents.[55]

The decision of whether to treat by the topical or the oral route is usually made on the basis of several factors, particularly the cure rate and the prevalence of unacceptable side effects (risk-benefit ratio). Optimal treatment of fungal infections depend on a thorough understanding of the differences in spectrum of activity, pharmacology, and pharmacokinetics of antifungal drugs and how they affect the individual patient.

The ideal antifungal agent must be active against the causative organism, penetrate infected tissues effectively, remain in these tissues in sufficient concentration to produce an antifungal effect, have short retention in serum and noncutaneous organs, and be safe. This combination of attributes permits short-duration regimens, minimizes side effects, and results in cost-effective treatments with a high degree of patient compliance.

REFERENCES

1. Greer DL: Dermatophytosis. In: Jacobs PH, Nall L (eds): Antifungal Drug Therapy: A Complete Guide for the Practitioner. New York, Marcel Dekker, 1990, pp 5–22.
2. Scher RK: Onychomycosis is more than a cosmetic problem. Br J Dermatol 130(Suppl):15, 1994.
3. Cohen PR, Scher RK: Geriatric nail disorders: diagnosis and treatment. J Am Acad Dermatol 26(4):521–531, 1992.
4. Roberts DT: Oral therapeutic agents in fungal nail disease. J Am Acad Dermatol 31:(3 Pr2):S78–S81, 1994.
5. Haneke E: Fungal infections of the nail. Seminars in Dermatology 10:41–53, 1991.
6. Arenas R: Aspectos clínico-epidemiológicos, micológicos y terapéuticos. Gac Med Mex 126:84–90, 1990.
7. Elewski BE, Hay RJ: International summit on cutaneous antifungal therapy: focus on tinea capitis. Boston, Massachusetts, November 11–13, 1994. Pediatr Dermatol 13:69–77, 1996.
8. Achten G, Wanet-Rouard J: The nail and its pathology: onychomycosis. In: Achten G (ed): Mycology 5. Schaffhausen, Switzerland, Cilag Ltd, 1981.
9. Elewski BE, Hay RJ: Update on the management of onychomycosis: highlights of the Third Annual Summit on Cutaneous Antifungal Therapy. Clin Infect Dis 23:305–313, 1996.
10. Gupta AK, Sibbald G, Lynde CW, et al: Onychomycosis in children: prevalence and treatment strategies. J Am Acad Dermatol 36:395–402, 1997.
11. Hennequin C, Bodemer C, Teillac D, De Porst Y: Onychomycosis in children. J Mycol Med 6:186–189, 1996.
12. Zaias N: Onychomycosis. Dermatol Clin 3:445–460, 1985.
13. André J, Achten G: Onychomycosis. Int J Dermatol 26:481–490, 1987.
14. Ramesh V, Reddy BSN, Singh R: Onychomycosis. Int J Dermatol 22:148–152, 1983.
15. Daniel RC III, Norton LA, Scher RK: The spectrum of nail disease in patients with human immunodeficiency virus infection. J Am Acad Dermatol 27:93–97, 1992.

16. Conant MA: The AIDS epidemic. J Am Acad Dermatol 31(Suppl): S47–S50, 1994.
17. Gupta AK, Lynde CW, Jain HC, et al: A higher prevalence of onychomycosis in psoriatics compared with non-psoriatics: a multicentre study. Br J Dermatol 136:786–789, 1997.
18. Dierckxsens C: Dermatophytoses of the foot: the role of tinea pedis in onychomycosis. Thesis (Pre-specialisatie Dermatologie, Dept Dermatologie, Prof Roseeuw D). Free University Brussels, Belgium, 1996.
19. Rabobee N, Aboobaker J, Peer AK: Tinea pedis et unguium in the muslim community of Durban, South Africa. Poster presented at the World Congress of Dermatology. Sydney, Australia, 1997.
20. Zaias N: Onychomycosis. Arch Dermatol 105:263–274, 1972.
21. Arrese JE, Piérard-Franchimont C, Greimers R, Piérard G: Fungi in onychomycosis: a study by immunohistochemistry and dual flow cytometry. J Eur Acad Dermatol Venereol 4:123–130, 1995.
22. Hay R, Baran R, Haneke E: Fungal (onychomycosis) and other infections involving the nail apparatus. In: Baran R, Dawber RPR (eds): Diseases of the Nails and Their Management, 2nd ed. Oxford, Blackwell Scientific Publications, 1994, pp 97–134.
23. Degreef H: Onychomycosis. Br J Clin Pract Supplement 71: 91–97, 1990 September.
24. Arrese JE, Piérard-Franchimont C, Piérard G: A review of the clinical and histological presentations of onychomycosis. Turk J Dermatopathol 2:175–178, 1993.
25. Baran R, Dawber RPR, Tosti A, Haneke E: Onychomycosis and its treatment. In: A Text Atlas of Nail Disorders: Diagnosis and Treatment. London, Martin Dunitz, 1996, p 155.
26. Haley L, Daniel RC III: Fungal infections. In: Scher RK, Daniels RC III (eds): Nails: Therapy, Diagnosis, Surgery. Philadelphia, WB Saunders, 1990, pp 106–119.
27. Noppakun N, Head ES: Proximal white subungual onychomycosis in a patient with acquired immune deficiency syndrome. Int J Dermatol 25:586–587, 1986.
28. Weismann K, Knudsen EA, Pedersen C: White nails in AIDS/ARC due to *Trichophyton rubrum* infection. Clin Exp Dermatol 13:24–27, 1988.
29. Hay RJ, Baran R, Moore MK, Wilkinson JD: *Candida* onychomycosis: an evaluation of the role of *Candida* in nail disease. Br J Dermatol 118:47–58, 1988.
30. Clayton YM: Scalp ringworm (tinea capitis). In: Verbov JL (ed): New Clinical Applications in Dermatology: Superficial Fungal Infections. Lancaster: MTP Press, 1986, pp 1–20.
31. Korstanje MJ, Staats CCC: Tinea capitis in northwestern Europe 1963–1993: etiological agents and their changing prevalence. Int J Dermatol 35:548–549, 1994.
32. Schwinn A, Ebert J, Brocker EB: Frequency of *Trichophyton rubrum* in tinea capitis. Mycoses 38:325–328, 1995.
33. Ginter G, Rieger E, Higl K, Propst E: Increasing frequency of onychomycoses: is there a change in the spectrum of infectious agents? Mycoses 39(Suppl 1): 118–122, 1996.
34. Summerbell RC, Kane J, Krajden S: Onychomycosis, tinea pedis, and tinea manuum caused by non-dermatophytic filamentous fungi. Mycoses 32:609–619, 1989.
35. Piérard GE, Arrese JE, Piérard-Franchimont C: Heterogeneity in fungal nail infections and life-threatening onychomycoses. Br J Dermatol 131(Suppl 1):80, 1994.
36. Zaias N: Autosomal dominant pattern of distal subungual onychomycosis by *T. rubrum*. J Am Acad Dermatol 34:302–304, 1996.
37. Barlow AJE, Chattaway FW, Holgate WC, Aldersley TA: Chronic paronychia. Br J Dermatol 82:448–452, 1970.
38. Gugnani HC, Nzelibe FK, Osunkwo IC: Onychomycosis due to *Hendersonula toruloidea* in Nigeria. J Med Vet Mycol 24:239–241, 1986.
39. English M, Atkinson R: Onychomycosis in elderly chiropody patients. Br J Dermatol 91:67–72, 1974.
40. Zaias N: Superficial white onychomycosis. Sabouraudia 52:99–103, 1966.
41. Aste N, Pau M, Biggio P: Tinea capitis in adults. Mycoses 39:299–301, 1996.
42. Piérard GE, Arrese JE, De Doncker P, Piérard-Franchimont C: Present and potential diagnostic techniques in onychomycosis. J Am Acad Dermatol 34:273–277, 1996.
43. Daniel RC III: The diagnosis of nail fungal infection. Arch Dermatol 127:1566–1567, 1991.
44. Suarez SM, Silvers DN, Scher RK, Pearlstein HH, Auerbach R: Histologic evaluation of nail clippings for diagnosing onychomycosis. Arch Dermatol 127:1517–1519, 1991.
45. Gupta AK, Scher RK, De Doncker P: Current management of onychomycosis: an overview. Dermatol Clin 15:121–136, 1997.
46. Nolting S: Non-traumatic removal of the nail and simultaneous treatment of onychomycosis. Dermatologica 169(Suppl 1):117–120, 1984.
47. Hay RJ: Onychomycosis: agents of choice. Dermatol Ther 11:161–168, 1993.
48. Hay RJ, Clayton YM: The treatment of patients with chronic mucocutaneous candidosis with ketoconazole. Clin Exp Dermatol 7:155, 1982.
49. De Doncker P, Decroix J, Piérard GE, et al: Antifungal pulse therapy for onychomycosis. Arch Dermatol 132:34–41, 1996.
50. Degreef HJ, De Doncker PRG: Current therapy of dermatophytosis. J Am Acad Dermatol 31(Suppl):S25–S30, 1994.
51. Haroon TS, Hussain I, Aman S, et al: A randomized double-blind comparative study of terbinafine for 1, 2 and 4 weeks in tinea capitis. Br J Dermatol 135:86–88, 1996.
52. Gupta AK, Alexis ME, Rabobee N, et al: Itraconazole pulse therapy is effective in the treatment of tinea capitis: an open multicenter study. Br J Dermatol 137:251–254, 1997.
53. Gupta AK, De Doncker P, Heenen M: An overview and assessment of the use of the antifungal agents itraconazole, terbinafine and fluconazole. In: Korting HC, Schafer-Korting M (eds): The Benefit/Risk Ratio: A Handbook for the Rational Use of Potentially Hazardous Drugs. Atlanta, CRC Press, 1996.
54. Hay RJ: Risk/benefit ratio of modern antifungal therapy: focus on hepatic reactions. J Am Acad Dermatol 29:S50–S54, 1993.
55. Del Rosso JQ: Advances in the treatment of superficial fungal infections: focus on onychomycosis and dry tinea pedis. J Am Osteopath Assoc 9:339–346, 1997.

7

Common Hair Loss Disorders

JERRY SHAPIRO

—

HARVEY LUI

By far the most common hair diseases are the noncicatricial alopecias, which occur in the following descending order of frequency: androgenetic alopecia (AGA), telogen effluvium, and alopecia areata (Table 7–1). At the University of British Columbia Hair Treatment, Research, and Transplant Centre, the relative incidences of these three entities are 20:7:1, respectively. Clinical differentiation of the common noncicatricial alopecias can occasionally be difficult, because they may appear alike until certain characteristic features become apparent.

▌ Androgenetic Alopecia

ETIOLOGY

AGA is caused by the combined effects of heritable and hormonal factors; the observed pattern of hair loss is the result of genetically determined end-organ sensitivity to androgens. The inheritance pattern does not appear to be mendelian but rather is polygenic and multiallelic,

TABLE 7-1 ■ Common Hair Loss Disorders

Factor	Androgenetic Alopecia	Telogen Effluvium	Alopecia Areata
Hair loss distribution	Focal balding pattern: Hamilton-Norwood (men) Ludwig (women)	Generalized	Usually patchy but can be generalized
Course	Gradual onset with progression	Onset abrupt; trigger factor	Onset abrupt; often waxes and wanes with relapses
Appearance	Thinning with or without bare patches; bare patches are gradual, not abrupt	Thinning with no bare patches	Thinning with abrupt bare patches
Shedding	Minimal	Prominent	Prominent
Age at onset	Onset at puberty or older	Onset at any age, but usually not childhood	Onset at any age, usually before 20 yr
Pull test	Usually negative	Positive; telogen hairs	Positive; dystrophic anagen and telogen hairs

with heritability from either parent.[1-3] Gene expression within a given follicle varies according to its embryonic scalp location, and this may account for the characteristic distribution of alopecia in AGA. During and after puberty, androgens trigger a cascade of events within genetically programmed follicles of the frontotemporo-parietal scalp that results in gradual transformation of terminal to miniaturized velluslike follicles and alteration of the hair cycle toward shorter anagen and longer telogen phases. These changes are mediated through specific interactions between androgens and their respective receptors and enzymes. Of particular note, androgen receptors are present within dermal papilla fibroblasts and are more abundant in balding than in nonbalding areas.[4] Signal transduction between the mesenchymally derived dermal papillae and epithelial follicular cells is mediated by regulatory growth factors, and these intrafollicular events culminate in the transformation of terminal to velluslike hair shafts in AGA. Not only is the number of androgen receptors higher in balding than in nonbalding scalps, but the receptors themselves also appear to be qualitatively different in terms of receptor protein expression.[5] Local androgen metabolism at the level of the follicle is yet another pathophysiological factor in AGA, as manifested by differential androgen-metabolizing enzyme activity in balding versus nonbalding scalp. 5α-Reductase converts testosterone to dihydrotestosterone (DHT), and both its activity and DHT levels are higher in balding versus nonbalding scalp biopsies.[6] Persons with a 5α-reductase genetic deficiency do not develop AGA. Finally, the P450 aromatase enzyme appears to be more prevalent in nonbalding scalp, where it may exert a protective effect on follicles by virtue of its ability to convert androgens to estrogens.[7] In summary, the quantity and quality of androgen receptors and the differential distribution of steroid hormone–metabolizing enzymes collectively determine whether a follicle will become part of an AGA picture (Table 7–2).

CLINICAL FEATURES

In men, thinning caused by AGA occurs on the top and front, with sparing of the back and sides of the scalp; bitemporal recession and vertex balding are characteristic features (see Table 7–1). Within affected areas of the scalp, there is uniform follicular miniaturization and

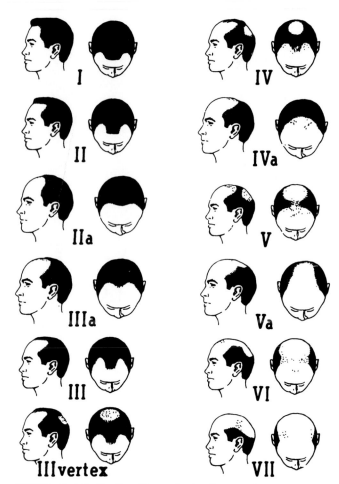

FIGURE 7–1 ■ Hamilton-Norwood classification. (From Norwood OT: Hair Transplant Surgery. Courtesy of Charles C Thomas, Publisher, Ltd., Springfield, Ill., 1984, p 6.)

TABLE 7-2 ■ Etiology of Androgenetic Alopecia

Genetic factors
Multiallelic, heritable from either parent

Hormonal factors
Androgen receptors
 Increased number of receptors in dermal papillae of balding scalp
 Receptors biochemically different in balding scalp
Enzymes for androgen interconversion
 5α-Reductase increased in balding scalp
 P450 aromatase decreased in balding scalp

velluslike hair production that eventually culminates in well-defined areas of balding. The incidence increases with age: 20% by age 20, 50% by age 50.[2] Hair loss typically begins after puberty, in concert with increasing levels of circulating androgens. Clinical staging classifications of AGA have been proposed by Hamilton[8] and by Norwood,[9] and a scheme that combines both classifications is the most widely accepted standard (Figs. 7–1 and 7–2). Hair loss in AGA is gradual and typically continuous, but cyclical patterns can be observed. In a young man presenting with AGA it can be difficult to accurately predict the ultimate extent of balding. However, if the age of onset is in the second decade of life, progressive disease is more likely. There is ethnic variability in that Asians, African-Americans, and North American Indians usually present with less extensive baldness, later onset, and preservation of the frontal hairline.[1]

In women, an oval area of thinning over the centroparietal area of the scalp is seen, and the frontal hairline margin usually remains intact. In contrast to men with AGA, in whom focally affected areas show uniform involvement of hair follicles, women tend to demonstrate a diffuse mosaic pattern of miniaturized hairs intermixed with coarse terminal hairs[3]; completely bald

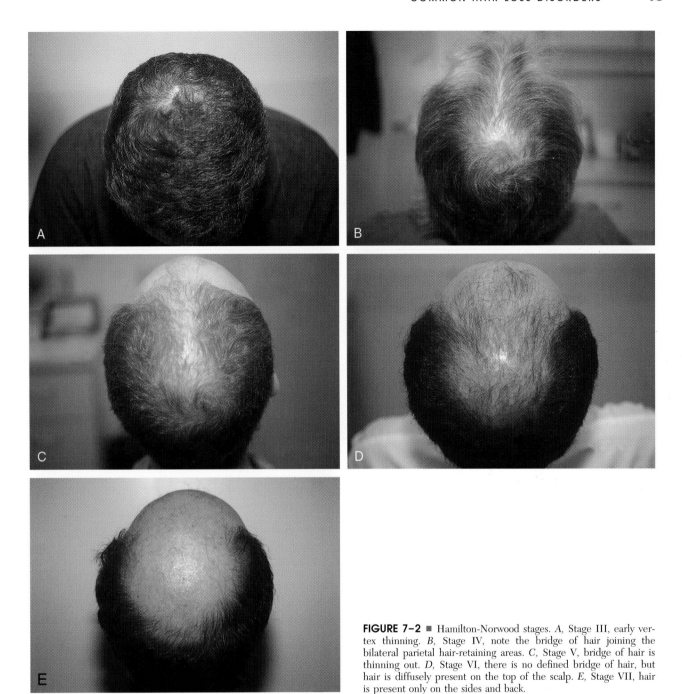

FIGURE 7–2 ■ Hamilton-Norwood stages. *A,* Stage III, early vertex thinning. *B,* Stage IV, note the bridge of hair joining the bilateral parietal hair-retaining areas. *C,* Stage V, bridge of hair is thinning out. *D,* Stage VI, there is no defined bridge of hair, but hair is diffusely present on the top of the scalp. *E,* Stage VII, hair is present only on the sides and back.

areas of scalp usually are not apparent. Because of this difference, it is important to compare part widths between the top and the back of the scalp when evaluating women with suspected AGA.[1] Ludwig divided AGA in women into three subtypes[10] (Figs. 7–3 through 7–5). Women usually notice that thinning begins in the middle twenties to early forties, whereas men usually experience AGA a decade earlier. In addition, AGA in women often first manifests during times of hormonal change, such as oral contraceptive initiation or discontinuation and the postpartum, perimenopausal, or postmenopausal periods. The prevalence of AGA is equal between men and women.[1] If a woman presents with deep frontal recession, it is important to exclude a hy-

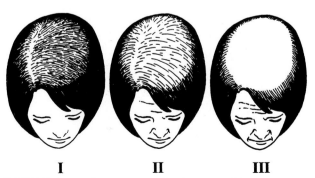

FIGURE 7–3 ■ Ludwig's patterns of androgenetic alopecia in women. (From Ludwig E: Classification of the types of androgenetic alopecia occurring in the female sex. Br J Dermatol 97:247–254, 1977.

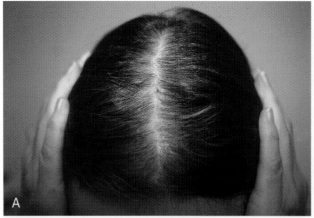

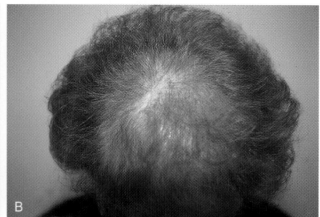

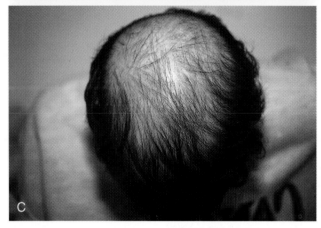

FIGURE 7-4 ■ Ludwig's pattern. A, Stage 1, thinning first noted over the centroparietal area. B, Stage 2, more thinning on the top of the scalp with retention of the frontal hair line. C, Stage 3, very little hair on the top of the scalp.

perandrogenic state. Although it is important to ask all women with AGA about other manifestations of hyperandrogenism (e.g., acne, hirsutism, infertility, menstrual abnormalities, galactorrhea), most patients do not exhibit any clinical signs of androgen excess, and routine laboratory testing for androgens is not recommended unless it is clinically indicated. There may be considerable overlap in the pattern of hair loss between the sexes, with women demonstrating a "male" pattern of hair loss and vice versa (Figs. 7–6 and 7–7).

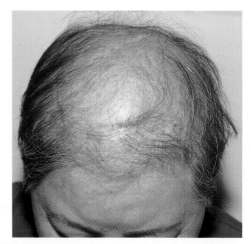

FIGURE 7-5 ■ Severe diffuse androgenetic alopecia in a woman.

HISTOLOGY

In affected follicles, the first histological change is perivascular degeneration of the lower third of the connective tissue sheath. Streamers are formed from the collapsed portions of the associated connective tissue sheath. The ratio of vellus to terminal hairs is increased owing to miniaturization, and the ratio of anagen to telogen hairs is decreased. There may also be mild upper dermal perifollicular lymphohistiocytic inflammation, but these changes are nonspecific and can be found in normal controls. Peribulbar or destructive inflammation is absent[2, 3] (Table 7–3).

TREATMENT

Accepted forms of therapy for AGA include minoxidil, hair transplantation, and antiandrogen therapy (Table 7–4). Finasteride is a novel antiandrogen that has recently been approved by drug regulatory agencies for use in men.

Minoxidil

Since 1988, topical minoxidil solution has been available for first-line therapy for AGA in the United States. All published data to date pertain to either the 2% solution (Rogaine)[11] or the 3% solution, with no significant differences being reported between these two concentrations. Fewer than 5% of men with Hamilton stage III–

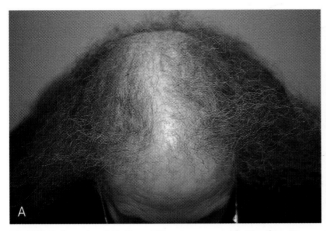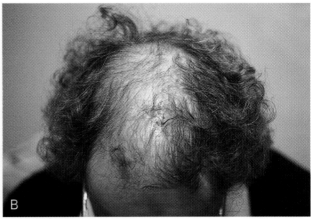

FIGURE 7-6 ■ *A* and *B,* Two different women with Hamilton-Norwood thinning stage VI.

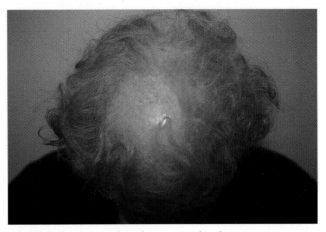

FIGURE 7-7 ■ Man with Ludwig stage II hair loss.

TABLE 7-3 ■ Histopathological Features of Common Hair Diseases

Androgenetic Alopecia	Telogen Effluvium	Alopecia Areata
Perivascular degeneration within lower third of the connective sheath Streamer formation Increased vellus-terminal ratio Miniaturization of follicles Increased telogen-anagen ratio	Increased telogen-anagen ratio (11%–30%) Terminal-vellus ratio unchanged (8:1)	Early phase: increased catagen and telogen hairs Peribulbar CD4-positive infiltrate Late phase: follicles miniaturized and peribulbar infiltrate scanty

TABLE 7-4 ■ Treatment of Common Hair Diseases

Androgenetic Alopecia	Telogen Effluvium	Alopecia Areata

Men
  Finasteride 1.0 mg/day
  Minoxidil 5% solution
  Hair transplantation
Women
  Minoxidil 5% solution
  Antiandrogens:
    Spironolactone
    Cyproterone acetate
    Flutamide
  Hair transplantation
	Identify and correct triggering factor (e.g., thyroid imbalance, nutritional deficiency, drugs)
	Minoxidil 5% solution for chronic telogen effluvium
		Adults
		  <50% hair loss
		    Intralesional corticosteroids
		    Minoxidil 5% solution ± corticosteroid cream or anthralin
		  >50% hair loss
		    Topical immunotherapy with diphencyprone
		    Psoralen with ultraviolet A
		    Minoxidil 5% solution ± corticosteroid cream or anthralin
		Children
		  Minoxidil 5% solution ± corticosteroid cream or anthralin

V AGA show dense regrowth with 2% minoxidil solution, and fewer than 25% exhibit moderate regrowth. Twice-daily use must be maintained indefinitely; once-daily application is less efficacious. With chronic therapy, peak hair counts are observed at 1 year,[12] after which they decrease but remain higher than at baseline after 5 years' follow-up. Among women with Ludwig stage I or II disease, 50% showed minimal regrowth and 13% had moderate regrowth.[1] The most common side effects of minoxidil are scalp irritation (7%) and facial hypertrichosis. A number of studies with the 5% solution are in progress, and one study that analyzed hair growth by weight showed significantly greater increases

with 5% compared with 2% minoxidil.[10] The currently available 2% minoxidil solution became an over-the-counter product in the United States in 1996; more recently the 5% minoxidil solution has been approved for over-the-counter use in men only.

Hair Transplantation

Follicles from the occipital scalp are genetically determined to produce terminal hairs, and they retain this phenotype when they are transplanted to other sites. This phenomenon is known as *donor dominance*, and because of it hair transplantation is possible. Hair trans-

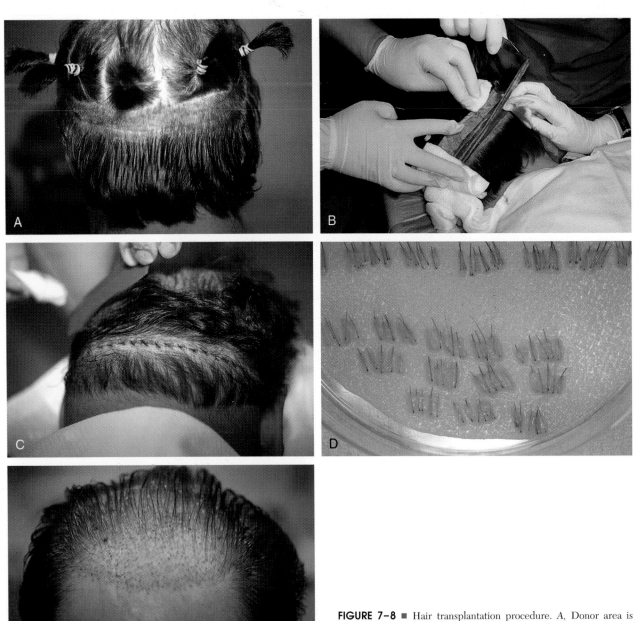

FIGURE 7–8 ■ Hair transplantation procedure. *A*, Donor area is prepared at the back of the scalp. *B*, Two strips are harvested from the donor site of the scalp. *C*, Donor area is sutured. *D*, Strips are cut into minigrafts (2 to 3 hairs each) or micrografts (1 to 2 hairs each). *E*, Grafts are placed into slits made on the anterior third of the scalp.

plantation techniques have been dramatically refined by the use of strip harvesting from the donor area (Fig. 7–8) and placement of minigrafts and micrografts onto the recipient sites. These two innovations have resulted in more natural-appearing hair transplants. Male patients usually require at least four sessions to fill in an area to adequate density, and there is usually a minimum of 5 months between sessions (Fig. 7–9). Women require fewer sessions because they generally have more hair baseline. In both men and women, surgical scalp reductions may be used in conjunction with grafting for extensive bald patches.

Antiandrogens

Pharmacological agents that block androgen secretion, interconversion, or binding to receptors can decrease androgenic effects on follicles, thereby helping to stabilize and reverse hair loss. The traditional antiandrogens in dermatology are androgen receptor blockers: spironolactone, cyproterone, and flutamide. These three agents have been used in the treatment of female, but not male, patients with AGA, because of side effects such as gynecomastia, decreased libido, and impotence.

Spironolactone is a competitive steroidal androgen receptor antagonist that is also a weak inhibitor of androgen biosynthesis. Doses of 100 to 200 mg/day are required to treat AGA. Side effects include breast tenderness and enlargement, menstrual irregularities, and fatigue. Minimal increases in serum potassium and mild reductions in blood pressure may occur. Small open trials have shown evidence of some clinical effect in AGA, but many clinicians do not consider spironolactone to be of major benefit.

Flutamide is a nonsteroidal androgen receptor antagonist that is less potent than spironolactone. Nevertheless, at higher doses good antiandrogenic effects can be achieved without steroid side effects. Flutamide has been used successfully for acne and hirsutism in women, and in one small study of female AGA patients mild benefit was demonstrated. Side effects include menstrual irregularities, dry skin, hot flushes, increased appetite, fatigue, headache, nausea, and gastrointestinal distress, chiefly diarrhea. Hepatotoxicity ($<1\%$) has been reported, with five deaths occurring in men who received the drug for prostate cancer. Concerns about hepatotoxicity necessitate monitoring of liver function 2 weeks after initiating therapy and then monthly thereafter. The flutamide dose for AGA in women is 250 mg given twice daily.

Cyproterone is an androgen receptor antagonist as well as a potent progestin. Although it is not approved by the US Food and Drug Administration, cyproterone is available in Europe and Canada. Oral doses of 50 to 100 mg/day are required in the treatment of AGA. Side effects include menstrual irregularities, weight gain, breast tenderness, loss of libido, depression, and nausea. Cyproterone, 50 to 100 mg/day on day 5 to 15 of the menstrual cycle, can be used in combination with an oral contraceptive such as Demulen 1/35. There are no large controlled studies. Cyproterone may help to stabilize the hair loss process, but it does not induce hair growth.

Finasteride is a 4-azasteroid compound that is a potent inhibitor of 5α-reductase. 5α-Reductase inhibitors block the conversion of testosterone to DHT. Two isozymes of 5α-reductase exist. Type 1 is the dominant form in the scalp and nongenital skin, and type 2 is dominant in genital skin and prostate. Finasteride primarily blocks the type 2 isozyme, which has been found in certain portions of the hair follicle. Oral finasteride causes marked suppression of circulating DHT without any change in circulating testosterone, cortisol, prolactin, sex hormone–binding globulin, thyroxine, estradiol, or glucose tolerance. Levels of luteinizing hormone and follicle-stimulating hormone rise approximately 10% but are still within normal limits. DHT levels in scalp biopsies are markedly decreased after daily doses of finasteride, 0.2 mg. A placebo-controlled study of finasteride in 1553 men aged 18 to 41 years with modified Hamilton-Norwood classification stages II v, III v, IV, or V monitored over 12 months showed 48% increased hair growth with finasteride, versus 7% in the placebo group.

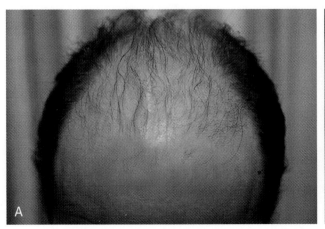
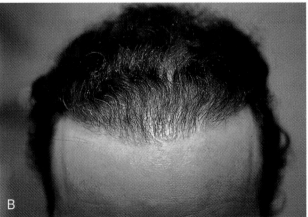

FIGURE 7–9 ■ Forty-year-old man with Hamilton-Norwood stage VII. *A,* Baseline before surgery. *B,* Results after four hair transplant procedures over 2 years.

A dose of 1 mg/day appears to be as effective as higher doses. Side effects are rare and have included decreased libido (1.8%), erectile dysfunction (1.3%), and decreased ejaculate volume (0.8%). Women of child-bearing potential should not take finasteride, because it can cause feminization of a male fetus. The use of finasteride on AGA in postmenopausal women is under investigation.[13]

Telogen Effluvium

ETIOLOGY

Telogen effluvium is caused by the abrupt synchronous induction of an abnormally high proportion of actively growing hair follicles into the resting telogen phase, with a corresponding decrease in anagen hairs. This process can be triggered by a wide variety of systemic metabolic derangements or physiological stresses, including thyroid dysfunction, iron deficiency, nutritional disorders, childbirth, fever, severe illness (malabsorption, renal failure, hepatic failure), surgery, and extreme stress. Drug therapy can also induce telogen effluvium. Common causative drugs include antidepressants, β-blockers, anticonvulsants, hormones, retinoids, anticoagulants, angiotensin-converting enzyme inhibitors, and cholesterol-lowering agents (Table 7–5).

CLINICAL FEATURES

Patients usually present with a history of abrupt generalized diffuse hair shedding and thinning over the entire scalp (see Table 7–1). Patients report finding increased hair on their pillows and combs and after shampooing (Figs. 7–10 and 7–11). The process may last from 6 months to several years. Whiting described "chronic telogen effluvium," in which hair loss lasts several years.[14] With a prolonged course of telogen effluvium, hair loss

TABLE 7-5 ■ Causes of Telogen Effluvium

Medications
Antidepressants
β-Blockers
Anticonvulsants
Hormones
Retinoids
Anticoagulants
Angiotensin-converting enzyme inhibitors
Cholesterol-reducing agents
Thyroid imbalance
Hypothyroidism
Hyperthyroidism
Iron deficiency
Nutritional deficiency
Childbirth
Severe illness
Malabsorption
Renal failure
Hepatic failure
Fever
Surgery
Extreme stress

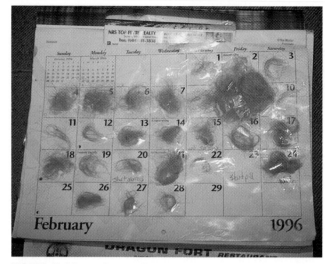

FIGURE 7-10 ■ Telogen effluvium hair lost daily collected by the patient.

is often cyclical. Patients usually present with a full head of hair, although bitemporal recession may be an early clinical sign (perhaps even more so than in AGA), because this area is visibly more sensitive to any decrease in hair density (Fig. 7–12). Hair volume is normally reduced at the temples owing to decreased hair shaft diameters. A hair pull test is positive throughout the scalp; usually more than 6 of 60 pulled hairs are easily extracted, provided the patient has not shampooed for 48 hours. Comparative assessment of part widths throughout the scalp shows uniform, marked decreases in hair density.

PATHOLOGY

Scalp biopsies may aid in the diagnosis; they usually are best taken from cosmetically less important areas, such as the posterior parietal area. The middle area is to be avoided, because a biopsy scar here may be more noticeable. The minimum recommended punch biospy size

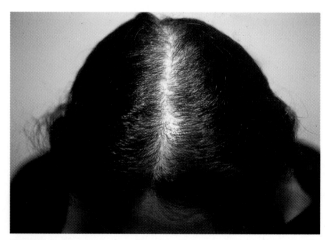

FIGURE 7-11 ■ Telogen effluvium: widening of the part can mimic androgenetic alopecia.

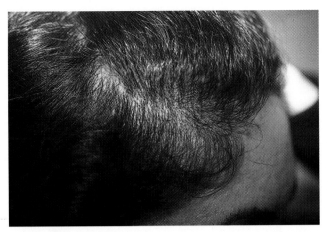

FIGURE 7-12 ■ Telogen effluvium may produce more obvious balding over the scalp.

is 4 mm, and the specimens should be sectioned transversely to maximize follicular yield. There is an increase in the proportion of telogen hairs (11% to 30%), and the ratio of terminal to vellus hairs is unchanged (8:1). The normal telogen count is typically 6% to 13%[2, 3] (see Table 7–3).

DIAGNOSIS

The differential diagnosis of telogen effluvium usually includes AGA and diffuse alopecia areata. AGA does not appear abruptly and is more patterned, with miniaturized hairs, negative pull test, and positive family history. AGA primarily involves thinning without much shedding, whereas telogen effluvium produces both thinning and shedding. Diffuse alopecia areata may mimic telogen effluvium, with abrupt onset, diffuse thinning, and a positive pull test. Clues pointing to alopecia areata include exclamation-point hairs, other well-circumscribed alopecia at other hair-bearing body sites, nail pitting, and a positive family history.

A detailed history is essential and should focus on possible triggering factors. Routine laboratory testing includes determination of serum ferritin and thyroid-stimulating hormone levels, and the need for any additional tests depends on the presence of other clinical signs and symptoms. A trichogram (forcible complete hair pluck of 40 to 60 hairs) to determine the telogen-anagen ratio may be helpful. However, by the time a patient presents to the physician, the hair shedding may be resolving, in which case there may be no significant increase in telogen hairs on trichographic analysis. The telogen-anagen ratio is significantly elevated just before the onset of effluvium (before the hairs have actually shed) and decreases markedly over the ensuing months. Another potential pitfall is the significant variability in telogen counts, which range from 4% to 37%.[3] In the absence of a baseline telogen-anagen ratio for a given patient, it may be hard to evaluate the significance of a measured ratio. These same considerations also apply to telogen-anagen ratios obtained by scalp biopsy. Nevertheless, a biopsy is useful for assessing the ratio of terminal to

vellus ratios, which are virtually unchanged from normal in telogen effluvium (8:1) but markedly reduced in both AGA and alopecia areata (1:1 to 2:1)[2, 3] (see Table 7–1).

TREATMENT

The treatment of choice is to reverse the underlying cause if it can be identified. Minoxidil may be beneficial because it helps to shorten the telogen phase and convert more hairs back into anagen. There are no published studies on the efficacy of minoxidil for telogen effluvium. We have used 5% minoxidil to treat chronic telogen effluvium for several years and believe that there is significant benefit in about 50% of cases in terms of decreased shedding and some regrowth (see Table 7–4).

Alopecia Areata

ETIOLOGY

The cause of alopecia areata is unknown, but it is considered to be a T cell–mediated autoimmune disease. Based on genetic factors, there appear to be subsets of patients with alopecia areata who are more susceptible either to developing disease in the first place or to developing more extensive disease once hair loss is established. Current research is focused on defining the genetic factors and elucidating the putative antigens or immunological triggers that attract T cells to hair follicles. The melanocyte, keratinocyte, bulb matrix, dermal papilla, and vascular endothelium have all been proposed as potential primary antigenic targets.

CLINICAL FEATURES

The lifetime risk for developing alopecia areata is 1.7%, and there is an equal incidence in men and women. Sixty percent develop their first patch before the age of 20 years (see Table 7–1). Alopecia areata can manifest with patchy scalp hair loss (Fig. 7–13) or with diffuse

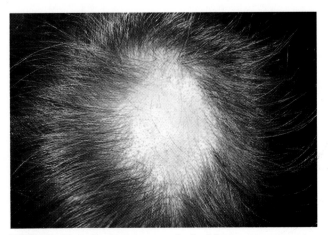

FIGURE 7-13 ■ Alopecia areata: patchy focal form.

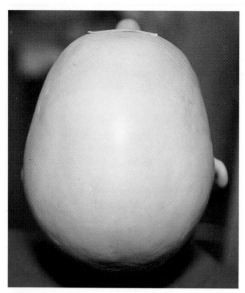

FIGURE 7–14 ■ Alopecia totalis.

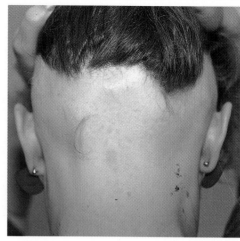

FIGURE 7–16 ■ Alopecia areata: ophiasis affecting the scalp periphery.

hair loss affecting the entire scalp (alopecia totalis, Fig. 7–14) or body (alopecia universalis, Fig. 7–15). A distinctive pattern known as *ophiasis,* which affects the periphery of the scalp, usually indicates a poorer prognosis (Fig. 7–16). Alopecia areata can affect any hair-bearing surface, and isolated loss of eyebrows, eyelashes, or beard hair can occur (Fig. 7–17). Hairs that taper proximally (exclamation-point hairs) are seen during active disease (Fig. 7–18). A pull test helps determine the location and extent of active disease by indicating areas of incipient hair loss. Nail abnormalities including pitting occur in 10% to 40% of patients. The more severe the condition, the greater the chance of nail involvement. Alopecia areata is capricious and its course is unpredictable. There is a 50% rate of spontaneous resolution without treatment in 1 year and a 10% overall

risk of the patient's developing severe chronic disease. A poorer prognosis has been observed in patients with atopy, ophiasis pattern of hair loss, long-standing hair loss, or disease onset before puberty.[14]

Atopy, thyroid disease, vitiligo, and a variety of other autoimmune diseases have been associated with alopecia areata, but no direct causal relations have been demonstrated. It is more likely that these correlations represent an autoimmune diathesis that may be predominantly genetically determined.

PATHOLOGY

In early or progressive disease, the numbers of catagen and telogen hairs are increased, implying an abbreviated anagen phase. Affected follicles do not progress beyond the early stages of anagen before being precipitated into catagen. The total number of follicles remains normal even in long-standing disease. The majority of affected hairs are surrounded by a cluster of peribulbar mononuclear cells. Most of these cells are CD4 positive. The

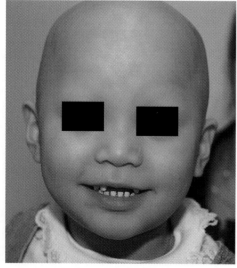

FIGURE 7–15 ■ Alopecia universalis.

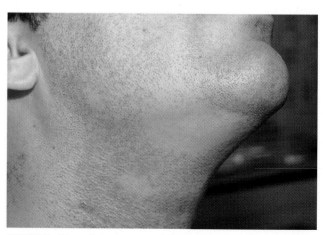

FIGURE 7–17 ■ Alopecia areata of the beard area.

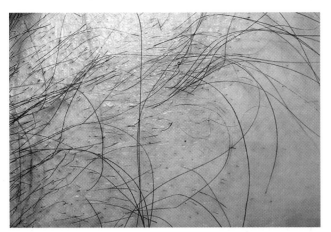

FIGURE 7–18 ■ Exclamation-point hairs are pathognomonic for alopecia areata.

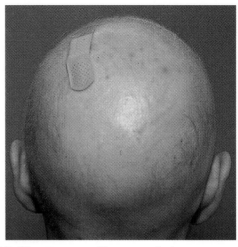

FIGURE 7–20 ■ Forty-year-old woman with alopecia universalis of 20 years' duration.

hair matrix is often infiltrated by inflammatory cells (Fig. 7–19), leading to intercellular edema. Long-standing disease differs in that follicles are miniaturized, with a scanty peribulbar infiltrate[3] (see Table 7–3).

DIAGNOSIS

The classic sign of alopecia areata is the presence of smooth patches that are virtually devoid of hair except for exclamation-point shafts (see Fig. 7–18). There may be a characteristic peach discoloration of the bare patches. The onset is abrupt, and there is marked shedding. The differential diagnosis is usually between telogen effluvium and AGA. In telogen effluvium, hair loss is generalized over the entire scalp, whereas in alopecia areata it usually is patchy. Hairs that are shed are either telogen or dystrophic anagen hairs in alopecia areata, but they are purely telogen hairs in telogen effluvium. Patients with AGA usually demonstrate the typical pattern of balding, and shedding is not prominent. The pull test usually is negative for AGA (see Table 7–1).

TREATMENT

Therapy for alopecia areata varies according to the extent of the condition and the age of the patient. Adults with less than 50% hair loss are first treated with intralesional corticosteroids. Other options include topical minoxidil in combination with either high-potency topical corticosteroid or anthralin. With hair loss greater than 50%, treatment consists of topical immunotherapy with weekly application of a contact sensitizer such as diphencyprone (DPCP). There is a 50% rate of hair regrowth with this treatment (Figs. 7–20 through 7–22), and growth is usually apparent by week 12. If a patient does not respond after 24 weeks, immunotherapy usually is discontinued. Side effects include eczema, cervical lymphadenopathy, and dyspigmentation (Figs. 7–23 through 7–25). Psoralen plus ultraviolet A

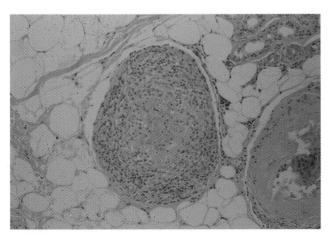

FIGURE 7–19 ■ Histopathology of alopecia areata: lymphocytes infiltrating the hair matrix. (Courtesy of Dr. Martin Trotter, Department of Pathology, University of British Columbia, Vancouver British Columbia, 100×.)

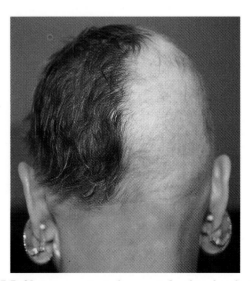

FIGURE 7–21 ■ Same patient after repeated unilateral application of diphencyprone for 24 weeks.

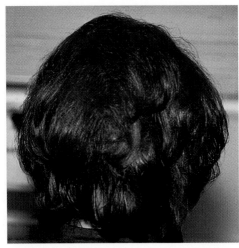

FIGURE 7–22 ■ Same patient after bilateral applications for 1 year.

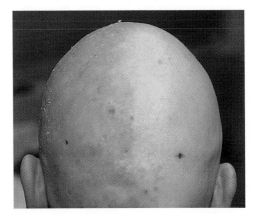

FIGURE 7–23 ■ Eczematous dermatitis is a side effect of diphencyprone application.

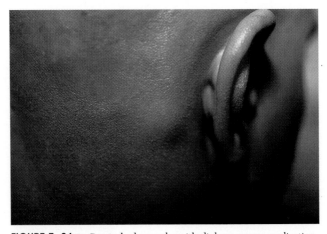

FIGURE 7–24 ■ Cervical adenopathy with diphencyprone application.

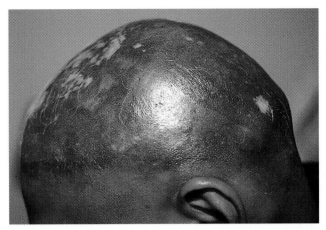

FIGURE 7–25 ■ Pigment changes with diphencyprone application.

(PUVA) is second-line treatment, with reported response rates varying between 10% and 50% and a high tendency to relapse. Combined minoxidil and topical corticosteroid or anthralin can also be considered in those with greater than 50% hair loss. Systemic corticosteroid therapy is another option that we rarely use because of the potential systemic side effects and high rates of relapse. Children are treated with 5% minoxidil, topical corticosteroid, or anthralin. DPCP has been used successfully in refractory cases in children 7 years of age or older (see Table 7–4).

It is critical that the psychological and emotional aspects of alopecia areata be addressed as part of any treatment regimen. A hair prosthesis may be necessary for the patient to function professionally* and socially. The National Alopecia Areata Foundation provides edu-

cational programs and support for patients and their families, with many local support groups throughout the United States and Canada.[15]

*National Alopecia Areata Foundation, 710 C Street, Suite 11, San Rafael, California, 94901-3853

REFERENCES

1. Olsen E: Androgenetic alopecia. In: Olsen E (ed): Disorders of Hair Growth. New York, McGraw-Hill, 1994, pp 257–284.
2. Whiting D, Howsden F: Color Atlas of Differential Diagnosis of Hair Loss. Cedar Grove, NJ, Canfield Publishing, 1996.
3. Sperling L: Evaluation of hair loss. Curr Prob Dermatol 8(3):2–30, 1996.
4. Randall V: The use of dermal papilla cells in studies of normal and abnormal hair follicle biology. Dermatol Clin 4:585–594, 1996.
5. Sawaya M: Purification of androgen receptors in human sebocytes and hair. J Invest Dermatol 98:92S–96S, 1992.
6. Dallob A, Sadick N, Unger W, et al: The effect of finasteride, a 5-alpha-reductase inhibitor, on scalp skin testosterone and dihydrotestosterone concentrations in patients with male pattern baldness. J Clin Endocrinol Metab 79:703–706, 1994.
7. Sawaya ME, Price VH: Different levels of 5α-reductase type I and II, aromatase, and androgen receptor in hair follicles of women and men with androgenetic alopecia. J Invest Dermatol 109:296–300, 1997.
8. Hamilton JB: Patterned loss of hair in man: types and incidence. Ann N Y Acad Sci 53:708–728, 1951.
9. Norwood OT: Male pattern baldness: classification and incidence. South Med J 68:1359–1365, 1975.
10. Ludwig E: Classification of the types of androgenetic alopecia occurring in the female sex. Br J Dermatol 97:247–254, 1977.
11. Price V: Symposium on Rogaine (topical minoxidil, 2%) in the management of male pattern hair baldness and alopecia areata: summary. J Am Acad Dermatol 16:749–750, 1987.
12. Price V, Menefee E: Quantitative estimation of hair growth: comparative changes in weight and hair count 5% and 2% minoxidil, placebo and no treatment. In: Van Neste D, Randall V (eds): Hair Research for the Next Millenium. New York, Elsevier Science, 1996, pp. 67–71.
13. Kaufman K, Olsen E, Whiting D, et al: Finasteride in the treatment of men with androgenetic alopecia. Journ Amer Acad Dermatol 39:578–589, 1998.
14. Whiting D: Chronic telogen effluvium. Dermatol Clin 14:723–732, 1996.
15. Shapiro J: Alopecia areata. Dermatol Clin 11:35–46, 1993.

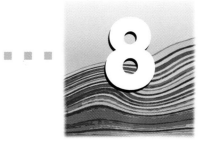

c h a p t e r

Hair Shaft Abnormalities

ULRIKE BLUME-PEYTAVI

—

NATHALIE MANDT

Hair shaft abnormalities may be of genetic origin, or they may be acquired structural defects or drug-induced changes (Table 8–1). *Genetic hair shaft abnormalities* can occur without other associated defects, but they also may be the leading symptom for an underlying genetic syndrome or a marker for a metabolic disorder leading to a genetically determined structural dysfunction. They can be classified as anomalies with increased fragility leading to hair loss and alopecia and as anomalies without increased fragility.[1, 2] *Acquired structural hair shaft defects* are caused mainly by physical and chemical manipulation, usually cosmetic manipulation. They can also be the consequence of drug-induced changes in the hair shaft. Morphological changes of hair shafts can also be nonspecific; that is, they can occur in a variety of diseases. Therefore, evaluation of a broad differential diagnostic spectrum is sometimes necessary (Table 8–2).

Genetic Hair Shaft Abnormalities

ABNORMALITIES WITH INCREASED FRAGILITY

Monilethrix
(Synonym: Beaded Hair)

Clinical Features

Monilethrix is a developmental defect of the hair shaft that is characterized by regular nodes and internodes with internodal fragility leading to breakage of hairs,

with varying degrees of alopecia. It is inherited as an autosomal dominant trait with high penetration but variable expressivity. Considerable variations in age of onset, severity, and course have been reported. Lanugo hair is usually present at birth but is soon replaced by dry, brittle, and lusterless moniliform hairs.[3] The beaded hair emerges from keratotic follicular papules, breaks spontaneously almost flush with the scalp or attains a maximum length of 0.5 to 2.5 cm, and leaves a stubblelike appearance (Fig. 8–1A). Some improvement has been reported in later life. Monilethrix occurs mainly on the scalp, but hairs of eyebrows and eyelashes, facial, pubic, and axillary hairs, and hairs of the arms and legs may also be affected (Fig. 8–1B). When the whole scalp is involved, patients are either totally bald or, more often, have a sparse covering of short, twisted, broken, lusterless hairs. Even in localized monilethrix, the noninvolved hair is seldom either thick or longer than 5 to 8 cm. Follicular keratosis is commonly associated, involving the scalp, face, and limbs but not necessarily corresponding in its distribution to areas with moniliform hairs. In addition, koilonychia has been reported in association with monilethrix. Generally, monilethrix is a genotrichosis occurring without other associated defects, but rare patients with physical retardation, juvenile cataracts, and other abnormalities of teeth and nails have been described.

Pathology

Light and polarizing microscopic examinations reveal uniform elliptical nodes and intermittent constrictions (internodes) along the hair shaft (Fig. 8–2). Transverse

TABLE 8-1 ■ Classification of Hair Shaft Abnormalities

Genetic hair shaft abnormalities

Abnormalities with increased fragility
  Monilethrix
  Pseudomonilethrix
  Trichorrhexis nodosa congenita
  Pili torti congenita
  Trichorrhexis invaginata
  Ribbonlike hair shaft in trichothiodystrophy
Abnormalities without increased fragility
  Pili annulati
  Pseudo–pili annulati
  Woolly hair
  Pili trianguli et canaliculi
  Pili bifurcati
  Pili multigemini

Acquired hair shaft abnormalities

Trichorrhexis nodosa acquisita
Pili torti in cicatricial alopecia
Acquired progressive kinking of the hair
Twisted and rolled body hairs with multiple, large knots
Bubble hair

Non–disease-specific hair shaft abnormalities

Bayonet hair
Longitudinal ridging and grooving
Trichoschisis
Tapered hair
Trichoclasis
Trichonodosis
Trichoptilosis
Weathering

Drug-induced changes

Pohl-Pinkus constriction
Synthetic retinoid–induced kinking and pili torti

TABLE 8-2 ■ Differential Diagnoses of Hair Shaft Abnormalities in Genetic Syndromes, Genetic Metabolic Disorders, and Acquired Defects of the Hair Shaft

Hair Structure Defect	Differential Diagnosis
Monilethrix	Pseudomonilethrix
Trichorrhexis nodosa or trichorrhexis nodosa–like	Proximal or distal trichorrhexis nodosa Argininosuccinic aciduria Pseudomonilethrix Trichothiodystrophy
Pili torti or pili torti–like	Menkes' disease Trichothiodystrophy Ectodermal dysplasias Bazex's syndrome Björnstad's syndrome Crandall's syndrome Hypotrichosis, hypercysteine hair, and glucosuria syndrome (HHG) Alopecia areata Cicatricial alopecia Drug-induced (etretinate)
Trichorrhexis invaginata	Netherton's syndrome
Ribbonlike hair shafts	Trichothiodystrophy, Tay's syndrome, BIDS, IBIDS, PIBIDS Neuroectodermal syndromes Marinesco-Sjögren syndrome
Pili annulati	Alopecia areata Woolly hair
Trichoschisis	Trichothiodystrophy Marinesco-Sjögren syndrome
Trichoptilosis	Pili torti Monilethrix Trichothiodystrophy Trichorrhexis invaginata

BIDS, brittle hair, intellectual impairment, decreased fertility, short stature syndrome; IBIDS, ichthyosis and BIDS; PIBIDS, photosensitivity and IBIDS.

sections of affected hair shaft at the node demonstrate a reduced number of cuticle cell layers, compared with the internodal regions. Scanning electron microscopy demonstrates normal imbricated scales in the node area but longitudinal ridging, and sometimes loss of normal scales and no medullary cavity, at the internodes. At the ultrastructural level, cytolysis and keratin tonofilament clumping (epidermolysis) are seen in the cortical cells of

the bulb of the hair follicle. Histological sections reveal wide and narrow beads of the cortex corresponding to the clinical necklacelike appearance (Fig. 8–3), but the morphological microscopic features of the hair follicle

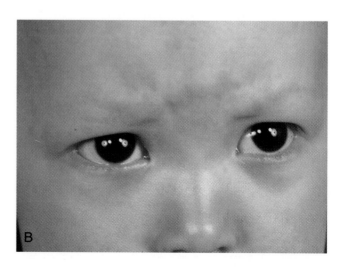

FIGURE 8–1 ■ Monilethrix. *A*, 14-month-old girl with scalp hair emerging from small keratotic follicular papules, breaking almost flush with the scalp or attaining maximum lengths of 1 cm. *B*, Involvement of eyebrows and eyelashes with only short stubble of tiny hairs.

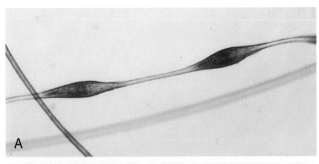

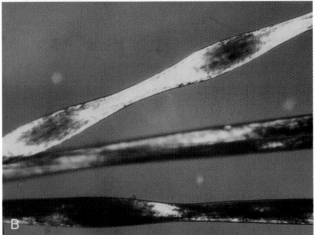

FIGURE 8–2 ■ *A,* Light and *B,* polarizing microscopic examination of longitudinal embedded hair reveals typical nodes and internodes resembling a pearl necklace.

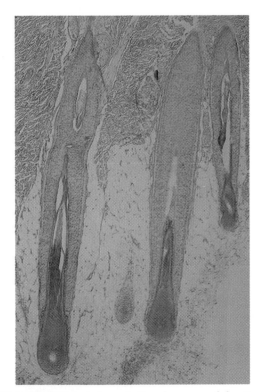

FIGURE 8–3 ■ Histological examination shows normal density of hair follicles and normal hair follicle architecture but wide and narrow beads of the cortex.

structure are apparently unchanged.[4] Monilethrix has been mapped by genetic linkage analyses to the type II keratin gene cluster on chromosome 12q13.[5, 6]

Treatment

Because there is no effective treatment, avoidance of hair trauma is a major principle in managing and counseling the patient. Reduction of hairdressing procedures permits the hair to grow to its maximum length. Systemic administration of retinoids (etretinate, acitretin) can induce some regrowth, but this effect is mainly a result of release of the follicular plug.[7] Although monilethrix exists throughout life, spontaneous improvement and improvement during pregnancy have been reported.

Pseudomonilethrix

Clinical Features

The name *pseudomonilethrix* was chosen to indicate the resemblance of this condition to classic monilethrix. It is a developmental defect characterized by irregular nodes along the hair shaft, with fragility and breakage of hair resulting in partial baldness.[8] It is inherited as an autosomal dominant trait with variable penetrance, mainly developing from the age of 8 years. However, artifactual induction must always be excluded. Spontaneous breakage of the hairs results in varying degrees of alopecia involving only the scalp. The hair is dry, brittle, irregular in length, and difficult to groom. Neither keratosis pilaris nor any other associated defects have been reported.

Pathology

The hallmark of pseudomonilethrix, observed by light microscopy, is the presence of nodes, 0.75 to 1 mm in length, interrupting the hair at irregular intervals. Internodes are of normal hair shaft thickness. On electron microscopy (magnifications up to 3000×), the "nodes" appear to be an optical illusion. Actually, the hair is indented at these regions, and the indentations extend beyond the normal diameter of the shaft. Irregular twists of 25 to 200 degrees without flattening of the shaft can be observed. Essentially, scales are normal along the whole hair shaft.

Trichorrhexis Nodosa Congenita

Clinical Features

In congenital trichorrhexis nodosa, hair shaft fragility is often the only abnormal clinical feature. However, other ectodermal defects occasionally are associated.[9] An autosomal dominant inheritance is suggested. The hair often appears normally thick and long at birth but becomes friable in the first year. Within a few months the abnormal fragility becomes evident as the hair breaks, leaving variable lengths of broken hair and even partial alopecia (Fig. 8–4A). The term *nodosa* is used primarily for historical reasons. It refers to the node that is sometimes seen with the naked eye at the site of this defect. The essential diagnostic feature is always the presence of the typical fracture, with release of individual cortical

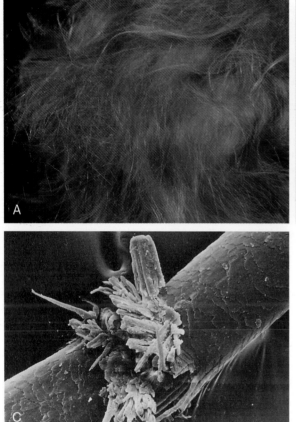

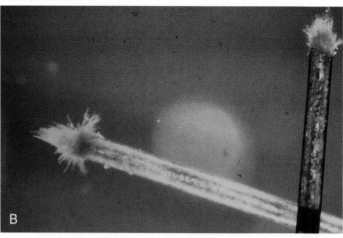

FIGURE 8-4 ■ Trichorrhexis nodosa congenita. *A,* Seven-year-old girl with blond, thin hair, variable lengths of broken hair, and even partial alopecia. *B,* Typical brushlike aspect at the extreme of the fracture nodule. *C,* Scanning electron microscopy illustrates the characteristic splayed-out spindle cells and their fragments pushed together after fracture. (*C,* Courtesy of Deutsches Wollforschungsinstitut an der Technischen Universitat, Aachen, Germany.)

cells and their fragments. Trichorrhexis nodosa is also found in infants with mental retardation and argininosuccinic aciduria. The hair defect, when present, is an important diagnostic clue to this rare syndrome, which is due to an inborn error of urea synthesis. In many of these children, the hair is dry, brittle, matted, and notable for its stubbly appearance.

Pathology

A hair shaft fracture, with individual cortical cells and their fragments splaying out, is indicative of trichorrhexis nodosa (Fig. 8–4*B*). In light microscopy, the defect resembles two brushes with their ends pushed together. Scanning electron microscopy reveals the characteristic fracture with splayed-out spindle cells and their fragments (Fig. 8–4*C*). When the break occurs, the brushlike end is clearly seen. A variety of processes, both congenital and acquired, can induce a structural flaw of hair keratin that is followed by this typical fracture defect. Abnormal amino acid composition has been reported.[10] No abnormal laboratory findings in familial or sporadic cases of congenital trichorrhexis nodosa have been noted. In contrast, in argininosuccinic aciduria, patients may present with other associated symptoms and related findings such as elevated amounts of argininosuccinic acid in urine, blood, and cerebrospinal fluid.

Treatment

In *trichorrhexis nodosa with argininosuccinase deficiency,* a low-protein, arginine-supplemented diet may

reverse grooving and abnormal polarization of hair shafts.[11]

Pili Torti Congenita

Clinical Features

Pili torti is characterized by a flattened hair shaft twisted through 180 degrees on its own longitudinal axis (Fig. 8–5*A*). The condition can be classified into two groups: a classic, early-onset Ronchese type and a late-onset Beare type. In addition, pili torti can be associated with copper deficiency (i.e., in Menkes' disease) or with ectodermal defects and syndromes (e.g., Bazex's, Crandall's, or Björnsted's syndrome; see Table 8–2). Acquired pili torti is discussed in a later section. Occasional irregular twists are also seen in normal hair and in hair shafts with other structural abnormalities (e.g., trichothiodystrophy, Netherton's syndrome; see Table 8–2), but these changes are better called pili torti–like.[12, 13]

Classic, early-onset pili torti is more common in women, primarily those with thin, blond hair. The hair may be abnormal from birth or it may become abnormal in the early years of life, starting on the temporal and occipital areas and occasionally affecting eyebrows and lashes. The pattern of inheritance is variable, and both autosomal dominant and recessive forms have been reported. The hair is spangled, dry, and brittle, breaks at different lengths, and may stand out from the scalp. It tends to be short, especially in areas subject to

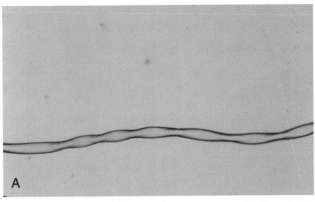 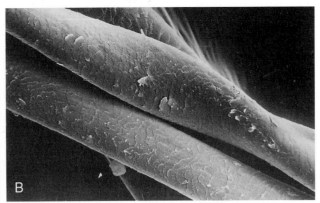

FIGURE 8-5 ■ Pili torti. A, Longitudinally embedded hair with typical twisting along the hair's longitudinal axis, showing B, twists through 180 degrees and sometimes loss of the cuticle in several areas, detectable by scanning electron microscopy. (B, Courtesy of Deutsches Wollforschungsinstitut an der Technischen Universitat, Aachen, Germany.)

trauma. The condition often improves over a number of years, particularly after puberty. Classic pili torti is part of a clinical syndrome with ectodermal abnormalities such as keratosis pilaris, widely spaced teeth, nail dystrophy, corneal opacities, and occasionally ichthyosis. In some pedigrees mental retardation and in a number of patients sensorineural hearing loss (cochlear type) have been reported in association. The latter emphasizes the importance of early auditory testing in children with this hair structure defect.

The *late-onset Beare type* tends to manifest as patchy scalp alopecia after puberty. In this autosomal dominant condition, affected hair is coarse, stiff, and jet-black. Eyebrows and lashes break off earlier during childhood, and sparse body hair may break off almost flush with the skin surface.

Pili torti with copper deficiency was first described by Menkes and colleagues in 1962. In Menkes' disease, an X-linked recessive disorder of copper metabolism, markedly decreased copper levels are found in the serum, brain, and liver of affected boys. Affected infants may

develop normally until the onset of symptoms, usually between the ages of 5 weeks and 5 months. Patients show characteristic white, steely hair and neurological symptoms such as seizures, delayed development, and muscular hypotony. The facial appearance is characteristic, with pale skin and plump cheeks, a bowed upper lip, and broken, twisted eyebrows. Prognosis is poor, and most of the patients die within the first 3 years of life (Fig. 8-6).

A rare type of pili torti is the so-called corkscrew hair, which shows a double twisting. It may be associated with ectodermal dysplasia and has also been reported as a classic symptom of scurvy, a result of prolonged ascorbic acid deficiency. In the latter case, corkscrew hairs together with perifollicular hemorrhages, large ecchymoses, and hemorrhagic gingivitis can be observed.

Pathology

In a hair mount, closely grouped twists of the flattened hair are readily seen. Each twist is 0.4 to 0.9 mm in width, and they occur in groups of 3 to 10 at irregular

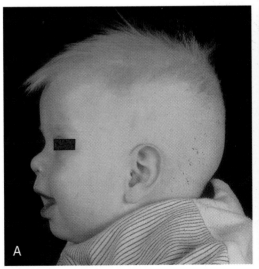 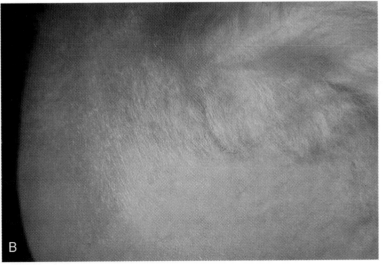

FIGURE 8-6 ■ A 15-month-old boy with Menkes' disease A, Pasty, pallid skin and white-yellow, depigmented, lusterless, stubby hair standing up in the frontal region but almost completely lost in the areas exposed to mechanical trauma. B, In the occipital region hair is short, broken, a few millimeters long, and twisted.

intervals along the shaft. Twists are almost always through 180 degrees, although some are through 90 degrees or 360 degrees. The hair shaft is somewhat flattened, and this fact can be appreciated particularly on scanning electron microscopy (Fig. 8–5B). Breaks occur in the shaft independent of the narrowness or the number of twists.[14] Under scanning electron microscopy scales are normal in pili torti. The only histological abnormality is some curvature of the follicle. The load-extension curve (breaking stress analysis) is comparable to that of merino sheep, with easy breakage.

In Menkes' disease, decreased serum levels of copper and ceruloplasmin are found. Careful analysis reveals accumulation of copper in the hair. Research supports the presumption that the genetic defect is located on the long arm of chromosome 13 (Xq13.3).[15] If Menkes' disease is suspected, a hair mount showing pili torti provides a simple, quick aid to early diagnosis. Occasional trichorrhexis nodosa fractures may be present.

Treatment

No effective treatment of pili torti exists. In *pili torti in Menkes' disease,* various therapeutic attempts with parenteral administration of copper-histidine complexes have been made, with rather discouraging results. However, when copper-histidine complexes are supplied before manifestation of neurological or developmental defects, prognosis can be influenced to a certain extent.[16]

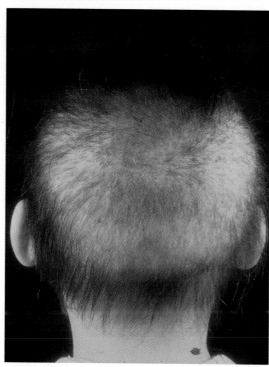

FIGURE 8–7 ■ A 12-year-old boy with Netherton's syndrome and bamboo hair leading to dry, lusterless appearance of the hair and partial alopecia with short, broken hair.

Trichorrhexis Invaginata
(Synonym: Bamboo Hair)

Clinical Features

The term *bamboo hair* refers to a distinctive hair shaft abnormality found in a rare, syndrome termed Netherton's syndrome that combines ichthyosiform skin changes, mainly consistent with ichthyosis linearis circumflexa Comel and frequently an atopic state. Available evidence suggests an autosomal recessive inheritance with a female prevalence of about 60%. The dermatosis usually appears in the first few days of life as redness and scaling affecting the face and other parts of the body. The hair defect appears in infancy and affects all hair to a certain degree. One or more nodes or nodular fractures irregularly distributed along the affected shafts provides the scalp hair a dry, lusterless appearance (Fig. 8–7). The abnormal, tuliplike invagination along the shaft (Fig. 8–8A) is responsible for the extreme fragility of the hair, not allowing the hair to reach its normal length. In some cases, the pathological findings are more prominent in vellus hairs than in terminal scalp hairs. Eyelashes and eyebrows are sparse or absent.

Pathology

Typical nodes resembling bamboo joints can be detected on longitudinal embedded hair by light microscopy; the proximal part of the defect is termed the *cup portion* and the distal part, the *ball portion* (Fig. 8–8B).

Ultrastructural studies of bamboo hair have confirmed the presence of a gross defect in keratinization, with abnormal invaginations in the keratogenous zone. Cortical microfibrils are markedly disorganized in a zigzag pattern in the invagination region. Electron microscopy can reveal additional abnormalities associated with Netherton's syndrome: twisting or caliber changes of the shaft, circumferential strictures, braidlike segments, tuliplike forms, and occasionally trichorrhexis nodosa.

Treatment

Successful treatment with systemic etretinate in patients with Netherton's syndrome has been reported.[17] The oral retinoid therapy did not heal the basic defect, but keratinization seemed to normalize and hair clinically improved.

Ribbonlike Hair Shaft in Trichothiodystrophy

Clinical Features

Trichothiodystrophy (TTD), or sulfur-deficient brittle hair, is a rare autosomal recessive disorder characterized by sulfur-deficient brittle hair, mental and physical retardation, and ichthyosis. Photosensitivity has been reported in 50% of the cases. Numerous clinical features may be present, producing a heterogenous syndrome. An autosomal recessive inheritance mode has been suggested.[18, 19]

Hair characteristics are key factors in recognizing pa-

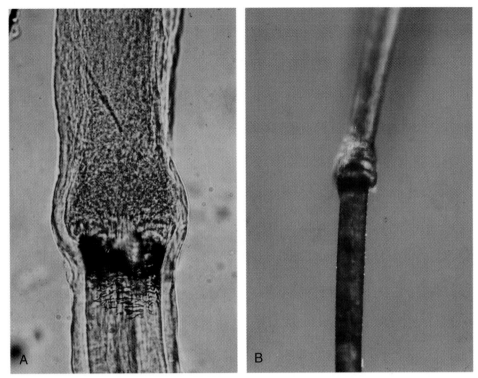

FIGURE 8–8 ■ Trichorrhexis invaginata. Abnormal tuliplike invagination along the shaft is detectable by light microscopy (A), showing the upper ball and the lower cup portion (B).

tients with a defect in synthesis of high-sulfur proteins. Scalp hair, eyebrows, and eyelashes are all brittle, short, uneven, and sparse. Patients with this condition have a typical facial appearance, with receding chin, protruding ears, and a slightly aged appearance. The voice may be raspy.[20] Sulfur-deficient brittle hair serves as an important clinical marker for a constellation of neuroectodermal syndromes. Various syndromes have been reported together with TTD (see Table 8–2), including BIDS (brittle hair, intellectual impairment, decreased fertility, short stature), IBIDS (ichthyosis and BIDS), and PIBIDS (photosensitivity and IBIDS).

Pathology

The hair has markedly low sulfur (cystine) content and presents characteristic light and polarizing microscopic features, the so-called tiger-tail pattern (Fig. 8–9). Light microscopy demonstrates in affected hairs an irregular, slightly undulating contour. In addition, the hair presents trichorrhexis nodosa–like fractures with less release of individual cortical cells and clean, transverse fractures. Trichoschisis may occur. The hair is usually notably flattened and may be folded like a ribbon or a shoelace; this is sometimes mistaken for pili torti. In polarizing light microscopy, the hair must be viewed between cross-polarizers and the hair axis must be aligned with one of the polarizer directions to reveal the striking bright and dark bands. Scanning electron microscopy of affected hair reveals severe cuticular and secondary cortical degeneration along almost the entire

hair shaft, with reduced or absent cuticle pattern and abnormal ridging and fluting.

Biochemical studies have shown that the abnormal hair has a lower cystine content than normal. Biochemical analysis has detected a deficient synthesis of the usual high-sulfur and ultra–high-sulfur proteins, with the appearance of new, low-molecular-mass proteins. A defect in a regulatory gene controlling functions in various tissues is supposed. A mutation of the *XPB/ERCC2* DNA repair transcription gene, producing a cellular de-

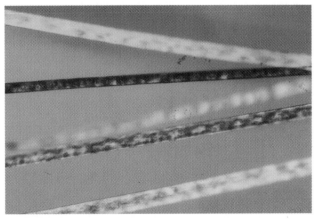

FIGURE 8–9 ■ Trichothiodystrophy. Light microscopy reveals in affected hairs an irregular, slightly undulating contour with a typical tiger-tail pattern that is detectable only by polarizing microscopy.

fect of DNA repair (as in xeroderma pigmentosum), may be associated with trichothiodystrophy.[21-22]

ABNORMALITIES WITHOUT INCREASED FRAGILITY

Pili Annulati
(Synonym: Ringed Hair)

Clinical Features

Pili annulati is a rare hair structure abnormality that may be sporadic or familial. In the latter type there is mainly an autosomal dominant pattern of inheritance. Usually the hair is strong and sound and there is no clinical problem with hair growth. In most cases, the diagnosis is made incidentally.[24] Close inspection of the hair reveals alternating bright and dark bands of 0.1 to 1.9 mm spaced in a random manner along the hair shaft, giving the hair a sandy color. The banded appearance of pili annulati is clinically detectable only in blond or lightly pigmented hair. The banding is obvious regardless of the direction from which light strikes the hair, but it is most clearly seen with longitudinal illumination. In contrast, brown hair absorbs most of the incident light and obscures the banding, even if it contains similar cavities. Occasionally, axillary hair is affected. Alopecia areata may be an additional finding; however, the significance of this coexistence is unknown. So far, no other associated abnormalities of skin or other organs have been reported, except for the association of pili annulati with woolly hair, anhidrotic ectodermal dysplasia, and blue nevi.[25-27]

Pathology

On a hair mount with transmitted light, characteristic alternating bright and dark bands are seen in the hair shaft. The bright appearance of the bands is caused by air-filled cavities within the cortex that scatter the light. The colors of the bands are reversed when seen with reflected light. Transmission electron microscopy shows small and large cavities randomly distributed within the cortex in the abnormal bands. Holes range in size from less than 1 μm to more than 10 μm in diameter. Scanning electron microscopy reveals an abnormal surface with cobblestonelike and fluted appearance. The affected hair appears longitudinally wrinkled and folded in bands that correspond to the cavity-bearing positions of the hair shaft. Electron histochemical studies suggested that hair cavities result from insufficient cortical material, which is the consequence of dissolution of the intermacrofibrillar material, possibly by chemical agents and water.[28] Breaking stress analysis is relatively normal, but when fractures occur they are located in the normal bands.

Treatment

Because fragility is seldom increased and this abnormality is most often detected only when deliberately sought, no therapy is necessary. The severity of the disease does not increase with age, but it also does not resolve spontaneously.

Pseudo-Pili Annulati

Clinical Features

This condition is an unusual variant of normal hair that is characterized by a strikingly banded appearance by reflected light. The hair is blond, strong, and normal apart from the unusual appearance. Such bright banding is conspicuous only in blond hair; brown hair, even if similarly twisted, absorbs most of the incident light. The sporadic bright highlights seen by reflected light in all normal blond hair are probably caused by the same phenomenon. In most cases, however, the twisting does not occur with the extensive periodicity seen in pili annulati. In contrast to pili annulati, the banded appearance is seen only if the light strikes the hair at right angles to the hair's long axis (transverse illumination).

Pathology

Examination of affected hair shafts by reflected light shows one of two features, depending on the position of the hair. Only if light strikes the hair at a right angle is banding seen. Any other angle does not demonstrate banding. If hair is rotated about its long axis, banding is seen only in certain positions. On polarizing light microscopy, with crossed polarizers and retardation plate, a pseudo-pili annulati hair presents alternating segments of color (i.e., a blue segment followed by a yellow segment). A hair mount with transmitted unpolarized light shows apparent variations in fiber diameter caused by twisting of the oval hair about its long axis, whereas the internal structure is entirely normal.

Woolly Hair

Clinical Features

The term *woolly hair* derives from sheep's wool, which is usually characteristically crimped. Human woolly hair is excessively curly, suggesting a woolly appearance, with a curl diameter of approximately 0.5 cm. The hair shaft may be twisted, sometimes breaking readily, with a brittle appearance, enabling the practitioner to sharply distinguish between affected and unaffected family members. The appearance of distinctly different, tight, curly hair occurs at birth or shortly after and is usually most severe during childhood, when it is often difficult to brush the hair. The condition may improve in adulthood. Woolly hair can be separated into three groups: autosomal dominant hereditary woolly hair, autosomal recessive familial woolly hair, and nongenetically determined woolly-hair nevus.

In autosomal dominant *hereditary woolly hair*, the hair color is usually the same as in unaffected family members. Occasionally the hair is unable to achieve long length, although hair growth rate appears to be normal and body hair is normal. Associated abnormalities of ectodermal origin have not been reported.

In autosomal recessive *familial woolly hair*, the patient presents with a distinctive clinical picture. The hair is usually lighter in color than that of unaffected family members and in some cases is whitish-blond. The hair

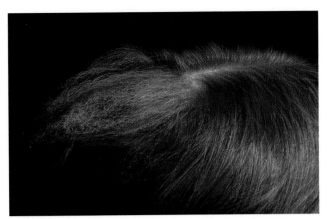

FIGURE 8-10 ■ Woolly-hair nevus. Typical circumscribed patches of fine, curly hair, lighter in color and smaller in diameter than the unaffected hair.

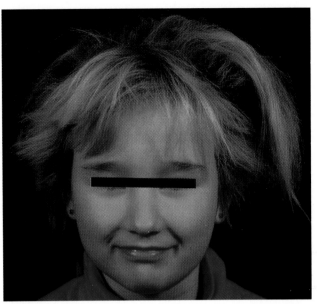

FIGURE 8-11 ■ Pili trianguli et canaliculi, or uncombable hair. In this 6-year-old girl, hair stands out from the scalp and is impossible to control by combing or brushing.

shaft diameter is markedly reduced. In some cases the tightly curled hair is present from birth, and in most cases the hair is unable to grow longer than a few centimeters.

Woolly-hair nevus occurs sporadically as one or more circumscribed patches of fine, curly hair within otherwise normal scalp hairs (Fig. 8–10). This rare, nonhereditary, circumscribed developmental defect of hair growth usually begins within the first 2 years of life. The affected hair shafts are often lighter in color and smaller in diameter than the unaffected hair. Ophthalmological examination is recommended in all cases of woolly-hair disease, because ocular anomalies have been reported in association. About 50% of the reported cases of woolly-hair nevus are associated with a linear, epidermal, or pigmented nevi.[29]

Pathology

Hair shaft microscopy demonstrates ovoid or elliptical cross-sections, 180-degree axial twisting of the hair, and occasionally trichorrhexis nodosa. The anagen hair bulb is commonly dystrophic, lacking a root sheath, but the anagen-telogen ratio is normal. In woolly hair, cuticular weathering or absence of cuticles can be detected by scanning electron microscopy.

Pili Trianguli et Canaliculi
(Synonym: Uncombable Hair, Spun Glass Hair)

Clinical Features

The term *uncombable hair* refers to a rare abnormality in which the peculiar appearance of "spun glass" is in part caused by reflection of light from variably oriented, flattened hair surfaces. Characteristic triangular or kidney-shaped hairs seen in cross-sections and longitudinal grooves are responsible for the frizzy, stand-away appearance of this uncombable hair (Fig. 8–11). The irregular hair shafts prevent adjacent hairs from lying flat or grouping to form locks and therefore provide the unruly appearance. The hair is often dry with a silvery blond color, normal in quantity and in length, and im-

possible to control by combing or brushing (see Fig. 8–11). Eyebrows and eyelashes are not involved. The hair shaft defect becomes obvious during the first years of life, and in some cases spontaneous improvement has been noticed. The abnormality may be familial, with probably an autosomal dominant inheritance mode. Most cases are isolated variants, but association with ectodermal dysplasia, progressive alopecia areata, atopic eczema, and ichthyosis vulgaris have been reported.[30]

Pathology

In this hair shaft abnormality, light microscopic examination may be normal, but examination under polarized light demonstrates a changing alignment of hair shafts. The characteristic feature can easily be demonstrated by the shrinkage tube technique or by electron microscopy, showing longitudinal grooves and triangular or kidney-shaped cross-sections.[31] The cause of this hair shaft malformation is suggested to be a misshapen dermal papilla that alters the shape of the inner root sheath, which hardens before the central forming hair in a kidney-shaped cross-section. The hair subsequently hardens, following the root sheath.

Treatment

No treatment is known, although biotin supplementation has been suggested. Use of a soft brush and hair conditioner applied to the hair after shampooing are recommended for facilitating management of the hair.

Pili Bifurcati

Clinical Features

Pili bifurcati refers to a rare anomaly in which the hair bifurcates at multiple irregular intervals along the hair shaft to form two separate, parallel branches (Fig. 8–

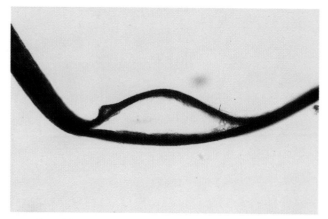

FIGURE 8-12 ■ Pili bifurcati. Splitting of a single hair shaft to form two parallel branches with subsequent fusing into a single hair shaft.

12), which later fuse to form a single shaft. The splitting and fusing of a single hair may be a variation of pili multigemini, and the term *pili gemini* may also be appropriate. Pili bifurcati has been reported in association with the mosaic trisomy 8 syndrome.[32]

Pathology

Typical features of pili bifurcati are seen in light microscopy and scanning electron microscopy. In the latter, two parallel branches, each vested with a complete circumferential cuticle, can be observed. Splitting and fusing occur at irregular intervals along the hair shaft.

Pili Multigemini

Clinical Features

Multigeminate hairs are usually found when the patient is examined for an unrelated problem. Pili multigemini is a rare developmental defect in which multiple hairs arises in tufts from a single pilosebaceous canal. Hairs are generally flattened, sometimes triangular in cross-section, sometimes also presenting longitudinal grooves. In adults this condition has been found in the beard,

and in children the abnormal hairs were found in the scalp. In some instances, the hair shaft may alternately split and unite, as in pili bifurcati.

Pathology

Biopsy specimen of the scalp in pili multigemini may reveal two to eight hairshafts with one dermal papilla, with all hair shafts emerging from a single pilosebaceous canal. Each hair is formed by a single branch of dermal papilla, which is surrounded by all layers present in the normal follicle except for the outer root sheath cells. The outer root sheath surrounds the entire follicle; therefore, transverse sections show an outer root sheath enclosing multiple hairs, each with its own inner root sheath.[33]

Acquired Hair Shaft Abnormalities

Trichorrhexis Nodosa Acquisita

Clinical Features

This is the most common cause of acquired hair fracture. There are at least three clinical varieties—proximal, distal, and circumscribed trichorrhexis nodosa—which may represent different biochemical defects; some may also represent a genetic weakness of hair keratin.

Proximal trichorrhexis nodosa presents a distinctive clinical picture. The hair is strikingly short (2 to 4 cm) over a large scalp area; however, the entire scalp is seldom involved, and generally, no associated alopecia occurs with hair breakage (Fig. 8–13A). The patients are invariably African-American, of all ages and both sexes, with fragile hair that breaks a few centimeters above the scalp surface. In many cases there is a family history of "short hair," but it is still unknown why proximal trichorrhexis nodosa develops in some persons after years of hair straightening or brushing, and not in others.

Distal trichorrhexis nodosa is seen primarily in Caucasian and Asian persons of both sexes. The hair is pri-

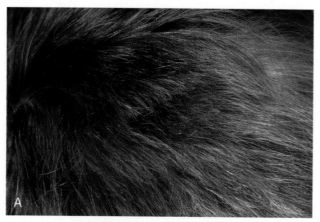

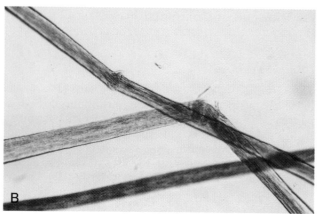

FIGURE 8-13 ■ Acquired proximal trichorrhexis nodosa. A, Short, broken segments close to the scalp surface. B, Multiple fractures detected by light microscopy.

marily affected with white specks or dots along the distal 10 to 15 cm of hair, often mistaken as dandruff. Acquired distal trichorrhexis nodosa occurs in otherwise normal hair as a result of cumulative cuticular damage, mainly as a consequence of intensive hair care and hair styling procedures. Repeated trauma (e.g., vigorous combing and brushing, prolonged sun exposure, chemical processing, repeated salt-water bathing, frequent shampooing) contributes to cuticular damage with subsequent loss of functional protective properties. Patients with distal trichorrhexis nodosa have dry, lusterless, and oddly faded hair in the affected areas. Hair breaks off distally at various lengths, with skimpy, ragged ends.

Circumscribed trichorrhexis nodosa occasionally occurs in the scalp hair, also in the mustache or beard, as a small, sharply demarcated patch. The affected hair looks oddly faded, lighter, and duller than the normal hair. Close inspection shows many white dots or specks along the shafts. In contrast to other types of trichorrhexis nodosa, a clear history of mechanical, chemical, or thermal injury is not always found. However, in the mustache or beard, the trauma of frequent twisting and manipulation may be sufficient to break these twisted fibers.

Pathology

Acquired proximal trichorrhexis nodosa can be analyzed by a hair mount showing short, broken segments close to the scalp surface (Fig. 8–13*B*). In addition to the typical hair shaft fractures, longitudinal splitting and greenstick fractures can be observed. The hair of African-American patients frequently forms spontaneous knots (trichonodosis, described in a later section), which further contributes to breakage of the weakened shaft.

Hair mount examination reveals in distal trichorrhexis nodosa the typical trichorrhexis nodosa fractures along the distal 10 to 15 cm of hair. Scanning electron microscopy demonstrates cuticular damage with a cuticle that is either completely worn down or in large portions torn away, leaving the underlying cortex unprotected. In other cases, the cuticle scales are present but the effects of chemical processing are obvious.

Treatment

Patients with proximal trichorrhexis nodosa are advised to stop all chemical and thermal hair straightening. A wide-toothed, round-tipped comb or a soft brush is recommended for minimal grooming of the hair. Hair conditioners are recommended, and a wig may be necessary until the hair grows longer. In distal trichorrhexis nodosa, the affected ends should be cut, and gentle and little combing or brushing is recommended. A cream rinse applied to the hair ends after shampooing minimizes tangling of the hair. Hot hair dryers should be avoided completely.

Pili Torti in Cicatricial Alopecia

Clinical Features

Irregular pili torti may occur within or at the edges of areas of cicatricial alopecia as a result of scarring dis-

eases such as lupus erythematosus, pseudopelade, congenital erythropoietic porphyria, and systemic sclerosis, presumably because of torsion of the follicle from perifollicular fibrosis. The twisted hairs are short, thick, and wiry within or surrounding the scarred skin. This appearance can be seen also at the edges of areas of aplasia cutis.

Pathology

Microscopic examination of affected hairs shows multiple twists of flattened hair shafts. The perifollicular fibrosis in cicatricial alopecia probably creates torsional forces that distort the hair follicle, followed by the growth of twisted hair.[34]

Acquired Progressive Kinking of the Hair

Clinical Features

In acquired progressive kinking of the hair, the appearance of tight, curly hair in an otherwise normal scalp is delayed until puberty or adulthood. Short, curly hair appears in circumscribed regions of the scalp, usually in the frontal and temporal areas, with an unruly and rough appearance. Occasionally, all scalp hair is involved. Affected hairs may be thinner or coarser than in unaffected scalp regions, and the hair color may be darker than normal. No associated abnormalities have been described. It has been suggested that this anomaly is a variant of "whisker hair" and is likely to progress in androgenetic alopecia.[35]

Pathology

The cause is unknown, but in some cases a shortened anagen has been documented.

Twisted and Rolled Body Hairs with Multiple, Large Knots

Clinical Features

Knotting of scalp hair (trichonodosis) is a frequent finding. Twisted and rolled body hairs differ clinically from common trichonodosis, in which only a single hair shaft is involved. In this disorder several different hair shafts roll together, resulting in large knots. This disorder is usually acquired, and sometimes these multiple knots are present in areas where rubbing is frequent. An inherited form with a probable autosomal inheritance pattern has also been suggested.[36]

Pathology

Light microscopy reveals central sticking and knotting of numerous hairs, resulting in one large knot. Scanning electron microscopy documents extreme rolling and twisting, with longitudinal fissures of hair shafts.

Bubble Hair

Clinical Features

Bubble hair has been described as an acquired hair shaft abnormality characterized by weak, dry, brittle hair that breaks easily. This reproducible hair shaft defect is caused by heat due to use of overheating hair dryers or any other hair care equipment that overheats. The disease clears spontaneously when thermal manipulation is discontinued.[37]

Pathology

The term *bubble hair* derives from the typical findings on light microscopy. The affected hair shows bubblelike areas in the hair shaft, and scanning electron microscopy indicates corresponding cavitary defects. Hair fibers may demonstrate a boomeranglike deformity containing small and large bubbles. Cross-sectional areas may show either a single large cavity or a reticulated, "Swiss cheese–like" loss of cells.

Non–Disease-Specific Hair Shaft Abnormalities

Bayonet Hair

Clinical Features

Bayonet hair is characterized by a thin, hypopigmented, threadlike tip and a hyperpigmented swelling or spindle. It has a double bend at its end and resembles a bayonet fixed to a rifle. The kinked hair has a slightly hypopigmented neck and a normal hair shaft. The spindle or swelling is 2 to 3 mm long, darker than the rest of the hair, and visible to the naked eye as well as palpable with the fingers. Bayonet hairs are barely longer than 8 cm. Patients usually are unaware of the presence of these hairs, because this anomaly is seen only if the hair has been neither cut nor broken. It is found in approximately 1% of scalp hairs in normal men and women and occurs more frequently in shed hairs, in the occipital hairline of balding men, and in patients with ichthyosis and seborrhea.

Pathology

On light microscopy the hair shows a distinct morphological pattern, with a thin, hypopigmented, threadlike tip followed by a hyperpigmented swelling or spindle, then a kinked shaft, followed by a slightly hypopigmented neck, and then a normal hair shaft. The spindle region contains pigment showing a wavelike pattern or clumps and irregularly arranged cuticle cells. Proximal to the spindle, the immediately succeeding neck is not necessarily present. If present, it is usually hypopigmented and thinner than the adjacent normal hair shaft.

Longitudinal Ridging and Grooving

Clinical Features and Pathology

This microscopic finding is commonly present in normal hair shafts, but it can reveal an underlying congenital defect such as monilethrix, Marie Unna hypotrichosis, pili torti, pili bifurcati, pili trianguli et canaliculi, trichothiodystrophy, and loose anagen hair syndrome.[38, 39]

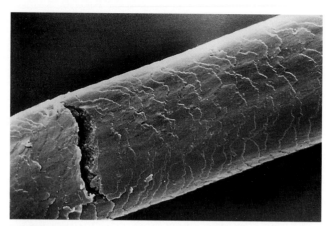

FIGURE 8–14 ■ Trichoschisis. Transverse fracture through the hair shaft with localized absence of cuticle cells. (Courtesy of Deutsches Wollforschungsinstitut an der Technischen Universitat, Aachen, Germany.)

Trichoschisis

Clinical Features and Pathology

A clean, transverse fissure or fracture through the hair shaft and localized absence of cuticle cells is called *trichoschisis* (Fig. 8–14). It generally results from trauma and is usually seen in the congenitally brittle hair of patients with trichothiodystrophy or Marinesco-Sjögren syndrome. Breakage occurs at the site of decreased high-sulfur matrix protein content in the exocuticle and in the A layer of cuticular cells.

Tapered Hair

Clinical Features and Pathology

A pencil-point tip is the characteristic finding in tapered hair. The emerging hair shaft shows an oblique fracture near the skin surface. Because of inhibition of protein synthesis in the hair root, a progressive narrowing of the hair shaft develops. This hair shaft defect can be seen with any process that intervenes in hair matrix cell division (e.g., anagen effluvium after cytostatic drugs, alopecia areata). It can also be observed after mechanical manipulation in trichotillomania and in acquired progressive kinking.

Trichoclasis

Clinical Features and Pathology

This transverse fracture is the classic greenstick fracture, in which the shaft is splinted in part by an intact cuticle. This abnormality is usually sporadic and can be observed after physical and chemical trauma.

Trichonodosis

Clinical Features and Pathology

Single- or double-knotted hair can be observed as a consequence of cosmetic procedures or friction from sticking to dresses or pillows, and it is most often ob-

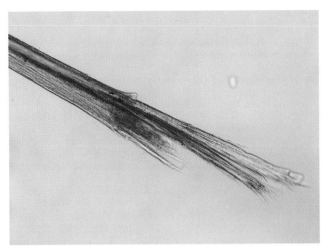

FIGURE 8–15 ■ Trichoptilosis. Longitudinal splitting of the hair shaft at its distal end, typically seen in excessive weathering or after mechanical trauma in trichotillomania.

served in short, curly hair. Hair shafts with a relatively thin diameter are most readily affected. Although no real hair shaft structure defects exist as a consequence of knotting, fractures of the shaft or loss of cuticular cells in close vicinity can be observed.

Trichoptilosis

Clinical Features and Pathology

Longitudinal splitting of the hair shaft at its distal end leads to the common split ends or frizzies (Fig. 8–15). It is caused by trauma or occurs with excessive weathering or as a consequence of excessive manipulation in trichotillomania, pruritic dermatoses, or excessive hair styling.

Weathering

Clinical Features and Pathology

This term is reserved primarily for all sorts of cosmetic manipulation, especially physical- and chemical-induced structural defects of the hair, principally at the ending tip. Hair styling, hair drying, perms, sun exposure, friction, and certain coiffure stylings lead to repetitive trauma to the hair. The damage to cuticular cells subsequently leads to loss of their cortex-protecting capacities and to breakage. Hair splitting at the hair tip is the typical finding on microscopy.

Drug-Induced Changes

Pohl-Pinkus Constriction

Clinical Features and Pathology

The hair shaft shows a decreased diameter that can be observed to be related in time to hair growth rate and

events such as drug administration (e.g., folic acid antagonists, other mitosis-inhibiting drugs), severe illness, or malnutrition. The number of affected hairs is variable, but apparently hair follicles in early anagen are most sensitive. These hair shaft "constrictions" are considered to be analogous to the transverse lines of the nails known as Beau's lines.[40]

Synthetic Retinoid-Induced Kinking and Pili Torti

Clinical Features and Pathology

Increased curling and kinking of scalp hair may be caused by etretinate or isotretinoin therapy. In these cases, scanning electron microscopic examination of kinking hair shows twists with sharp-edged defects and splitting of cuticle cells in several hair shafts in patients receiving long-term etretinate therapy.[27] In addition, pili torti has been reported in patients taking isotretinoin.[41]

Diagnosis

The diagnostic procedure to characterize and classify genetic or acquired hair structure abnormalities demands careful evaluation and a complete clinical exami-

TABLE 8-3 ■ Diagnostic Workup and Management of Hair Shaft Abnormalities

Clinical diagnosis
History of patient and family (design pedigree if possible)
Clinical examination
  Pull test
  Physical examination, including scalp and body hair, distribution, pattern, color, nail involvement, teeth, bone development, sweating behavior (i.e., search for signs of ectodermal dysplasia)
  Laboratory tests depending on the differential diagnosis: serum ferritin, copper, copper oxidase, total sulfur content, paper chromatographic estimation of blood and urine amino acids

Diagnostic methods
To analyze hair structure
  Hair mount examination by light and polarizing microscopy
  Scanning or transmission electron microscopy, or both
  Skin biopsy examination by histology and immunohistochemistry
To analyze hair growth activity
  Trichogram
  Phototrichogram
To analyze mechanical stability and physical properties of hair
  Elastic deformation
  Stress strain analysis (load elongation)
  Elasticity modules
To analyze biochemical composition of affected hair
  Amino acid analysis by chromatography, spectroscopy
  Elemental analysis by neutron activation analysis (e.g., copper, sulfur)
  Tests on fractionated chemical components (oxidation reduction tests)
  Keratin analysis
To analyze molecular biological aspects of the disease
  Genetic linkage analyses (e.g., microsatellite markers) and others

nation (Table 8–3). Frequently, hair shaft abnormalities are the trichological manifestation of a genetic syndrome or a phenotypic marker for an underlying metabolic defect, and they therefore may provide an important diagnostic clue to systemic disease.[1]

The procedure for correct diagnosis comprises a panel of different methods, because no single test or examination technique can be representative for the entire person. To recognize hair shaft abnormalities, methods to analyze hair structure are mandatory. Light and polarizing microscopic examination of longitudinal embedded hair shafts permits easy recognition of a large number of the main hair structure abnormalities. Three or four short, selected segments of hair cut flush with the scalp surface are placed side by side on a microscope slide and covered by a coverslip. Two to three drops of a suitable mounting medium are placed at the edge of the coverslip and spread across the slide by capillary action. The mounting medium should be balsam or a synthetic equivalent.

Hair is a three-dimensional fiber, whereas a microscope shows only a two-dimensional picture. A twisted hair may appear to vary in diameter when it is viewed microscopically. Consequently, twisted hair is often misdiagnosed as monilethrix. Scanning electron microscopy or transmission electron microscopy can be a helpful additional tool for certain difficult cases. In a few indications, skin biopsy helps to reveal the diagnosis. Additional methods, such as tests for mechanical stability and physical properties of the investigated hair or analysis of its biochemical composition, may be helpful in selected cases and for investigation of the underlying etiology or pathology of the defect. Clinical and experimental research is needed to further understand the underlying mechanism. In certain cases, possible therapeutic consequences can be pointed out, mainly in genotrichoses caused by faulty amino acid metabolism.

The exact diagnosis is most important in genetic hair shaft abnormalities, to exclude possible associated defects and to allow precise genetic counseling of the patient and family. In severe genetic diseases, a correct prenatal diagnosis (e.g., in trichothiodystrophy based on DNA repair measurements in trophoblasts or amniotic cells) may be a very helpful tool.[42]

Early and precise recognition and classification of acquired hair structure defects is fundamental for counseling the patient regarding future hair care and cosmetic procedures. Only on this basis can the acquired hair structure defects be successfully approached.

REFERENCES

1. Blume U, Föhles J, Gollnick HPM, Orfanos CE: Genotrichoses: clinical manifestations and diagnostics techniques. In: Burgdorf WHC, Katz SI (eds): Dermatology Progress and Perspectives. Proceedings of the 18th World Congress of Dermatology. The Parthenon Publishing Group, New York, Casterton, London, England, 1993, pp 204–206.
2. Orfanos CE: Genetische Anomalien des Haares: Die Genotrichosen und ihre Klassifkation. Z Hautkr 10:S22, 1990.
3. Richard G, Itin P, Lin JP, Bon A, Bale SJ: Evidence for genetic heterogeneity in monilethrix. J Invest Dermatol 107:812–814, 1996.
4. De Berker DAR, Ferguson DJP, Dawber RPR: Monilethrix: a clinicopathological illustration of a cortical defect. Br J Dermatol 128:327–331, 1993.
5. Winter H, Rogers MA, Langbein L, et al: Mutations in the hair cortex keratin hHb6 cause the inherited disease monilethrix. Nat Genet 16:372–374, 1997.
6. Stevens HP, Kelsell DP, Bryant SP, et al: Linkage of monilethrix to the trichocyte and epithelial keratin gene cluster on 12q11–q13. J Invest Dermatol 106:795–797, 1996.
7. Sivasundram A: A case of monilethrix treated with etretinate. Dermatology 190:89, 1995.
8. Bentley-Phillips B, Bayles MAH: A previously undescribed hair anomaly (pseudomonilethrix). Br J Dermatol 89:159–167, 1973.
9. Wolff HH, Vigl E, Braun-Falco O: Trichorrhexis congenita. Hautarzt 26:576–580, 1975.
10. Rushton DH, Norris MJ, James KC: Amino-acid composition in trichorrhexis nodosa. Clin Exp Dermatol 15:24–28, 1990.
11. Kvedar J: Dietary management reverses grooving and abnormal polarization of hair shafts in argininosuccinase deficiency. Am J Med Genet 40:211–213, 1991.
12. Moreau-Cabarrot A, Bonafe JL, Hachich N, et al: Follicular atrophoderma, basal cell proliferation and hypotrichosis (Basex-Dupre-Christol syndrome). A study in 2 families. Ann Dermatol Venereol 121:297–301, 1994.
13. Petit A, Dontewille MM, Bardon CB, Civatte J: Pili torti with congenital deafness (Björnstad's syndrome): report of three cases in one family suggesting autosomal dominant transmission. Clin Exp Dermatol 182:184–187, 1993.
14. Maruyama T, Toyoda M, Kanei A, Morohashi M: Pathogenesis in pili torti: morphological study. J Dermatol Sci 7(Suppl):S5–S12, 1994.
15. Tumer Z, Tommerup N, Tonnesen T, Kreuder J, Craig IW, Horn N: Mapping of the Menkes locus to Xq13.3 distal to the X-inactivation center by an intrachromosomal insertion of the segment Xq13.3-q21.2. Hum Genet 88:668–672, 1992.
16. Christodoulou J, Danks DM, Sarkar B, et al: Early treatment of Menkes disease with parenteral histidine: long-term follow-up of four treated patients. Am J Med Genet 76:154–164, 1998.
17. Haas OA, Martins da Cunha A, Gadner H, Stingl G, Kornmuller R: The Netherton syndrome: clinical characteristics, differential diagnosis and new ways of therapy. Pediatr Padol 19:153–159, 1984.
18. Crovato F, Borrone C, Rebora A: Trichothiodystrophy—BIDS; IBIDS and PIBIDS? Br J Dermatol 108:257, 1983.
19. Meynadier J, Guillot B, Barneon G, Djian B, Levy A: Trichothiodystrophy. Ann Dermatol Venereol 114:1529–1536, 1987.
20. Price VH: Trichothiodystrophy: update. Pediatr Dermatol 9:369–370, 1992.
21. Mondello D, Nardo T, Giliani S, et al: Molecular analysis of the XP-D gene in Italian families with patients affected by trichothiodystrophy in xeroderma pigmentosum group D (XP-D). Mutat Res 314:159–165, 1994.
22. Stefanini M, Lagomarsini P, Giliani S, et al: A new nucleotide-excision repair gene associated with trichothiodystrophy. Am J Human Genet 53:817–821, 1993.
23. Taylor EM, Broughton BC, Botta E, et al: Xeroderma pigmentosum and trichothiodystrophy are associated with different mutations in the XPD (ERCC2) repair/transcription gene. Proc Natl Acad Sci U S A 94:8658–8663, 1997.
24. Amichai B, Grunwald MH, Halevy S: Hair abnormality present since childhood: pili annulati. Arch Dermatol 132:575–578, 1996.
25. Dawber R: Investigations of a family with pili annulati with blue naevi. Trans St Johns Hosp Dermatol Soc 58:51–58, 1972.
26. Kopysc Z, Barczyk K, Krol E: A new syndrome in the group of euhidrotic ectodermal dysplasia. Pilodental dysplasia with refractive errors. Hum Genet 70:376–378, 1985.
27. Moffitt DL, Lear JT, de Berker DA, Peachy RD: Pili annulati coincident with alopecia areata. Pediatr Dermatol 15:271–273, 1998.
28. Ito M, Hashimoto K, Sakamoto F, Sato Y, Voorhees JJ: Pathogenesis of pili annulati. Arch Dermatol Res 280:308–318, 1988.
29. Amichai B, Grunwald MH, Halevy S: A child with a localized hair abnormality: woolly hair nevus. Arch Dermatol 132:573–574,577, 1996.
30. Itin PH, Buhler U, Buchner SA, Guggenheim R: Pili trianguli et

canaliculi: a distinctive hair shaft defect leading to uncombable hair. Dermatology 187:296–298, 1993.

31. Mallon E, Dawber RP, De Berker D, Ferguson DJ: Cheveux incoiffables: diagnostic, clinical and hair microscopic findings, and pathogenic studies. Br J Dermatol 131:608–614, 1994.

32. Breslau-Siderius LJ, Beemer FA, Boom BW: Pili bifurcati: occuring in association with mosaic trisomy 8 syndrome. Clin Dysmorphol 5:275–277, 1996.

33. Cambiaghi S, Barbareschi M, Cambiaghi G, Caputo R: Scanning electron microscopy in the diagnosis of pili multigemini. Acta Derm Venereol 75:170–171, 1995.

34. Kurwa AR, Abdel-Aziz A-HM: Pili torti—congenital and acquired. Acta Derm Venereol (Stockh) 53:385–392, 1973.

35. Schauder S, Tsambaos D, Nikiforidis G: Curling and kinking of hair caused by etretinate. Hautarzt 43:509–513, 1992.

36. Itin PH, Bircher AJ, Lautenschlager S, Zuberbuhler E, Guggenheim R: A new clinical disorder of twisted and rolled body hairs with multiple, large knots. J Am Acad Dermatol 30:31–35, 1994.

37. Detwiler SP, Carson JL, Woosley JT, Gambling TM, Briggaman RA. Bubble hair: case caused by an overheating hair dryer and reproducibility in normal hair with heat. J Am Acad Dermatol 30:54–60, 1994.

38. Baden HP, Kvedar JC, Magro CM: Loose anagen hair as a cause of hereditary hair loss in children. Arch Dermatol 128:1349–1353, 1992.

39. Hamm H, Traupe H: Loose anagen hair of childhood: the phenomenon of easily pluckable hair. J Am Acad Dermatol 20:242–248, 1989.

40. Tosti A, Misciali C, Bardazzi F, Fanti PA, Varotti C: Telogen effluvium due to recombinant interferon alpha-2b. Dermatology 184:124–125, 1992.

41. Hays SB, Camisa C: Acquired pili torti in two patients treated with synthetic retinoids. Cutis 35:466–468, 1985.

42. Sarasin A: Prenatal diagnosis in trichothiodystrophy patients defective in DNA repair. Br J Dermatol 127:485–491, 1992.

BIBLIOGRAPHY

Abramovits-Ackerman V: Cutaneous findings in a new syndrome of autosomal recessive ectodermal dysplasia with corkscrew hairs. J Am Acad Dermatol 27:917–921, 1992.

Blume-Peytavi U, Gollnick HM, Föhles J, Pineda-Fernandez MS, Blankenburg G, Orfanos CE. Anhidrotic ectodermal dysplasia: defective expression pattern leading to faulty keratinization. Hautarzt 45:494–497, 1994.

Blume-Peytavi U, Föhles J, Gollnick H, Wortmann G, Schulz R, Orfanos CE. Hypotrichosis, hair structure defects, hypercysteine-hair and glucosuria: a new genetic syndrome? Br J Dermatol 134:319–324, 1996.

Ghorbani AJ, Eichler C: Scurvy. J Am Acad Dermatol 30:881–883, 1994.

Price VH: Structural abnormalities of the hair shaft. In: Orfanos CE, Happle R (eds): Hair and Hair Diseases. 1990; Berlin, Springer pp. 363–417.

Rogers M: Hair shaft abnormalities: part I. Australas J Dermatol 36:179–184, 1995.

Trueb RM: Ectodermal dysplasia with corkscrew hairs: observations of probable autosomal dominant tricho-odonto-onychodysplasia with syndactyly. J Am Acad Dermatol 30:289–290, 1994.

Hirsutism and Hypertrichosis

MARY GAIL MERCURIO

Hirsutism

ETIOLOGY

In women, testosterone is the major circulating androgen; it is derived in approximately equal quantities from the adrenal gland and the ovary and also arises from peripheral conversion of androgen precursors. In conditions in which the adrenal gland produces excessive testosterone, levels of the adrenal androgen precursor, dehydroepiandrosterone, and its sulfated form, dehydroepiandrosterone sulfate (DHEAS), are increased. Sex hormone binding globulin (SHBG) acts as a sink for circulating testosterone, limiting the concentration available to exert an effect on peripheral tissues. The hair follicle is a target tissue capable of responding divergently to endogenous androgens. Paradoxically, the same androgen stimulus may cause regression of hair growth on the scalp and stimulation of hair growth on the face, suggesting a differential response to androgens by the hair follicle based on anatomical location and depending on specific high-affinity receptor molecules.[1] Enzymes in the hair follicle play an important role in androgen biology, particularly in the conversion of testosterone to the more potent dihydrotestosterone (DHT) by 5-α reductase.

DHT is the major nuclear androgen in many sensitive tissues, including the skin, where it is ultimately responsible for the conversion of fine vellus hairs to terminal hairs resulting in hirsutism. In the presence of excessive circulating androgen precursors resulting from adrenal/pituitary or ovarian overproduction, there is increased production of DHT. In addition, some persons have enhanced 5-α reductase activity in the hair follicle, re-

sulting in greater conversion of *normal* circulating androgen levels to DHT. It is possible that women with idiopathic hirsutism fall into this latter category. It has been shown that the activity of 5-α reductase in genital skin is higher in hirsute women than in normal women.[2] The DHT metabolite, 3α-androstanediol glucuronide, has been identified as a specific marker of skin 5-α reductase activity.[3]

CLINICAL FEATURES

A thorough history and physical examination are essential to the evaluation of hirsutism. The history should include details about onset of hair growth and rate of progression. Family history, including hair growth patterns and country of origin, are important in the diagnosis of familial disorders. Menstrual irregularities, infertility, galactorrhea, or thyroid dysfunction should be investigated. A drug history should be performed to identify the athlete self-administering androgenic compounds and the woman taking prescription medications with androgenic side effects. Idiopathic hirsutism is a diagnosis of exclusion, and the history is very helpful in making this diagnosis (Table 9–1). Hirsutism that first

TABLE 9-1 ■ Features Suggestive of Idiopathic Hirsutism

Pubertal onset of hirsuitism
Slow progression of hirsuitism
Family history of hirsuitism
Regular menstrual periods
No virilization
No infertility

TABLE 9-2 ■ Features Compatible
with Neoplasm

Onset of hirsutism outside peripubertal period
Sudden onset of hirsutism
Rapid progression of hirsutism
Severe hirsutism (Ferriman-Gallwey score >15)
Signs of virilization
Signs of Cushing's syndrome

TABLE 9-4 ■ Causes of Hirsutism

Ovarian
  Polycystic ovary syndrome
  Virilizing neoplasm
  Hyperthecosis
Adrenal
  Congenital adrenal hyperplasia
  Cushing's syndrome
  Virilizing neoplasm (adenoma, carcinoma)
Pituitary
  Cushing's disease
  Prolactinoma
  Acromegaly
Exogenous
  Testosterone
  Anabolic steroids
  Oral contraceptives
  Danazol
Increased peripheral androgen activity (idiopathic hirsutism)

appears well before or well after puberty or that progresses rapidly is compatible with a neoplasm (Table 9–2). The woman who presents with hirsutism must be approached compassionately, taking into account an often profoundly low self-esteem related to a perceived loss of femininity.

The Ferriman-Gallwey grading scheme is a semiquantitative tool for scoring the degree of hirsutism. Nine key anatomical sites are graded on a scale of 0 (no terminal hair) to 4 (frankly virile), for a maximum score of 36. A score of 8 or more denotes hirsutism. There exists no clear distinction between physiological and pathological hirsutism. Caucasian women of Mediterranean ancestry have heavier hair growth and a higher incidence of hirsutism than those of Nordic ancestry, and Asians have the least. Cultural and social pressures may influence a woman to seek medical attention for the hair growth even though its quantity is normal based on heritage. Physicians treating patients for one manifestation of androgen excess should have a high index of suspicion for others. Because women may be embarrassed by androgenic changes, they often conceal them so that they are not readily apparent. Additional findings that should be sought include recalcitrant acne and androgenetic alopecia; more ominous would be any signs of virilization, such as clitoromegaly, voice deepening, loss of female body contour, or male pattern alopecia see (Table 9–2). A pelvic examination is indicated in patients with amenorrhea or signs of virilization.

In most patients with hirsutism an appropriate history and physical examination can sufficiently exclude any underlying pathology. However, other features of hyperandrogenism or any signs of virilization necessitate a more elaborate diagnostic evaluation (Table 9–3). Initial laboratory testing to exclude serious disease consists of immunoassays for serum testosterone and DHEAS. These two tests alone can detect almost all androgen-producing tumors. Testosterone levels exceeding 200 ng/dL are highly suggestive of an adrenal or ovarian tumor. A DHEAS value exceeding 700 μg/dL is indicative of an adrenal source. When a neoplasm is sus-

pected, diagnostic imaging is useful to confirm its location. Mild to moderately elevated testosterone and DHEAS are more compatible with a functional disorder such as polycystic ovary syndrome (PCOS) or late-onset congenital adrenal hyperplasia (CAH). A thorough history and physical examination facilitate selection of the most appropriate secondary tests to confirm or exclude these diagnoses, such as measurement of 17-hydroxyprogesterone for late-onset CAH or luteinizing hormone and follicle-stimulating hormone for PCOS or ovarian failure. Prolactin level and thyroid function should be assessed as part of the evaluation for amenorrhea.

DIAGNOSIS

There are a number of conditions that can result in androgen excess, and a useful scheme for categorization is based on the androgen source (Table 9–4).

OVARY. PCOS is the most common ovarian cause of hirsutism. A common constellation of findings in women with this heterogeneous disorder includes hirsutism, dys-

TABLE 9-3 ■ Signs of Virilization

Male pattern alopecia
Voice deepening
Clitoromegaly
Muscle enlargement
Breast atrophy
Increased libido

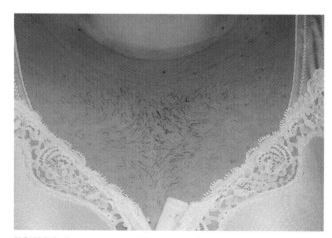

FIGURE 9–1 ■ A 34-year-old woman with polycystic ovary syndrome. She also has amenorrhea and android obesity in addition to the hirsutism.

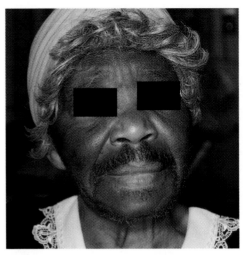

FIGURE 9–2 ■ A 68-year-old woman with an androgen-secreting ovarian arrhenoblastoma.

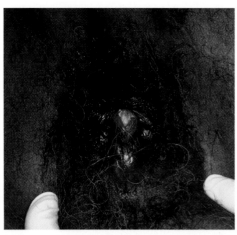

FIGURE 9–4 ■ Same patient as in Figures 9–2 and 9–3, demonstrating clitoromegaly. Clitoral enlargement is defined by the "clitoral index" (vertical × horizontal dimension of the glans), with values greater than 35 mm² being considered abnormal. This patient's index was 120 mm².

functional uterine bleeding, infertility, acne, obesity, and polycystic ovaries (Fig. 9–1). Metabolic alterations are found in many patients with PCOS that result in premature cardiovascular disease from dyslipidemias and frank diabetes.[4] The anovulatory ovaries increase the risk of endometrial cancer. A variant of PCOS is HAIR-AN syndrome, which is characterized by hyperandrogenism, insulin resistance, and acanthosis nigricans. In the setting of androgen-producing ovarian tumors, which are uncommon and usually benign, the hirsutism develops rapidly and virilization generally coexists (Figs. 9–2 through 9–4).

ADRENAL. CAH is the most common adrenal cause of hyperandrogenism. In most cases the defect is identified at birth, but a less severe form, late-onset CAH, may manifest initially at the time of puberty with a highly

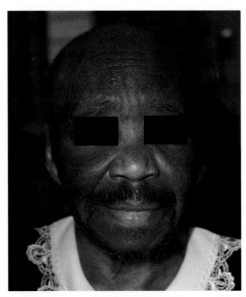

FIGURE 9–3 ■ Same woman as in Figure 9–2, without her wig, demonstrating *male-pattern* androgenetic alopecia.

variable clinical presentation. It is an autosomal recessive disorder most prevalent among women of Ashkenazi Jewish heritage. The adrenal defect is characterized by partial deficiency of 21-hydroxylase, resulting in accumulation of 17-hydroxyprogesterone. Levels of 17-hydroxyprogesterone should be obtained in the morning during the follicular phase of the menstrual cycle. In all forms of enzyme-deficiency adrenal hyperplasia, maintenance of normal cortisol production is attempted at the expense of increased androgen production. The hirsutism usually appears at about the time of puberty as an idiopathic hirsutism. Virilizing adrenal tumors are rare and often malignant, and signs and symptoms of virilization develop rapidly in this setting. Cushing's syndrome is the persistent oversecretion of cortisol. It may be caused by pituitary secretion of corticotropin (ACTH), a primary adrenal tumor, or ectopic ACTH production. The hirsutism is usually accompanied by other findings, including hypertension, muscle weakness, easy bruising, and truncal weight gain.

PITUITARY. Prolactin-secreting adenomas are the most common pituitary tumor, and the patient usually presents with symptoms of amenorrhea or galactorrhea. Elevated prolactin may be a reaction to drugs such as metoclopramide, phenothiazines, butyrophenones, or marijuana. Acromegaly and Cushing's disease are other pituitary causes of hirsutism.

IDIOPATHIC HIRSUTISM. Idiopathic hirsutism is a diagnosis of exclusion. Genetics is the dominant factor in these women, so it is important to glean information on hair growth in close female relatives. The aberration appears to be caused by enhanced cutaneous conversion of 5α-reductase. The onset of abnormal hair growth in these patients occurs at the time of puberty, and a gradual, continued increase is often noted into the third decade (Fig. 9–5). Abrupt changes in hair growth or distribution pattern do not occur. If abrupt changes are seen in the pattern of hair growth or if the hirsutism appears before or after puberty, another cause is likely.

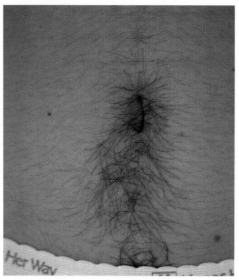

FIGURE 9–5 ■ A 26-year-old woman with idiopathic hirsutism. Her sister and mother have a similar pattern of hair growth.

Peripubertal onset is also compatible with late-onset CAH and PCOS.

MISCELLANEOUS. Postmenopausal women who are not receiving hormone replacement therapy commonly show *gradual* development of hirsutism with simultaneous thinning of pubic and axillary hair (Fig. 9–6). At menopause, cyclical estradiol production ceases but ovarian androgen production persists, resulting in an increasing ratio of androgen to estrogen due to physiologic ovarian failure. Hirsutism may be caused by or accentuated by certain drugs, including anabolic steroids, testosterone, danazol, and oral contraceptives. Certain oral contraceptives containing progestins with higher intrinsic androgenic activity are the primary culprits.

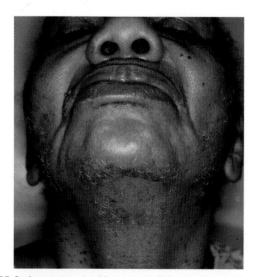

FIGURE 9–6 ■ A 62-year-old woman with postmenopausal hirsutism. The facial hair gradually appeared after menopause without any additional signs of hyperandrogenism.

DIFFERENTIAL DIAGNOSIS

Hirsutism must be distinguished from hypertrichosis, which represents diffuse increased vellus hair growth involving areas of the body that are *not* androgen dependent (see later discussion).

TREATMENT

After successful exclusion of neoplastic sources of androgen excess, pharmaceutical intervention can be implemented. Limitations of treatment are important to discuss with the patient before therapy begins. The choice of treatment for hirsutism is governed by underlying cause, age, contraceptive needs, and coexistence of metabolic aberrations that must be addressed. It is usually the visible effects of androgen excess that are most alarming to the patient, but it is the metabolic abnormalities that have the greatest long-term health implications and may require separate intervention. Suppression of ovarian androgen production can be achieved with oral contraceptives. An alternative approach to hormonal therapy is based on competition with the androgen receptor or inhibition of 5-α reductase, or both. Adrenal hyperplasia is managed with low-dose exogenous glucocorticosteroids to suppress ACTH and thereby inhibit androgen production. No treatment has yet been shown to be optimal. In many instances obesity directly contributes to the condition owing to increased production of androgens or decreased SHBG, or both, and weight reduction can improve the hirsutism.[5]

ORAL CONTRACEPTIVES. Oral contraceptives are a safe therapeutic modality commonly used in women with androgen-mediated disorders including hirsutism, acne, and androgenetic alopecia. They reduce ovarian androgen production by gonadotropin suppression and decrease androgen availability by elevating SHBG. Virtually all of the available oral contraceptives today are a combination of estrogen and progestin. A product that is relatively estrogenic would provide antiandrogen benefits but at the expense of clotting risks. Although the newer oral contraceptive formulations have less estrogen (30 to 35 μg), they are less androgenic by virtue of improved progestin components. Concerns about the safety of oral contraceptives have declined since these low-dose combinations were introduced, especially in regard to lipid metabolism and cardiovascular disease risks.

The so-called third-generation agents (desogestrel, norgestimate) are preferred because of their enhanced ability to elevate SHBG, reducing the unbound fraction of testosterone, the major culprit in androgenic effects.[6] Use of oral contraceptive preparations containing these progestins results in clinical improvement of such symptoms as acne and hirsutism.[7, 8] Among the least favorable progestins for androgenic disorders are levonorgestrel, norgestrel, and norethindrone. Oral contraceptives may represent the first line of treatment in women with androgenic disorders; they can be used alone or in combination with specific antiandrogens. Ortho Tri-Cyclen, which contains norgestimate, is labeled for the indication of acne and is the first oral contraceptive approved for the treatment of an androgenic disorder.[9, 10] Adequate counseling about side effects and noncontraceptive health benefits before treatment with an oral contraceptive begins is essential to minimize noncompliance.

SPIRONOLACTONE. Antiandrogens are substances that prevent androgens from expressing their activity at target sites. None of the antiandrogens is labeled for use in treatment of an androgenic disorder. Spironolactone is an aldosterone antagonist used as a diuretic and antihypertensive agent. Its antiandrogenic effect results both from competition with DHT for intracellular androgen receptor binding sites and interference with adrenal testosterone biosynthesis.[11] The antiandrogenic side effects of gynecomastia and decreased libido preclude its use in men. Women should begin with a single morning dose of 25 or 50 mg/day, gradually increasing to 100 mg twice daily, with monitoring of potassium levels.

Hyperkalemia does not ordinarily occur with normal renal function, but prescribing of several agents that raise potassium levels must be done with caution. Starting with a low dose reduces the incidence of side effects, which are dose related. The drug is usually well tolerated, the most common adverse effects being irregular menstrual bleeding and breast tenderness. These adverse effects can usually be mitigated by concomitant use of an oral contraceptive, preferably a third-generation agent with a more favorable androgenic profile. Fatigue and dizziness due to orthostatic hypotension from mild volume depletion, polyuria, and polydypsia are less common side effects.

Several studies of the antiandrogenic effects of spironolactone have been performed in women with hirsutism, in whom regression of hair growth has been demonstrated by decreasing Ferriman-Gallwey scores.[12–14] Because spironolactone could cause feminization of a male fetus, it should be given only to women who are using effective contraception methods. Improvement is gradual with drug treatment because of the hair growth cycle. Of the dermatological disorders, acne shows the quickest response, followed by hirsutism; androgenetic alopecia is slowest to respond, often taking longer than 1 year before any appreciable benefit is seen. Dual-agent therapy with oral contraceptives plus spironolactone is more effective than either agent alone and is very well tolerated. Topically applied medication would be a great advance. In preliminary studies a topically applied blocker of androgen receptors, RU58841, appears to show promise in stimulating balding scalp hair growth and has theoretical usefulness in the treatment of hirsutism.[15]

FINASTERIDE. Finasteride is the newest drug in the hirsutism treatment armamentarium. Finasteride is a 5-α reductase (type II) inhibitor that selectively blocks DHT biosynthesis. It profoundly reduces DHT levels without other hormonal effects. Finasteride was first introduced in 1989 in a 5-mg dose (Proscar) for the treatment of benign prostatic hypertrophy.[16] Because of its selective inhibition of conversion of testosterone to DHT, the side-effect profile is extremely promising, with no clinically significant changes in circulating testosterone or other routine laboratory safety measurements. Extensive use of this drug in the treatment of patients with benign prostatic hypertrophy has established its excellent safety profile; the side effects are related primarily to sexual function, including decreased libido, impotence, and decreased seminal volume, which are seen in a small percentage of patients.

Finasteride in a 1-mg dose (Propecia) has been shown to grow hair in men with androgenetic alopecia, and it has been approved by the US Food and Drug Administration for this indication.

The first randomized, controlled trial of finasteride in women involved 136 postmenopausal subjects with androgenetic alopecia. The results were disappointing, showing no significant difference in mean hair count between women receiving 1-mg finasteride and those receiving placebo. It remains possible that finasteride will be more effective in younger women.[17] Although it is not presently indicated for the treatment of hirsutism, studies have shown that finasteride is effective in lowering the Ferriman-Gallwey hirsutism scores of patients with moderate to severe idiopathic hirsutism and is well tolerated.[18–20] The drug is contraindicated in pregnancy because it is known to cause urogenital deformations in male offspring of pregnant animals.

Determination of a patient's suitability for treatment with a 5-α reductase inhibitor may be based on levels of 3α-androstenediol glucuronide, the DHT metabolite reflective of 5-α reductase activity that is an indicator for potential efficacy of enzyme inhibition in women with idiopathic hirsutism.[21]

PHYSICAL METHODS. Available physical methods of hair camouflaging and removal include chemical depilation, shaving, electrolysis, and the newest option, laser therapy. Electrolysis remains the only permanent form of hair removal, but this process is tedious, painful, and inefficient, requiring multiple treatments. A topical anesthetic, called EMLA for "eutectic mixture of local anesthetic," is a helpful adjuvant for reducing the discomfort associated with electrolysis. Emerging laser technology is being directed toward permanent hair removal; the systems presently available produce prolonged but not completely permanent cessation of hair growth, and efforts still need to be directed toward enhancing efficacy and minimizing adverse cosmetic effects such as pigmentary changes. Physical methods may be used alone or concomitantly while awaiting effects of pharmacotherapy. The combination of preventing new hair growth with a systemic agent and physically removing the old hair yields the most expeditious results. There is clearly a need for a more effective treatment for the many distressed women with hirsutism.

Hypertrichosis

Hypertrichosis is an overgrowth of hair not localized to androgenetic sites. The hair is usually vellus in nature.[22]

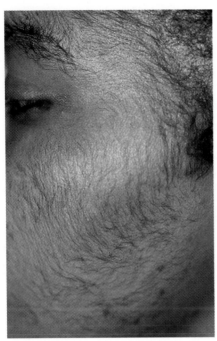

FIGURE 9-7 ■ Facial hypertrichosis in a 42-year-old woman taking oral minoxidil for hypertension.

GENERALIZED ACQUIRED HYPERTRICHOSIS

This pattern of hair growth can result from use of drugs such as cyclosporine, phenytoin, diazoxide, penicillamine, hexachlorobenzene, glucocorticoids, and minoxidil—the hair-stimulation properties of which have been exploited for the topical treatment of androgenetic alopecia (Fig. 9-7). The pathophysiology of drug-induced hypertrichosis is unknown. Metabolic disturbances, including anorexia nervosa and hypothyroidism, may also result in hypertrichosis. Acquired hypertrichosis lanuginosa may be a manifestation of a variety of malignancies and usually occurs with advanced disease.

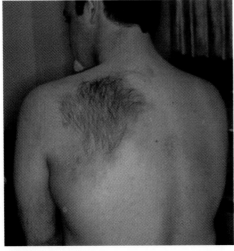

FIGURE 9-8 ■ Becker's nevus in a 32-year-old man.

GENERALIZED CONGENITAL HYPERTRICHOSIS

Congenital hypertrichosis lanuginosa is a very rare autosomal dominant condition characterized by excessive diffuse lanugo hair growth that may be present at birth or arise during the first few months of life. Other hereditary syndromes with lanugo hypertrichosis as a feature include *Cornelia de Lange's*, *Rubinstein-Taybi*, *Crow-Fukase (POEMS)*, and *Hurler's syndromes*. Congenital generalized hypertrichosis may be a feature of maternal drug ingestion syndromes, including fetal hydantoin syndrome and fetal alcohol syndrome.

LOCALIZED ACQUIRED HYPERTRICHOSIS

Chronic irritation, inflammation, topical steroid use, or occlusion beneath a cast may lead to local transformation of vellus to terminal hairs. Becker's nevus is an area of pigmentation and hypertrichosis most commonly appearing on the shoulder region of young men (Fig. 9-8). Porphyria cutanea tarda and variegate porphyria may show a localized hypertrichosis over the malar region, and in congenital erythropoietic porphyria the growth may be more generalized.

LOCALIZED CONGENITAL HYPERTRICHOSIS

Localized hypertrichosis over the sacral region may be a marker for an underlying occult neural abnormality. Dermal tumors such as congenital smooth-muscle hamartomas and congenital nevi may have overlying hypertrichosis. Hairy elbows is a rare anomaly characterized by progressive excessive growth of hair on the elbows.

REFERENCES

1. Rittmaster RS, Loriaux DL: Hirsutism. Ann Intern Med, 106:95–107, 1987.
2. Serafini P, Lobo RA: Increased 5-α reductase activity in idiopathic hirsutism. Fertil Steril 43:74–78, 1985.
3. Lobo RA: Investigating the cause of hirsutism and acne in women. Clin Chem 41:12–13, 1995.
4. Haseltine F, Wentz AC, Redmond GP, Wild RA: Androgen and women's health. Clinician 1994; 12(3):1–32
5. Frisch RE: Body weight, body fat and ovulation. Trends Endocrinol Metab 2:191–197, 1991.
6. Speroff L, DeCherney A: Evaluation of a new generation of oral contraceptives: The Advisory Board for the New Progestins. Obstet Gynecol 81:1034–1047, 1993.
7. Cullberg G, Hamberger L, Mattson LA, et al: Effects of a low-dose desogestrel-ethinylestradiol combination on hirsutism, androgens and sex hormone binding globulin in women with polycystic ovarian syndrome. Acta Obstet Gynecol Scand 54:195–202, 1985.
8. Lemay A, Dewailly DS, Grenier R, et al: Attenuation of mild hyperandrogenic activity in postpubertal acne by a triphasic oral contraceptive containing low doses of ethinyl estradiol and D,L-orgestrel. J Clin Endocrinol Metab 71:8–14, 1990.
9. Redmond G, Olson W, Lippman J, et al: Norgestimate and ethinyl estradiol in the treatment of acne vulgaris: a randomized, placebo-controlled trial. Obstet Gynecol 89:615–622, 1987.
10. Lucky A, Henderson T, Olson W, et al: Effectiveness of norgestimate and ethinyl estradiol in treating moderate acne vulgaris. J Am Acad Dermatol 37:746–754, 1997.

11. Corvol P, Michaud A, Menard J, et al: Antiandrogenic effect of spironolactone: Mechanism of action. Endocrinology 97:52–63, 1975.
12. McMullen GR, Van Herle AJ: Hirsutism and the effectiveness of spironolactone in its management. J Endocrinol Invest 16:925–932, 1993.
13. Cumming DC, Yang JC, Rebar RW, Yen SSC: Treatment of hirsutism with spironolactone. JAMA 247:1295–1299, 1982.
14. Shapiro G, Evron S: A novel use of spironolactone: treatment of hirsutism. J Clin Endocrinol Metab 51:429–435, 1980.
15. Sawaya ME: RU58841, a new therapeutic agent affecting androgen receptor molecule interaction in human hair follicles. In: Van Neste DJ, Randall VA (eds). Hair Research for the Next Millennium. Amsterdam, Elsevier, 1996, pp 355–357.
16. Rittmaster RS: Finasteride. N Engl J Med 330:120–125, 1994.
17. Kaufman KD, Olsen EA, Whiting D, et al: Finasteride in the treatment of men with androgenetic alopecia. J Am Acad Dermatol 39:578–589, 1998.
18. Ciotta L, Marletta E, Sciuto A, et al: Clinical and endocrine effects of finasteride, a 5-α reductase inhibitor, in women with idiopathic hirsutism. Fertil Steril 64:299–306, 1995.
19. Castello R, Tosi F, Perrone F, Negri C, Muggeo M, Moghetti P: Outcome of long-term treatment with the 5α-reductase inhibitor finasteride in idiopathic hirsutism: clinical and hormonal effects during a 1-year course of therapy and 1-year follow-up. Fertil Steril 66:734–740, 1996.
20. Wong IL, Morris RS, Chang L, Spahn M, Stanczyck FZ, Lobo RA: A prospective randomized trial comparing finasteride to spironolactone in the treatment of hirsute women. J Clin Endocrinol Metab 80:233–238, 1995.
21. Hughes CL: Hirsutism. In: Olsen EA (ed). Disorders of Hair Growth: Diagnosis and Treatment. New York, McGraw-Hill, 1994, pp 337–352.
22. Olsen EA: Hypertrichosis. In: Olsen EA (ed). Disorders of Hair Growth: Diagnosis and Treatment. New York, McGraw-Hill, 1994, pp. 322–332.

Cicatricial Alopecias

LEONARD C. SPERLING

Traditionally, alopecia (hair loss) has been divided into scarring (cicatricial) and nonscarring types. "Scarring" implies that normal tissue has been replaced by fibrous tissue. However, in some cases of alopecia, follicles seem to simply disappear without noticeable alteration in tissue architecture. The broadest definition of scarring alopecia includes all forms of alopecia in which hair follicles are permanently lost[1]; in contrast, nonscarring alopecia is potentially reversible.

However, this simple definition blurs the traditional distinction between scarring and nonscarring alopecia.[1, 2] Long-standing traction alopecia, androgenetic alopecia, and alopecia areata can result in permanent loss (disappearance) of some follicles, yet they are classified as forms of nonscarring alopecia.[3] Actually, these diseases are biphasic, causing reversible (nonscarring) alopecia during a prolonged early phase and permanent alopecia during a much later phase. This chapter is devoted to the traditional forms of scarring alopecia, which tend to result in follicular destruction even in early or mild disease.

Scarring alopecia comprises two very different groups of disorders.[2] In primary scarring alopecia, the hair follicle appears to be the major target of the destructive process, and there is relative sparing of other structures. This chapter is devoted to the primary scarring alopecias.

Secondary scarring alopecia[1, 2] is another subset of conditions resulting in diffuse scarring throughout the dermis. Deep burns, radiation dermatitis, cutaneous malignancies, sclerosing dermatoses such as morphea, and certain chronic infections fall into this group. In these conditions, the hair follicles are probably innocent bystanders in a widespread destructive process. A discus-

sion of these disorders is beyond the scope of this chapter.

The classification of scarring alopecia is confused. Different authors have applied different definitions and diagnostic criteria to the same nosological entities. A major difficulty is that for most conditions the cause is unknown.

Central, Centrifugal Scarring Alopecia

The term *central, centrifugal scarring alopecia* (CCSA) was coined to incorporate several variations of inflammatory, scarring alopecia. The clinical entities grouped under CCSA have clinical and histological patterns that appear to segregate them, but they may all have a single, unifying (and as yet unidentified) cause. The variations in these patterns may be a result of racial differences or of the well-recognized differences in immune response among individuals. Hansen's disease may represent an analogous situation. Although *Mycobacterium leprae* is responsible for both tuberculoid and lepromatous leprosy, to the uneducated but observant eye they appear to be very different diseases. Individual immune response and not etiology accounts for the difference in clinical and histological features.

The patterns of scarring alopecia grouped under CCSA include pseudopelade, the follicular degeneration syndrome (FDS), folliculitis decalvans, and tufted folliculitis. These subtypes of CCSA have the following features in common: (1) they are chronic and progressive, with eventual spontaneous burnout after years or decades; (2) they are predominantly centered on the crown or vertex; (3) they progress in a roughly symmetrical fashion, with most disease activity limited to a peripheral zone of variable width, surrounding a central alopecic zone; and (4) in both, clinical and histological evidence of inflammation is found in the active, peripheral zone.

PATTERNS

Pseudopelade

The term *pseudopelade* has become so confusing that it constitutes a major impediment to the rational discussion and understanding of scarring alopecia. Traditional pseudopelade, that is, *pseudopelade of Brocq* as described by Brocq,[4] is a term that is well established in the literature and is discussed later in this chapter. The term pseudopelade has been borrowed to describe a form of CCSA that differs from the condition described earlier in the century (Brocq's pseudopelade). The following paragraphs are a discussion of the *modern* concept of pseudopelade, essentially a synonym for CCSA.

Pseudopelade includes[5] (and is thought by some authors[6] to be synonymous with) FDS, a condition described in more detail later. Even authors who favor the concept of modern pseudopelade do not describe a distinctive clinical picture.[7] There may be single or multiple, round or irregularly shaped patches of complete or nearly complete alopecia, most commonly located on or near the vertex or crown; variable degrees of erythema, follicular papules, and perifollicular scaling at the periphery of the bald spots; variable amounts of polytrichia (multiple hair shafts emerging from a single orifice); and a paucity of pustules[8] (Fig. 10–1). The majority of patients are men.

Modern pseudopelade is better defined histologically than clinically. Based on transverse and vertical sections, the diagnostic histological features include[1, 6] variably dense lymphocytic perifollicular inflammation, primarily at the level of the infundibulum; eccentric infundibular epithelial atrophy (thinning); frequent eccentricity of the

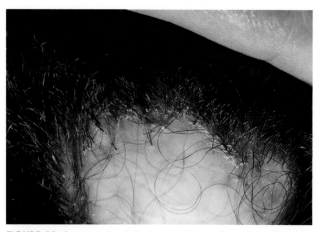

FIGURE 10–1 ■ Pseudopelade variant of central, centrifugal scarring alopecia on the crown of a Caucasian woman.

follicular canal; occasional fusion of infundibula (polytrichia); concentric lamellar fibroplasia (onion skin–like fibrosis) around affected follicles; and, in advanced lesions, total destruction of the follicular epithelium with retained hair shaft fragments and granulomatous inflammation. Interface alteration of the follicular epithelium and the absence of perifollicular and intrafollicular pustules are pertinent negative findings.[1, 6] These features are similar to those found in the later (nondiagnostic) stages of FDS (see Fig. 10–5) in the next section.[9] This is hardly surprising when some authors equate FDS with modern pseudopelade.[6]

Follicular Degeneration Syndrome

Originally called "hot comb alopecia" by LoPresti, Papa, and Kligman,[10] the condition was renamed *follicular degeneration syndrome* in 1992.[9] Several authors[1, 11, 12] would include FDS under the heading of modern pseudopelade. FDS has some distinctive clinical and histological features and therefore is described separately from other forms of CCSA.

Most patients with FDS are African-American adults, and FDS is the most common form of scarring alopecia in any population that includes significant numbers of African-Americans. Among African-Americans, FDS is responsible for more cases of scarring alopecia than all other forms combined. A few cases of CCSA involving Caucasians have shown the typical histological findings of FDS, with clinical findings more suggestive of modern pseudopelade. This suggests a relationship between these two forms of CCSA, and it is unclear (and perhaps unimportant) whether cases in Caucasians should be labeled FDS or modern pseudopelade.

The majority of patients with FDS are women, with a female-male ratio of about 3:1.[9, 13] The average age at presentation is 36 years for women and 31 years for men, although most patients have had progressive disease for years or decades before they seek medical attention. The disease invariably begins and remains most severe on the crown or vertex of the scalp, gradually expanding in a centrifugal fashion. The amount of hair loss is disproportionate to the symptoms, which may be absent. Most patients note only mild, episodic pruritus or dysesthesia of even markedly alopecic areas.

The crown or vertex of the scalp shows a symmetrical zone of partial or complete alopecia. When inflammation is subtle, androgenetic alopecia may be incorrectly diagnosed (Fig. 10–2). The follicular orifices between remaining hairs are obliterated, and the scalp is smooth and shiny, evidence of scarring alopecia. However, on palpation the involved scalp skin is often soft, supple, and nontender. Except for the obliteration of follicular openings, the scarring in FDS is more evident histologically than clinically.

A few isolated hairs, some showing polytrichia, may be stranded in the otherwise denuded central zone. Early or mild disease may manifest as a partially bald patch only a few centimeters in diameter. Long-standing or severe disease can result in hair loss covering the entire crown of the scalp. As the examiner moves from the center of the alopecic patch, a gradual increase in

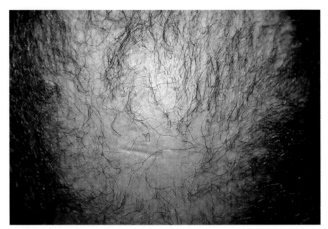

FIGURE 10-2 ■ Follicular degeneration syndrome. Central, centrifugal scarring alopecia on the crown of an African-American woman. Her disease is indolent and slowly progressive and was initially misdiagnosed as androgenetic alopecia.

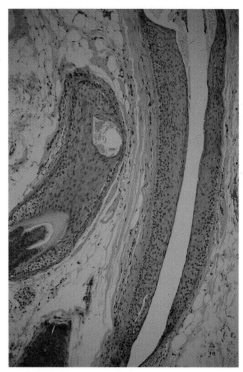

FIGURE 10-4 ■ Follicular degeneration syndrome. Two follicles from a normal-appearing portion of the scalp show loss of the inner root well below the isthmus.

hair density is noted, merging imperceptibly with the surrounding normal scalp. In this transitional zone, a few inflammatory, follicular papules may be found (Fig. 10–3). Even "normal" scalp skin may show small foci of alopecia and an occasional follicular papule or some perifollicular scaling. Pustules and crusting may be found in the minority of patients with rapidly progressive disease or bacterial superinfection. Such patients are often incorrectly labeled as having folliculitis decalvans.

If the central, bald zone is sampled, the histological findings will be those of a burnt-out, scarring alopecia. The most productive area for biopsy is the peripheral, partially alopecic fringe, but even clinically normal scalp may be diseased at the microscopic level. Not every follicle in a given area is involved simultaneously. A 4-mm punch biopsy specimen may contain only one or two diagnostic follicles. This is because the involved follicles are selectively destroyed, leaving behind relatively normal follicles. Although an occasional vertical section may sample an involved hair, in most cases

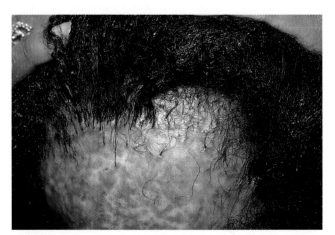

FIGURE 10-3 ■ Follicular degeneration syndrome. The central, scarred zone healed with considerable dyspigmentation in this inflammatory case.

transverse sections at several levels are required to establish a definitive diagnosis.

The most distinctive and controversial histological finding is premature desquamation of the inner root sheath (IRS).[7, 14] Normally, the IRS desquamates and disappears within the middle to upper isthmus,[15] which is located in the upper half of the dermis. In FDS, the IRS of an involved follicle desquamates in the lower half of the dermis, sometimes as low as or below the dermosubcutaneous junction (Fig. 10–4). This finding can be observed in follicles that are otherwise normal. Premature IRS desquamation can occasionally be seen in other conditions in which follicles are subject to marked inflammation and degenerative changes.[7] However, as an early, isolated, and characteristic finding, premature IRS desquamation is unique to FDS and is linked to the pathogenesis of the disease.[9, 13]

In clinically abnormal scalp skin, involved follicles also demonstrate some or all of the histological features already described for modern pseudopelade (Fig. 10–5). These advanced histological changes are secondary to chronic inflammation of those follicles expressing premature IRS desquamation. The immunofluorescent findings in patients with FDS have not been studied.

Hot combs are not in common use today and cannot be implicated as a pathogenetic factor. Virtually all women with FDS are using or have used chemical hair relaxers for styling purposes, but few men have used anything except pomades. Progression of the disease is observed by patients even after all chemical treatments are discontinued. Caustic cosmetics may aggravate the

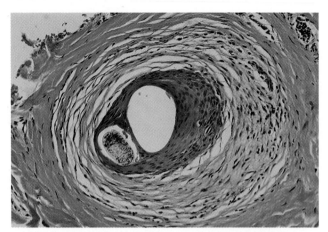

FIGURE 10–5 ■ Infundibular atrophy, impending infundibular fusion, and lamellar fibroplasia are evident in this case of follicular degeneration syndrome. Histological findings would be identical in modern pseudopelade. Only clinical findings and evidence of premature desquamation of the inner root sheath (not evident on this section) separate these two similar forms of central, centrifugal scarring alopecia.

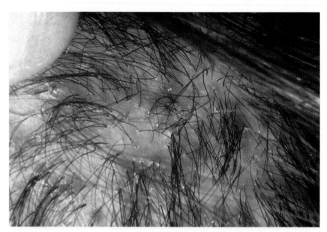

FIGURE 10–6 ■ Caucasian patient with folliculitis decalvans. Follicular pustules and perifollicular erythema and scaling improved with the use of potent topical corticosteroids. This is probably a pustular variant of pseudopelade.

disease or hasten its progression but cannot fully explain its pathogenesis.[9]

Folliculitis Decalvans

Folliculitis decalvans is a clinical pattern that is probably common to a heterogeneous group of disorders.[16] Like other forms of CCSA, it is a chronic, inflammatory form of alopecia characterized by peripheral extension and central, cicatricial healing.[8] It is often asymptomatic and usually resistant to therapy. Lesions can be multifocal, but they eventually merge into one larger patch, usually located on the crown or vertex. Unfortunately, the term *folliculitis decalvans* is often used by clinicians as a catchall designation for any chronic, inflammatory form of scarring alopecia of uncertain nosology. This use of the term is discouraged.

One feature distinguishes folliculitis decalvans from modern pseudopelade, namely the presence of pustules at the active periphery of the lesion (Fig. 10–6). Some would argue that the presence of peripheral pustules is required for diagnosis.[8] The reality is that pustular lesions come and go during the course of the disease. The pustules of folliculitis decalvans are a manifestation of bacterial superinfection or of the immune response of the patient[16] to degenerating follicular components. Both are altered by therapy, and a short course of antibiotics or systemic corticosteroids can turn folliculitis decalvans into a nonpurulent condition that clinically and histologically is identical to modern pseudopelade or FDS (Fig. 10–7). In other words, folliculitis decalvans may simply be a pustular variant of modern pseudopelade or FDS.

Because the definition of folliculitis decalvans requires the presence of pustules, it is not surprising that the microscopic description of folliculitis decalvans includes intrafollicular and perifollicular neutrophilic infiltrates.[1, 6] However, if nonpustular lesions at the active periphery are sampled or if the biopsy is performed during a

period of suppressive therapy, the histological picture is that of chronic, perifollicular inflammation with variable degrees of follicular epithelial disintegration. These features are similar to those found in other forms of CCSA. If enough lesions and patients are sampled, all the histological changes described for modern pseudopelade and FDS can be found in folliculitis decalvans.

Tufted Folliculitis

Polytrichia (tufts of hair shafts emerging from a single orifice, with fibrosis separating individual tufts) can be found in several forms of scarring alopecia, including modern pseudopelade, folliculitis decalvans, FDS, folliculitis keloidalis, dissecting cellulitis, and kerion. The condition, called *tufted folliculitis*,[17, 18] most likely represents a variant of CCSA, such as folliculitis decalvans or modern pseudopelade.[7, 16]

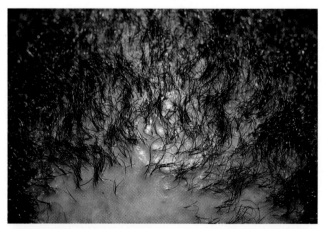

FIGURE 10–7 ■ African-American patient with folliculitis decalvans. The periphery of the scarred zone was studded with tender, follicular pustules that cleared with a course of oral corticosteroids. This probably represents a pustular variant of the follicular degeneration syndrome.

TREATMENT

Treatments of the various forms of CCSA are considered together. Therapy is largely empirical because there is no known cause and because controlled or long-term studies have never been performed. The key to successful treatment is continuity of care. Patients tend to shuttle from one care provider to another in their search for an experienced physician or a certain cure. No single regimen works well for all patients, and a solitary visit to any given provider usually ends in disappointment. However, persistent and sufficiently aggressive therapy delivered by a single, concerned physician can result in marked improvement and slowing of disease progression. The goal is not cure but slowing of disease progression until spontaneous "burnout" occurs. This may take months or years, and patience is required.

Therapy is directed largely at two interrelated components of the disease: follicular inflammation and bacterial superinfection. Disruption of the integrity of the follicular epithelium allows resident flora to gain access to the dermis, and pathogenic bacteria such as *Staphylococcus aureus* can establish a foothold. Therefore, short courses of antibiotics directed at pathogens and long-term suppressive therapy directed at resident flora are usually helpful. The effect of these antibiotics may be anti-inflammatory as well as antimicrobial.[16] Oral tetracycline and topical clindamycin or erythromycin are useful for long-term treatment.

Suppression of inflammation can be achieved with corticosteroids. For severe and rapidly progressive disease, a short course of systemic corticosteroids (over a few weeks to months) is warranted. This should be supplemented with topical and intralesional corticosteroids. Intralesional therapy should be repeated with gradually decreasing dose and frequency until the condition is under control. The fear of temporary skin atrophy is not warranted when the alternative is permanent hair loss and progressive disease.

Patients who are using chemical irritants such as hair relaxers, permanents, and bleaches should be warned that these treatments may exacerbate the condition.

In progressive, treatment-resistant disease, alternative therapies may be considered. Hydroxychloroquine has been tried with variable success in cases of modern pseudopelade.[7] Given the tendency for neurophilic inflammation in folliculitis decalvans, dapsone may be worth trying. Because of its utility in dissecting cellulitis, oral isotretinoin has been tried in highly inflammatory forms of CCSA, but with only occasional success. None of these modalities has been studied prospectively in a controlled fashion.

Folliculitis Keloidalis Nuchae (Acne Keloidalis Nuchae)

The term *folliculitis keloidalis nuchae* (FKN) is favored over acne keloidalis because the disease bears little clinical or histological resemblance to acne vulgaris. Most cases involve young adult African-American men, but

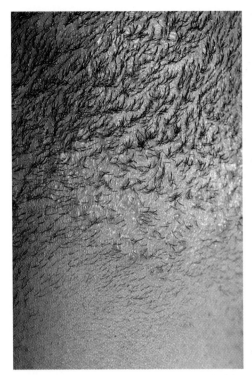

FIGURE 10–8 ■ Early papular lesions of folliculitis keloidalis nuchae.

African-American women and occassionally persons of other racial groups can also be affected.[19]

Early lesions are folliculocentric, slightly erythematous, firm papules found most commonly on the lower occiput (Fig. 10–8). The hair shaft emerging from an early papule or pustule of FKN does not curve back and re-enter the skin, and there is neither clinical nor histological evidence suggesting a relationship with pseudofolliculitis barbae.[20] In severe cases, lesions can extend up the entire occiput onto the vertex and crown. One form of CCSA is distinguished by lesions that are clinically and histologically similar to those of FKN but are centered and most dense on the vertex and crown (Fig. 10–9). Whether this is the same condition as FKN has

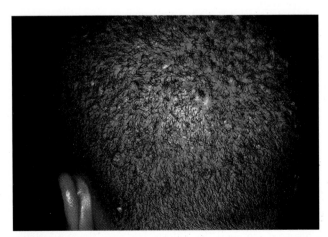

FIGURE 10–9 ■ In this patient, lesions identical to those of typical folliculitis keloidalis nuchae are centered and most severe on the vertex, with minimal nuchal involvement.

yet to be established, but certainly overlap cases with numerous lesions on the vertex and crown as well as on the occiput are not uncommon.

In severe and advanced disease, lesions coalesce into large, hypertrophic scars; hence, the designation *keloidalis*. Hair follicles and associated shafts become trapped within a matrix of fibrous tissue, leading to a foreign-body reaction, sinus tract formation, bacterial superinfection, and further follicular damage. Pustular lesions are common in this stage and represent bacterial superinfection or a brisk immune response to foreign bodies within the dermis. Eventually the follicles and naked hair shafts trapped within the hypertrophic, fibrotic tissue disintegrate and a hairless but noninflamed hypertrophic scar remains as the residual of burnt-out disease.

The histopathology of early lesions, which are most indicative of pathogenesis, is that of a primary folliculitis and perifolliculitis,[21] with each papule representing only one or two involved follicles. Most commonly, a dense infiltrate of lymphocytes and plasma cells surrounds the involved follicles, predominantly at the level of the lower infundibulum and isthmus.[21] There is epithelial atrophy and concentric, lamellar fibroplasia, most prominent at the level of the isthmus. Lymphocytes invade the follicular epithelium, a sign of true folliculitis. In many cases, however, the inflammatory infiltrate of early lesions is predominantly neutrophilic rather than lymphocytic. The fact that clinically identical lesions of FKN can be affected by either acute (neutrophilic) or chronic (lymphoplasmacytic) inflammation has frustrated attempts to classify the disease and clarify its cause.

In more advanced lesions, there is a variable degree of follicular disintegration, with dilatation of the follicular canal, thinning of the follicular wall, and extrusion of the shaft into the dermis. This incites intense lymphoplasmacytic inflammation of the midportion of the follicle. In such follicles, a neutrophilic infiltrate is seen within and surrounding the infundibulum and isthmus, and granulomatous inflammation occurs around the deeper portions of the follicle. Sebaceous glands tend to disappear early in the course of the disease and may represent an early focus of follicular inflammation and destruction.[21]

In advanced, keloidal lesions, there are numerous "naked" hair shafts trapped within a dense fibrotic matrix and a variable mixture of associated granulomatous, lymphoplasmacytic, and neutrophilic inflammation. Continuity between naked hair shafts in the dermis and the cutaneous surface provides a continual nidus for bacterial superinfection. Eventually, hair shafts are dissolved or are completely buried beneath the surface, leading to a decrease in inflammation.

Treatment of early or mild disease is similar to the empirical therapy for CCSA. The treatment of large, keloidal, inflamed plaques is surgical excision below the level of the hair bulbs (Figs. 10–10 and 10–11).[20, 22] Intralesional corticosteroids and superficial tissue removal are temporizing measures in advanced disease. They are doomed to failure because the underlying problem (trapped hair shaft and follicular components) is not addressed by these modalities.

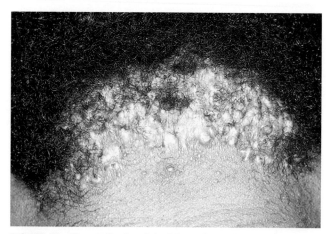

FIGURE 10–10 ■ Folliculitis keloidalis nuchae. Chronic inflammation in response to degenerating follicular components, trapped hair shaft fragments, and secondary bacterial infection has resulted in hypertrophic scarring.

Dissecting Cellulitis (Perifolliculitis Capitis Abscedens et Suffodiens)

Dissecting cellulitis, first described in Germany by Hoffman[23] in 1908 and in the United States by Wise and Parkhurst[24] in 1921, is a rare but distinctive disease. The disease most commonly affects young adult men, especially African-American men. Dissecting cellulitis is part of the follicular occlusion triad that includes hidradenitis suppurativa and acne conglobata, but it often occurs alone.

Lesions begin[25] as multiple, firm scalp nodules, most commonly on the crown, vertex, and occiput. The nodules rapidly develop into boggy, fluctuant, oval, linear ridges that eventually release a purulent discharge (Fig. 10–12). Lesions eventually interconnect so that pressure on one fluctuant area may result in a discharge of pus from perforations several centimeters distant. Despite

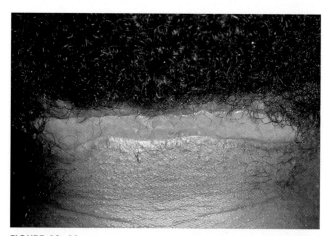

FIGURE 10–11 ■ Same patient as in Figure 10–10, photographed 4 weeks after excision of hypertrophic scarring, with secondary intention healing. A flat, supple scar was the long-term result.

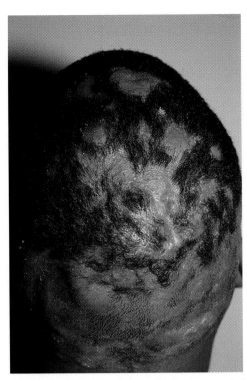

FIGURE 10–12 ■ Dissecting cellulitis. This case responded to retinoid therapy.

massive, deep inflammation, there can be surprisingly little pain, and patients often seek help because of alopecia and a foul-smelling discharge.

The disease waxes and wanes for years but eventually leads to dense dermal fibrosis, sinus tract formation, permanent alopecia, and hypertrophic scarring. Rarely, squamous cell carcinoma may arise in the setting of long-standing disease.[26]

The earliest histological finding may be acneiform dilatation of the follicular infundibulum, with perifollicular neutrophilic inflammation.[1] The term *dissecting cellulitis* is a misnomer because the condition is a suppurative folliculitis, not a cellulitis.[27] Follicular epithelium is invaded by inflammatory cells, and there is subsequent disruption of the epithelium and follicular destruction. If fluctuant nodules and sinuses are sampled, large perifollicular and middle-to-deep reticular dermal abscesses composed of neutrophils and often copious plasma cells are found.[1] At this stage, numerous intact and seemingly normal follicles seem surrounded by acute and chronic inflammation. Eventually, chronic abscesses become lined with squamous epithelium derived from the overlying epidermis, and true sinus tracts result. As follicles are completely destroyed, inflammation subsides and is replaced by dense fibrosis of the dermis and the superficial fat.

Dissecting cellulitis is a notoriously treatment-resistant disease. Although fluctuant lesions of dissecting cellulitis are often sterile, systemic antibiotics often cause a transient and partial improvement. This may be due to a component of bacterial superinfection or a direct anti-inflammatory action of some antibiotics, such as the tet-

racyclines. Chronic antibiotic therapy is seldom useful and may predispose the patient to gram-negative folliculitis.[25] Incision and drainage of lesions should be avoided because it does not alter the course of the disease and causes additional scarring. Intralesional and systemic corticosteroids are dependably helpful but can cause side effects if used in high doses for prolonged periods.

Before the availability of retinoids, radiation therapy was the only effective treatment for severe, refractory disease.[24] Systemic retinoids such as isotretinoin, 1 to 2 mg/kg per day for 20 or more weeks, may cause significant or total, long-lasting remission, similar to the response seen in acne conglobata.[25] Higher doses for longer periods than those used in acne are often needed. However, response to retinoids is not dependable, and treatment failures are seen. If the disease goes into remission, excision of hypertrophic scars and persistent sinus tracts can be performed 6 to 12 months after retinoid theraphy is stopped.[25]

Pseudopelade of Brocq

The term *pseudopelade of Brocq*, a source of much confusion over the past several decades, should probably be abandoned. Traditional pseudopelade of Brocq is not a disease but a pattern of scarring alopecia as described by Brocq.[4] It is an end-stage or clinical variant of various other forms of scarring alopecia[16] and a diagnosis of exclusion. The same pattern of hair loss can be seen in burnt-out discoid lupus erythematosus (DLE), lichen planopilaris, and other forms of scarring alopecia. If a definitive diagnosis of DLE, lichen planopilaris, or another form of scarring alopecia (such as modern pseudopelade or FDS) can be made based on clinical, histological, or immunofluorescent features, then the term *pseudopelade of Brocq* cannot be used. A "primary" form of traditional pseudopelade may exist, but this has yet to be established with certainty.

Pseudopelade of Brocq is a pattern of alopecia that is rarely encountered. The typical patient is a Caucasian adult who is surprised to discover discrete, asymptomatic areas of scalp hair loss (Fig. 10–13). In many patients, the disease is slowly progressive[8] in that new areas of alopecia develop over a period of months to years. However, the condition often worsens in spurts, with periods of activity followed by dormant periods. This is distinctly different from the slow but steady disease progression seen in the other forms of CCSA described previously. Disease progression in pseudopelade eventually terminates spontaneously.[28]

Unlike CCSA, traditional pseudopelade results in irregularly shaped and often widely distributed and clustered alopecic patches on the scalp (see Fig. 10–13). Cases with exclusive crown or vertex involvement may actually represent examples of burnt-out CCSA.

The individual lesion is hypopigmented ("porcelain white" is the classic description) and slightly depressed (atrophic). Lesions are often irregularly shaped, in contrast to the round or oval patches usually seen in alope-

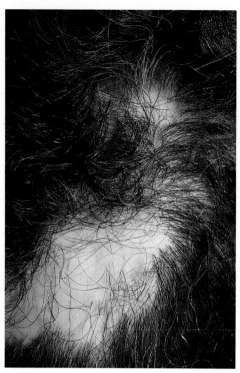

FIGURE 10–13 ■ Traditional pseudopelade of Brocq in a 50-year-old Caucasian woman. Her hairdresser was the first to note these lesions, which showed the histological pattern of a burnt-out scarring alopecia.

cia areata and most cases of CCSA. The classic description of "footprints in the snow"[28] refers to dermal atrophy that causes a slight depression below the surrounding normal scalp. However, many cases of pseudopelade do not demonstrate atrophy. Usually only mild erythema and slight perifollicular scaling are present, and often there is no clinical evidence of inflammation. Some authors[29] argue that the presence of any inflammation excludes traditional pseudopelade from the clinical differential diagnosis. Typical of many forms of scarring alopecia, a few isolated hairs may remain within an otherwise smooth, shiny, denuded patch.

The histopathological findings of traditional pseudopelade have yet to be clearly defined.[28] The criteria established by Pinkus,[30] based on his own experience and the writings of several other authors, are not correlated in any way with clinical features. The pseudopelade described by Pinkus is a histological, not a clinical, entity. In most cases of traditional pseudopelade, the active lesion is elusive and the typical histological findings are those of a burnt-out scarring alopecia.

The histological findings of "pseudopelade" in more recent descriptions[1, 6, 7] apply to the pseudopelade pattern of CCSA rather than the pseudopelade of Brocq. It would not be surprising to find an occasional case of pseudopelade of Brocq demonstrating the typical histological findings of CCSA. Traditional pseudopelade is, after all, the end stage of several different forms of scarring alopecia. A prospective study of pseudopelade of Brocq with sound clinical correlation has yet to be performed.

Lichen Planopilaris

An indisputable case of lichen planopilaris includes the triad of typical lichen planus lesions, spinous or acuminate follicular papules, and scarring alopecia of the scalp (Graham Little–Piccardi–Lassueur syndrome).[31, 32] Not all three features of classic lichen planopilaris may be present, and the condition may be confined to the scalp. The term *lichen planus of the scalp* or *follicular lichen planus* can be used when other components of the lichen planopilaris syndrome are absent.

Lichen planopilaris may be an insidious disease evolving over years, or the course may be fulminant, with marked permanent hair loss occurring within a few months. Physical findings vary depending on the severity of the disease and the rapidity of progression in a given patient. Unless the disease has burnt out, the common feature clinically is evidence of inflammation in the setting of scarring alopecia. Inflammation may manifest as erythema and scaling of the affected scalp; perifollicular scaling; spiny, keratotic follicular papules; erythematous or violaceous, follicular papules; or a combination of these (Fig. 10–14). Scarring is manifested by hairless, dilated follicular ostia plugged with keratinous debris (follicular plugging); several shafts exiting from a single ostium (polytrichia); and total obliteration of follicular ostia.

Patients with indolent disease may be asymptomatic, but itching and tenderness are often present. Patients with lesions of lichen planus on the skin or oral mucosa may have symptoms related to these lesions. The pattern of scalp hair loss is variable. Hair loss may be confined to one or more circumscribed areas, or it may affect most of the scalp. Most commonly there are several asymmetrical, scattered foci of partial hair loss, but the patterns seen in traditional pseudopelade of Brocq and the pseudopelade pattern of CCSA can also develop (Fig. 10–15). Therefore the diagnosis of lichen planopilaris cannot be made solely by clinical examination. His-

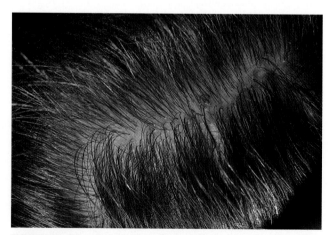

FIGURE 10–14 ■ Lichen planopilaris. Foci of involvement, characterized by perifollicular erythema, scaling, and hair loss, were scattered throughout the scalp.

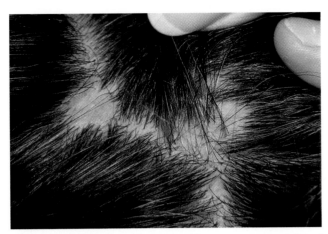

FIGURE 10–15 ■ Lichen planopilaris. This pattern is suggestive of traditional pseudopelade, but the patient had classic clinical and histological features of the Graham Little syndrome.

tological correlation and recognition of other manifestations of the lichen planopilaris syndrome (if present) are required for definitive diagnosis.

Typical lichen planopilaris shows a bandlike mononuclear cell infiltrate obscuring the interface between follicular epithelium and dermis.[2] Vacuolar alteration at the interface and wedge-shaped hypergranulosis within affected infundibula is typical. The epithelial-adventitial junction often shows prominent dyskeratosis with individually necrotic, polygonal basal keratinocytes.[1] Colloid or Civatte bodies are occasionally found as part of the interface alteration. Inflammation affects the upper portion of the follicle (infundibulum and isthmus) most

severely but may extend down the length of the follicle (Fig. 10–16). Perivascular and perieccrine lymphocytic infiltrates of the middle and deep dermis that are typical of DLE are absent in lichen planopilaris.[1] Occasionally, interfollicular changes of lichen planus are found; when present, they strongly support a diagnosis of lichen planopilaris.

Eventually the infundibulum becomes distended and plugged with keratinous debris. Perifollicular fibrosis and chronic inflammation (without distinct interface changes) may be seen at this later stage of disease. Although these changes are often seen in patients with long-standing lichen planopilaris, they are not diagnostic and can be observed in other forms of inflammatory, scarring alopecia.

In time, the follicle is entirely destroyed. At first, retained hair shaft fragments and a granulomatous response are observed, but eventually the follicle is replaced by a column of connective tissue. This represents another end-stage phenomenon that is shared by all forms of permanent hair loss.

Grouped globular immunofluorescence, usually immunoglobulin M (IgM), especially when found adjacent to the follicular epithelium, is the characteristic pattern seen in lichen planopilaris.[29] Linear deposits of immunoreactants are typical of DLE. This distinction can be important, because lichen planopilaris and DLE may resemble each other both clinically and histologically in the setting of scarring alopecia.

Treatment can be difficult, and controlled studies are lacking.[7] Potent topical and intralesional corticosteroids are usually tried first but may be ineffective. High-dose oral corticosteroids are usually helpful, but their use is risky in chronic, progressive disease. Antimalarials such as hydroxychloroquine may be effective, and the use of immunomodulators such as cyclosporine has been considered,[7] but long-term safety and efficacy have not been determined.

FRONTAL FIBROSING ALOPECIA

This condition has been reported in several Australian, postmenopausal, Caucasian women[33]; it has yet to be reported in the United States. Patients are elderly women (mean age, 67 years) with progressive hair loss along the frontal fringe and the eyebrows. The histopathological features are similar to those found in lichen planopilaris, and the condition has been interpreted as a distinct subtype of lichen planopilaris.[33] However, lesions of lichen planus are not found in these patients, and the lichenoid inflammation does not affect the interfollicular epidermis. As is true for lichen planopilaris, therapy is difficult.

Chronic Cutaneous Lupus Erythematosus

The term *chronic cutaneous lupus erythematosus* (CCLE) is preferred to discoid lupus erythematosus because it is more inclusive. CCLE usually occurs in

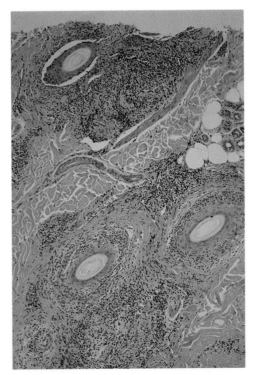

FIGURE 10–16 ■ Lichen planopilaris.

adults and is more common in women. Although lesions of CCLE are often found in patients with systemic lupus erythematosus (SLE), most patients with CCLE do not have systemic disease. Among patients with skin disease only, about 50% have scalp lesions,[34] and very few of these cases ever progress to SLE.[35] Although itching or tenderness is common, the condition may be asymptomatic. The presence of lesions outside the scalp greatly simplifies diagnosis.

Scalp involvement may resemble that seen in classic DLE lesions, with alopecia, erythema, epidermal atrophy, and dilated, plugged follicular ostia. Central hypopigmentation and peripheral hyperpigmentation are characteristic of lesions in dark-skinned persons. Plaques of CCLE may merge to form large, irregularly shaped zones of scarring alopecia (Fig. 10–17). However, some patients with CCLE present with clinically noninflammatory alopecia[29] resembling traditional pseudopelade or alopecia areata. Long-standing, burnt-out disease confined to the scalp may be impossible to differentiate from traditional pseudopelade or lichen planopilaris.

Eventual progression of CCLE to SLE is uncommon but possible.[34] An antinuclear antibody (ANA) titer is the only test required if signs and symptoms of SLE are absent, and it is seldom positive except in patients with widespread disease. If the ANA titer is negative, the laboratory evaluation is complete. If it is positive, the patient requires long-term follow-up to screen for evidence of progression to systemic disease.

Histologically, vacuolar interface alteration of the epidermis and follicular epithelium is typical, although the epidermis may be spared in scalp lesions. The interface change of CCLE tends to be vacuolar rather than lichenoid and lacks the dense, bandlike lymphocytic infiltrate of lichen planopilaris (Fig. 10–18). Dyskeratosis and colloid (Civatte) bodies are occasionally seen, but less commonly than in lichen planopilaris. However, moderate-to-dense, superficial and deep chronic inflammation, often including plasma cells, is seen in both perivascular and periadnexal locations. Perifollicular inflammation is most severe at the level of the infundibulum, and inflammatory cells may invade the follicular

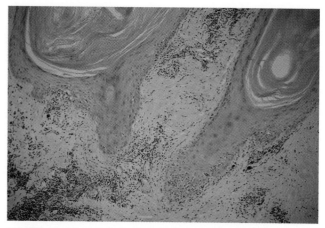

FIGURE 10–18 ■ Well-developed, chronic, cutaneous lupus erythematosus (discoid LE). Keratinous plugging of the follicular ostia, vacuolar interface change, and a combination of periadnexal (follicles and sweat glands) and perivascular lymphoplasmacytic inflammation are present.

epithelium.[1] Similar inflammation may be found in and around the follicular tracts below follicles that have entered the telogen phase or have been destroyed. Increased dermal mucin is often present and is helpful in differentiating CCLE from lichen planopilaris.[1, 6] The presence of a focally thinned epidermis, numerous plasma cells, and a thickened basement membrane and the absence of wedge-shaped hypergranulosis also support a diagnosis of CCLE over lichen planopilaris.[2]

Granular deposits of IgG and C3 (rarely IgM or IgA) at the dermoepidermal junction or at the junction of the follicular epithelium and dermis are typical of CCLE.[36] Globular deposits of IgM representing colloid bodies may be present, but not as commonly as in lichen planopilaris.

Treatment of scalp CCLE is discussed in detail by Newton and colleagues.[25] Sun protection (hats, sunscreens, and sun avoidance) and potent topical and intralesional corticosteroids are tried first. Systemic corticosteroids should be avoided[25] in this very chronic and slowly progressive disease. Antimalarials are more dependably effective in CCLE than all other forms of scarring alopecia. Isotretinoin can also be considered in refractory disease.

Pressure-induced Alopecia

Most cases of pressure-induced alopecia are associated with surgical operations, and the condition is often referred to as *postoperative alopecia*. The term *pressure-induced alopecia* would also encompass cases caused by trauma, coma, or drug overdose. Pressure-induced alopecia is usually temporary (nonscarring) but is included in this chapter because numerous cases of permanent (scarring) hair loss have been reported.

The typical patient is an adult who has recently undergone a prolonged surgical procedure, especially one requiring tracheal intubation.[37] The condition has also been described in children. Within the first postopera-

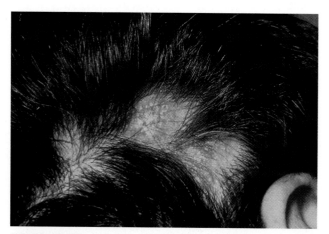

FIGURE 10–17 ■ Chronic, cutaneous lupus erythematosus (discoid LE). Irregularly shaped plaques are beginning to merge into a large, alopecic zone.

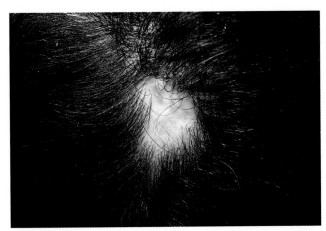

FIGURE 10–19 ■ Pressure-induced (postoperative) alopecia. This central zone of scarring alopecia showed no regrowth 2 years after the causative event.

tive week, the patient notes tenderness and swelling in a localized area on the occiput. The affected (occipital) area is erythematous and edematous. Crusting and ulceration may supervene in severe cases. Within 3 to 4 weeks, and as early as 2 weeks, hair loss is noted. During the next several weeks, the affected area becomes increasingly bald, most severely in the central portion of the lesion. Over several months, there is partial to complete hair regrowth. Permanent hair loss, when it occurs, is confined to the central portion of the lesion (Fig. 10–19).

Histological findings vary as lesions evolve. Early lesions show intravascular thrombosis, edema, follicular necrosis, and perivascular inflammation without vasculitis.[38] During the active shedding phase, dermal fibrosis, chronic dermal inflammation, and numerous catagen hairs are seen.[37] After the hair loss is complete, a moderate to severe obliterative vasculitis in the deep dermis and fat, a perivascular lymphocytic infiltrate, deep dermal fibrosis, and atrophic follicles may be present.[39]

ACKNOWLEDGMENT

The author wishes to thank Dr. Alvin R. Solomon for reviewing the chapter and providing helpful comments.

REFERENCES

1. Templeton SF, Solomon AR: Scarring alopecia: a classification based on microscopic criteria. J Cutan Pathol 21:97–109, 1994.
2. Ackerman AB: Histologic Diagnosis of Inflammatory Skin Diseases. Philadelphia, Lea & Febinger, 1978, pp 702–713.
3. Sperling LC, Lupton GP: The histopathology of non-scarring alopecia. J Cutan Pathol 22:97–114, 1995.
4. Brocq L, Lenglet E, Ayrignac J: Recherches sur l'alopecie atrophiante, variete pseudopelade. Ann Dermatol Syphilol (France) 6:1–32, 97–127, 209–237, 1905.
5. Whiting DA, Howsden FL: Color Atlas of Differential Diagnosis of Hair Loss. Cedar Grove, NJ, Canfield Publishing, 1996.
6. Solomon AR: The transversely sectioned scalp biopsy specimen: the technique and an algorithm for its use in the diagnosis of alopecia. Adv Dermatol 9:127–157, 1994.
7. Headington JT: Cicatricial alopecia. In: Whiting DA (ed): Update on Hair Disorders, Philadelphia, WB Saunders, 1996, 773–782.
8. Laymon CW: The cicatricial alopecias. J Invest Dermatol 8:99–122, 1947.
9. Sperling LC, Sau P: The follicular degeneration syndrome in black patients: "hot comb alopecia" revisited and revised. Arch Dermatol 128:68–74, 1992.
10. LoPresti P, Papa CM, Kligman AM: Hot comb alopecia. Arch Dermatol 98:234–238, 1968.
11. Price VH: Hair loss in cutaneous disease. In: Baden HP (ed): Symposium on Alopecia, vol. 6. New York, HP Publishing Co., 1987, pp 3–11.
12. Whiting DA: Current Concepts: The Diagnosis of Alopecia. Kalamazoo, Michigan, Upjohn, 1990, p 24.
13. Sperling LC, Skelton HG, Smith KJ, Sau P, Friedman K: The follicular degeneration syndrome in men. Arch Dermatol 130:763–769, 1994.
14. Gibbons G, Ackerman AB: Follicular degeneration syndrome? Dermatopathology Practical and Conceptual 1;197–200, 1995.
15. Sperling LC: Hair anatomy for the clinician. J Am Acad Dermatol 25:1–17, 1991.
16. Dawber RPR, Van Neste D: Hair and scalp disorders: common presenting signs, differential diagnosis, and treatment. Philadelphia, JB Lippincott, 1995, p 124.
17. Pufol RM, Matias-Guiu X, Garcia-Patos V, de Moragas JM: Tufted-hair folliculitis. Colin Exp Dermatol 16:199–201, 1991.
18. Dalziel KL, Telfer NR, Wilson CL, Dawber RP: Tufted folliculities. a specific bacterial disease? Am. J Dermatopathol 12:37–41, 1990.
19. Dinehart SM, Tanner L, Mallory SB, et al: Acne keloidalis in women. Cutis 44:250–252, 1989.
20. Kantor GR, Ratz JL, Wheeland RG: Treatment of acne keloidalis nuchae with carbon dioxide laser. J Am Acad Dermtol 14:263–267, 1986.
21. Herzberg AJ, Dinehart SM, Kerns BJ, Pollack SV: Acne keloidalis: transverse microscopy, immunohistochemistry and electron microscopy. Am J Dermatopathol 12:109–121, 1990.
22. Glenn MJ, Bennett RG, Kelly AP: Acne keloidalis nuchae: treatment with excision and second-intention healing. J Am Acad Dermatol 33:243–246, 1995.
23. Hoffman E: Perifolliculitis capitis abscedens et suffodiens: case presentation. Derm Ztschr 15:122, 1998.
24. Wise F, Parkhurst HJ: A rare form of suppurating and cicatrizing disease of the scalp. Arch Dermatol Syphilol 4:750–768, 1921.
25. Newton RC, Hebert AA, Freese TW, Solomon AR: Scarring alopecia. Dermatol Clin 5:603–618, 1987.
26. Curry SS, Gaither DH, King LE: Squamous cell carcinoma arising in dissecting perifolliculitis of the scalp. J Am Acad Dermatol 4:673–678, 1981.
27. Ackerman AB: Histologic diagnosis of inflammatory skin diseases: an algorithmic method by pattern analysis. Baltimore, Williams & Wilkins, 1988, p 175.
28. Ronchese F: Pseudopelade. Arch Dermatol 82:336–343, 1960.
29. Elston DM, Bergfeld WF: Cicatricial alopecia (and other causes of permanent alopecia). In: Olsen EA (ed): Disorders of Hair Growth. New York, McGraw-Hill, 1994, pp 285–313.
30. Pinkus H: Differential patterns of elastic fibers in scarring and non-scarring alopecias. J Cutan Pathol 5:93–104, 1978.
31. Feldman S: Lichen planus et acuminatus atrophicans. Arch Dermatol Syphilol 5:102–113, 1922.
32. Matta M, Kibbi A-G, Khattar J, Salman SM, Zaynoun ST: Lichen planopilaris: a clinicopathologic study. J Am Acad Dermatol 22:594–598, 1990.
33. Kossard S, Lee M-S, Wilkinson B: Postmenopausal frontal fibrosing alopecia: a frontal variant of lichen planopilaris. J Am Acad Dermatol 36:59–66, 1997.
34. Callen JP: Chronic cutaneous lupus erythematosus. Arch Dermatol 118:412, 1982.
35. Callen JP: Systemic lupus erythematosus in patients with chronic cutaneous (discoid) lupus erythematosus. J Am Acad Dermatol 12:278, 1985.
36. Jordan RE: Subtle clues to diagnosis by immunopathology: scarring alopecia. Am J Dermatopathol 2:157–159, 1980.
37. Boyer JD, Vidmar DA: Postoperative alopecia: a case report and literature review. Cutis 54:321–322, 1994.
38. Lawson N, Mills N, Oscher J: Occipital alopecia following cardiopulmonary bypass. J Thorac Cardiovasc Surg 71:342–347, 1976.
39. Abel R, Lewis G: Postoperative (pressure) alopecia. Arch Dermatol 81:34–42, 1960.

Tumors of Hair and Nails

...

TUMORS OF THE NAIL APPARATUS

PHILIPPE ABIMELEC

Overview

ETIOLOGY

More than 70 tumors of the nail apparatus have been described. They can originate from the epidermis, dermis, subcutaneous tissues, or bone.

CLINICAL FEATURES

Tumors of the nail apparatus may be localized in the nail bed, nail matrix, hyponychium, posterior or lateral nail folds, perionychium, or bony phalanx. Most of the time the tumor is single, a polydactylous process may be seen with Bowen's disease, warts, glomus tumors, myxoid cysts, and onychomatrichomas. Depending on their location, they may be revealed as a tumor or tumefaction, granulation tissue, onycholysis, a subungual hyperkeratosis, a nail bed erosion or ulceration, a longitudinal nail groove, macular or longitudinal pigmentation, nail plate overcurvature, a nail plate fissure, nail plate destruction, pachyonychia, clubbing, periungual pigmentation or scaling, paronychia, or pain. The main characteristics of the most common tumors are listed in Table 11–1.

PATHOLOGY

Each tumor has a specific pathology; see discussions of individual tumors.

DIAGNOSIS

Diagnostic tests may include biopsy and histology, radiographs, and magnetic resonance imaging (MRI).

TREATMENT

Surgical removal of the tumor with pathological examination is usually advised.

Epidermal Tumors

KERATINOCYTIC/ONYCHOCYTIC TUMORS

Benign

Subungual Corn (Heloma, Onychoclavus)

ETIOLOGY. Corns are localized areas of hyperkeratosis that are caused by repeated microtrauma induced by faulty biomechanics, toe deformities, or ill-fitting shoes.[1]

141

TABLE 11-1 ■ Locations and Manifestations of the Most Common Tumors of the Nail Apparatus

Location or Manifestation	Wart	Bowen's Disease/Squamous Cell Carcinoma	Malignant Melanoma of the Nail Apparatus	Nail Matrix Nevus	Glomus Tumor	Myxoid Cyst	Subungual Exostosis	Pyogenic Granuloma
Hand	++	++	++	++	++●	++●	+	+
Foot	++	+	++	++	+		++●	++
Pain	+	+	+		++●	+	++	+
Desquamation		++●						
Fissuring/ bleeding		++●	+			+		
Subungual hyperkeratosis	++	++					++	
Longitudinal melanonychia		+	++●	++●				
Hutchinson's sign			++●	+				
Chromonychia	+	+	++		++●		+	+
Longitudinal nail groove	+					++●		
Nail destruction	+	++	+		+			
Onycholysis	+	++●	+		+		++	+
Paronychia		+	+			++		++
Tumor/ Tumefaction	++	++●	+		+	++●	++●	++●

+, rare; ++, usual; ●, characteristic.

PATHOLOGY. There is a large conical, parakeratotic plug within the epidermis.

DIAGNOSIS. Pain is accentuated by footwear and walking. Subungual lesions are located at the distal third of the nail bed or in the hyponychium. There is a yellow, red, or black localized area of onycholysis. The nail plate over the lesion may be thinned or fissured.[1]

DIFFERENTIAL DIAGNOSIS. Hematoma, foreign body, wart, Bowen's disease, keratoacanthoma, or malignant melanoma may sometimes be considered. These diagnoses are easily ruled out by microscopic examination of the excised corn.

TREATMENT. Removal of the corn is easily performed with a scalpel after sectioning of the overlying nail plate. Correction of faulty biomechanics or toe deformities and counseling about shoe wear are necessary to avoid recurrences.

Epidermoid Inclusion/Epidermoid Cyst/ Implantation Cyst

ETIOLOGY. These lesions are caused by traumatic implantation of epidermis into the dermis or subcutaneous tissues.[2]

PATHOLOGY. The cyst is filled with horny material arranged in laminated layers; its wall is composed of epidermis.

DIAGNOSIS. Cutaneous cysts are frequently located in the periungual skin. Subungual epidermal cysts are usually asymptomatic and associated with fingernail clubbing. Bone cysts usually manifest as painful swelling of

the terminal phalanx.[2] Radiography is useful when it shows a localized zone of osteolysis.

DIFFERENTIAL DIAGNOSIS. A great number of tumors may be considered. The diagnosis becomes evident perioperatively.

TREATMENT. Surgical excision of the cyst, including its entire lining, is necessary.

Onychomatricoma

ETIOLOGY. It is a recently described matrical tumor.[3]

PATHOLOGY. There is an epithelial proliferation related to the nail matrix or surrounding epidermis.

DIAGNOSIS. Onychomatrichomas may be single or multiple. They occur in elderly persons and manifest as longitudinal xanthonychia or melanonychia, splinter hemorrhages, and transverse nail plate overcurvature (Fig. 11–1).[3] Paronychia and tumefaction of the proximal nail fold may occur. The nail plate is thickened.

DIFFERENTIAL DIAGNOSIS. The presentation is unlike that of other disorders. The perioperative aspect is diagnostic, showing the proximal nail plate with multiple holes storing the filamentous digitations of the tumor.

TREATMENT. Surgical excision is the treatment of choice.

Distal Subungual Keratosis

ETIOLOGY. Distal subungual keratosis is a typical fingernail nail bed onychocytic tumor of unknown cause.[4]

PATHOLOGY. Localized, multinucleate, distal keratosis

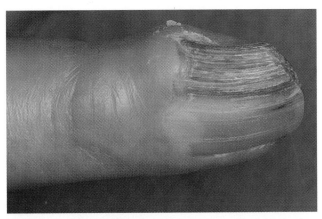

FIGURE 11-1 ■ Onychomatricoma. Large longitudinal black chromonychia is associated with pachyonychia, transverse nail plate overcurvature, onychorrhexis, and posterior nail fold tumefaction.

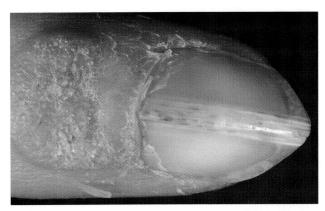

FIGURE 11-3 ■ Wart. This wart of the posterior nail fold and matrix is responsible for the longitudinal leukonychia and proximal splinter hemorrhages.

shows papillomatosis and acanthosis of the distal nail bed. The presence of numerous multinucleated cells is characteristic.[4] The keratogenous zone is thickened and devoid of a granular layer. There are often a few dyskeratotic cells.[4]

DIAGNOSIS. The lesion manifests as a monodactylous, longitudinal, pink-to-red, 1- to 5-mm longitudinal band. Splinter hemorrhages may be seen at the distal third of the lesion, and there may be a distal triangular onycholysis or fissure[4] (Fig. 11-2). A filiform hyperkeratosis emerging from the hyponychium may sometimes be observed.

DIFFERENTIAL DIAGNOSIS. Glomus tumor, subungual wart, Bowen's disease, and Darier's disease should be included in the differential diagnosis. Histopathological examination of the lesion is necessary to exclude Bowen's disease.

TREATMENT. Excision of the lesion is not mandatory. Recurrences are frequent if excision is not complete.

Warts

ETIOLOGY. Ungual warts are benign tumors induced by various subtypes of human papillomaviruses (HPV).[5]

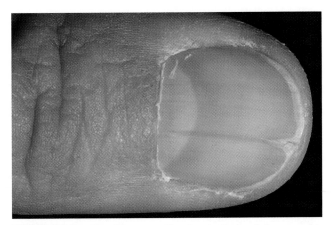

FIGURE 11-2 ■ Distal keratosis. Fine longitudinal red chromonychia is associated with distal triangular onycholysis and fissure.

PATHOLOGY. The histological features of common warts include acanthosis, papillomatosis, and parakeratosis. Vacuolated cells (koilocytes) are found in the upper epidermis.

DIAGNOSIS. When the nail apparatus is involved, the periungual skin is usually the first site of infection. Any other part can secondarily be involved. Nail bed involvement may lead to onycholysis and subungual keratosis. In the case of posterior nail fold infection, longitudinal grooving may rarely appear, and contiguous matrix involvement may be responsible for longitudinal leukonychia (Fig. 11-3). Lateral nail plate destruction is rare. Distal phalangeal bone erosion may be secondary to long-standing verruca vulgaris.

Most of the time, the diagnosis is readily made on clinical grounds. Early squamous cell carcinoma (SCC) may be indistinguishable from a common wart. Biopsy and histopathological examination is mandatory in the immunocompromised host, in atypical warts, and in long-standing warts that are unresponsive to conventional treatments. HPV subtyping should be obtained if the patient's immune status is suspect.

DIFFERENTIAL DIAGNOSIS. The main differential diagnosis is early SCC.

TREATMENT. A few points should be highlighted: treatments do not eliminate latent or subclinical infection, and aggressive, potentially scarring procedures should be avoided for asymptomatic warts.[6]

In cases of matrix or nail bed involvement, nail plate section and avulsion is a prerequisite.

Therapeutic modalities are numerous, and most necessitate repeated treatments at 2- to 6-week intervals.[6] The most widely used first-line treatments are cryotherapy and keratolysis. Various caustics, electrosurgery, and curettage are time-honored alternatives. Carbon dioxide laser vaporization and intralesional injections of bleomycin (not approved by the U.S. Food and Drug Administration) give excellent results in expert hands. Use of etretinate or acitretin may be considered for multiple refractory warts. Evolving treatments include interferons, photodynamic therapy, various types of lasers, and induction of delayed-type hypersensitivity.[6] Inappropriate treatments include fluorouracil under occlusion and intralesional injections of bleomycin at concentrations higher than 0.5 U/mL.

Malignant

Bowen's Disease and Squamous Cell Carcinoma

ETIOLOGY. Bowen's disease is an SCC in situ. Left untreated, 3% to 5% of the patients may develop invasive SCC.[7]

There is emerging evidence that SCC of the nail apparatus is linked to oncogenic subtypes of HPV that are generally associated with neoplasms of the anogenital tract—mostly HPV-16.[8] Exposure to x-rays has been associated with digital SCC; arsenic, trauma, and chronic infections have also been cited as possible etiological factors.

PATHOLOGY. The epidermis is acanthotic with marked parakeratotic hyperkeratosis. Anaplasia and disarray involves its entire thickness. Many epidermal cells are atypical, dyskeratotic, multinucleated, pyknotic, or necrotic or contain large hyperchromatic nuclei. Mitoses are noted.[7]

Invasive SCC shows irregular masses of epidermal squamous cells that proliferate downward into the dermis, subcutaneous tissues, or even bone.

DIAGNOSIS. There is often a long delay in diagnosis (5 to 7 years). Lesions are most often diagnosed in the sixth decade. The fingers (thumbs especially) are more commonly affected than the toes. Lesions are often monodactylous, but polydactylous Bowen's disease has been reported.

The following clinical features have been associated with early-evolving SCC: scaling and onycholysis that are disproportional to the verrucous changes,[7] periungual pigmented scaling (Fig. 11–4), lateral onycholysis with erosion of the nail bed (Fig. 11–5), and longitudinal melanonychia. Other features of digital SCC may include periungual swelling and acropachy, hyperkeratotic tumors and plaques, crusts, nail plate dystrophy, and

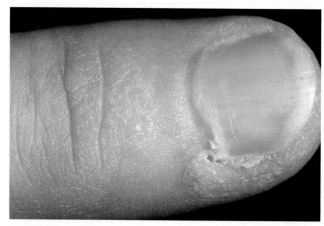

FIGURE 11–5 ■ Bowen's disease. Distolateral onycholysis with periungueal scaling.

paronychia. An adequate biopsy specimen should be obtained to make the correct diagnosis.

When a diagnosis of SCC of the nail apparatus is made, the following steps are recommended: (1) radiography of the affected digit to evaluate bone invasion; (2) complete cutaneous and digital examination to search for a polydactylous process; (3) HPV subtyping; (4) genital examination of the patient and the patient's sexual partners[8]; and (5) investigation of the patient's immune functions.[8]

The prognosis of SCC is encouraging despite the frequent delay in diagnosis. Evolution is mostly local, and there is a very low risk of distant metastasis.

DIFFERENTIAL DIAGNOSIS. The following diagnoses may be discussed: chronic paronychia, ingrown nail, keratoacanthoma, malignant melanoma, pyogenic granuloma, subungual exostosis, and verruca vulgaris.

TREATMENT. As for warts, no mode of treatment ensures eradication of oncogenic HPV. For most authors, Mohs' micrographic surgery is the treatment of choice.[7] Patients with early SCC may benefit from laser vaporization. SCC invasive to the bone requires amputation of the distal phalanx. After surgery, patients should undergo regular follow-up examinations.

MELANOCYTIC TUMORS

Longitudinal Melanonychia

ETIOLOGY. Longitudinal melanonychia (LM) manifests as a tan, brownish, or black longitudinal stripe of the nail plate that results from increased melanin deposition.[9] Pseudo-LM, which results from dyschromia of the nail bed, may simulate this condition (i.e., splinter hemorrhages, onychomycosis, foreign bodies). LM has numerous causes (Table 11–2) that may often be recognized by a careful medical history, clinical examination, and selected diagnostic tests. Because LM has been recognized as an early sign of malignant melanoma, a biopsy should be performed when its cause is not apparent.[9]

PATHOLOGY. In a study concerning "idiopathic" mono-

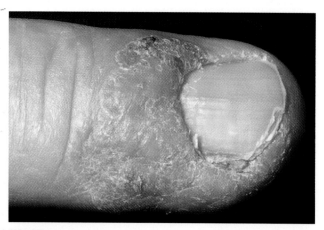

FIGURE 11–4 ■ Bowen's disease. Posterior nail fold pigmented scaling is associated with fissuring of a lateral nail sulcus.

TABLE 11–2 ■ Possible Causes of Longitudinal Melanonychia (LM)

Polydactylous LM	Monodactylous LM
Drugs and chemicals	Neoplastic
Antibiotics: cyclines, sulfona-	Melanocytic
mide	Malignant melanoma
Antimalarials	Melanocytic hyperplasia
Antineoplastic drugs	Nevus
β-blocking agents: timolol	Nonmelanocytic
Heavy metals: arsenic, gold,	Bowen's disease
mercury	Myxoid cyst
Ketoconazole	Wart
Phenothiazine	Pseudo-LM
Psoralen	Hemorrhage
Zidovudine	Foreign body
Endocrine	Onychomycosis
Corticotropin therapy	
Tumors producing corticotropin	
or melanocyte-stimulating	
hormone	
Addison's disease	
Hyperthyroidism	
Pregnancy	
Ethnic	
Dark-skinned persons	
Genetic	
Peutz-Jeghers syndrome	
Infectious	
Onychomycosis	
Inflammatory	
Lichen planus	
Lichen striatus	
Metabolic and nutritional	
Hemochromatosis	
Hemosiderosis	
Kwashiorkor	
Vitamin B_{12} deficiency	
Miscellaneous	
Laugier-Hunziker syndrome	
Carpal tunnel syndrome	
Radiation	
Trauma	
Acute	
Chronic: self-inflicted,	
onychomania	

dactylous melanonychia in Caucasians,[10] histopathology showed melanocyte activation in two thirds of the patients, nevus in 22%, melanocyte hyperplasia in 8%, and malignant melanoma in 5%.

DIAGNOSIS. The diagnosis of LM requires the following steps:

• Careful medical history, clinical examination, and adequate diagnostic tests to exclude medical causes known to produce LM or pseudo-LM.
• Punch biopsy of the matrical origin of any adult monodactylous melanonychia that does not receive adequate explanation.
• When there is a high index of suspicion for a malignant melanoma (age ≥50, large band >5 mm, Hutchinson's sign, recent enlargement or modification), complete surgical excision of the lesion.
• For polydactylous melanonychia or monodactylous melanonychia in a child, follow-up and photographing at regular intervals of any single band that is clinically

suspected to be malignant melanoma with biopsy in case of color modifications or gradual enlargement.
• Complete surgical excision if the biopsy shows an increase in the number of melanocytes.[10]

DIFFERENTIAL DIAGNOSIS. The many causes that may be responsible for LM are listed in Table 11–2.

TREATMENT. Treatment of neoplastic melanonychia is reviewed later.

Benign Melanocytic Tumors

Melanocytic Nevus and Lentigo of the Nail Apparatus

ETIOLOGY. Melanocytic nevus of the nail apparatus is a benign neoplasm derived from melanocytes.

PATHOLOGY. Junctional nevus shows melanocytes arranged in nests at the dermoepidermal junction.[10] Compound nevus shows melanocytes that are present both in nests at the dermoepidermal junction and in aggregates at the papillary dermis.[10] Lentigo shows melanocyte hyperplasia, with an increase in the number of melanocytes among basal onychocytes.[10]

DIAGNOSIS. The clinical aspects of nail matrix nevus (NMN) are often indistinguishable from those of malignant melanoma.[10] NMN may be congenital or acquired. Among adults, NMN appears in the third decade. The thumb and the great toe are affected in about two thirds of cases. NMN manifests as a monodactylous LM (Fig. 11–6) that is most often wide (mean width 4 mm, totally black nail in 15% of the patients).[10] The color is dark brown in two thirds of the cases, sometimes with linear streaks of hyperpigmentation; a light brown color is noted in one third of the patients.[10] Nail plate alterations, Hutchinson's sign, and gradual enlargement or fading are more rarely reported.[10]

DIFFERENTIAL DIAGNOSIS. The clinical differential diagnosis of NMN is that of LM.

TREATMENT. Because it is not possible to adequately differentiate NMN from early evolving malignant mela-

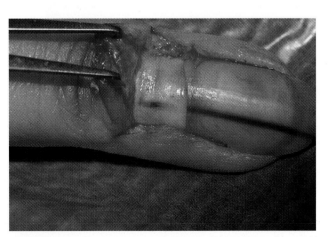

FIGURE 11–6 ■ Nevus. Fine longitudinal melanonychia. Reflection of the posterior nail fold permits an easy visualization of the lesion, which is then excised.

noma of the nail apparatus (MMNA) on clinical grounds or on partial biopsy, the diagnostic steps proposed in the LM diagnosis section should be followed to ascertain that LM is produced by an increase in the number of melanocytes. When histology of the punch biopsy shows melanocyte hyperplasia or a nevus, a complete surgical excision of the suspected NMN is usually recommended in adults.[10]

Malignant Melanoma of the Nail Apparatus

ETIOLOGY. MMNA is a malignant neoplasm derived from melanocytes. MMNA represents 2% to 3% of all melanomas in Caucasians and about 20% of those in dark-skinned races.

PATHOLOGY. Histological types of MMNA, in order of descending frequency, are acral lentiginous malignant melanoma, superficial spreading malignant melanoma, and nodular malignant melanoma.

DIAGNOSIS. MMNA is most frequently diagnosed in the sixth decade; women are more frequently affected than men. The thumb and great toe are most often concerned.[11–14] Much attention has been drawn to early detection of MMNA. Clinically, malignant melanoma in situ of the nail apparatus manifests as a large LM (≥7 mm) (Fig. 11–7) or a nail that is totally black. The diagnosis is rarely made when the band is thin. Pigmentation of the periungual tissue, Hutchinson's sign, is frequent but inconstant and not pathognomonic.[15] Progressive widening of the band is an almost constant feature. A band width that is greater proximally than distally indicates a rapid growth rate (Fig. 11–8). Light brown bands may be seen, but the color of the band is more often dark, with variegated colors and multiple fine, linear streaks of denser hyperpigmentation.[14] Brown-black

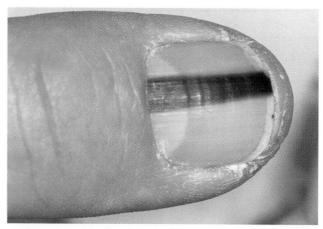

FIGURE 11–8 ■ Malignant melanoma (acral lentiginous malignant melanoma; Breslow tumor thickness, 0.6 mm). There is a large longitudinal melanonychia that is wider at its base, a good indicator of rapid growth.

macular pigmentation of the nail may indicate malignant melanoma of the nail bed. Late signs may include destruction of the nail plate or fissure, tumor, granulation tissue (pigmented or not), ulceration of the nail bed associated with onycholysis or destruction of the nail plate, infection, bleeding, or pain.[14] Amelanotic malignant melanoma accounts for 15% to 25% of MMNAs (Fig. 11–9). The prognosis of these lesions is essentially related to their Breslow tumor thickness and Clarke level of invasion. Because of the typical delay in diagnosis, tumors are usually thick at presentation, and as a consequence the mortality rate is high.

DIFFERENTIAL DIAGNOSIS. In cases of LM, the many causes of benign LM and pseudo-LM should be kept in mind. The most constant features that differentiate malignant melanoma from benign LM are onset in the sixth decade, width greater than 5 mm, progressive enlargement, and Hutchinson's sign. Diagnosis of amelanotic melanoma is difficult; it should be suspected in case

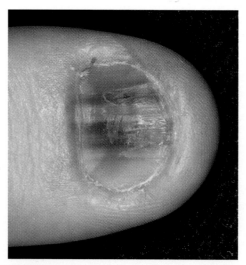

FIGURE 11–7 ■ Malignant melanoma in situ. Typical aspect of malignant melanoma of the thumb, very large longitudinal melanonychia with variegated colors and multiple hyperpigmented streaks. There is no Hutchinson's sign.

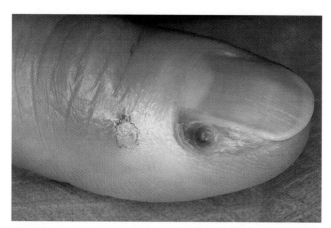

FIGURE 11–9 ■ Amelanotic nodular malignant melanoma (Breslow tumor thickness, 2.8 mm). Pyogenic granuloma–like nodular melanoma.

of monodactylous onycholysis, pyogenic granuloma of the nail apparatus, ingrown nail, and chronic nail infection.

TREATMENT. Early diagnosis and surgical removal of MMNA is necessary to improve currently poor survival rates. Initial assessment, staging, and follow-up are similar to that for melanomas at other skin sites. Wide local surgical excision of the lesion is recommended. There are no clear surgical guidelines. For malignant melanoma in situ, we recommend complete excision of the nail apparatus to the underlying bone, followed by a full-thickness graft. For invasive malignant melanoma, amputation of the digit or toe is required. In one study,[11] there was no difference in survival between patients treated with local proximal interphalangeal joint amputation compared with those having more proximal amputations; another work seems to confirm this view.[12] Provided that adequate excision of the lesion is performed, the level of amputation is chosen to obtain the best functional outcome. Therapeutic lymphadenectomy is advised when there is clinical evidence of metastatic disease in regional lymph nodes.

Dermal and Subcutaneous Tumors

TUMORS OF THE SUPPORTING TISSUES

Benign

Fibromas

ETIOLOGY. Fibromas are benign tumors of the connective tissue. Acral fibrokeratoma (AFK), Koenen's tumor, and dermatofibroma are the main forms that have been described.[16] AFK may be post-traumatic; Koenen's tumors develop in almost half of patients with tuberous sclerosis; dermatofibroma appears spontaneously.[16]

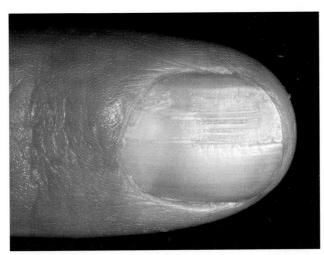

FIGURE 11–10 ■ Acral fibrokeratoma (AFK). There is a longitudinal, irregular grooving of the superficial nail plate, indicating matrix and dorsal nail fold AFK before its exteriorization from the undersurface of the proximal nail fold.

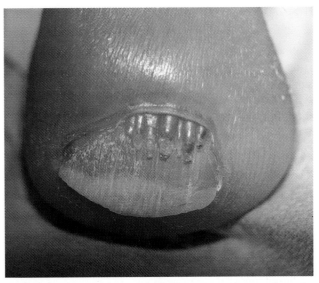

FIGURE 11–11 ■ Typical acral fibrokeratoma originating from the matrix and dorsal nail fold.

PATHOLOGY. The tumor is composed to varying degrees of collagen, fibroblasts, and capillaries. Slight differences are recognized among the three types of fibromas.

DIAGNOSIS. AFKs and dermatofibromas may be localized on the periungual skin, in the nail matrix and dorsal nail fold, or in the nail bed.[16]

Nail matrix and dorsal nail fold (Figs. 11–10 and 11–11) is the most common location for these three types of fibromas. The elongated, conical, flesh-colored tumor (which has been compared with a garlic clove in appearance) emerges from the undersurface of the proximal nail fold. Matrix compression may induce nail plate thinning or a longitudinal groove.[16]

Nail bed AFK and dermatofibroma appear as nodular tumors uplifting the nail plate.[16]

Periungual AFK appears as a keratotic papule or nodule with a peripheric collarette. Periungual dermatofibromas look similar but lack the peripheral epidermal collarette (Fig. 11–12).[16]

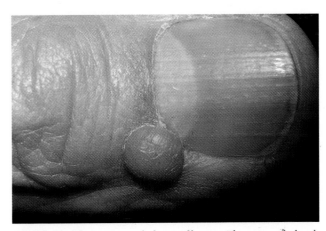

FIGURE 11–12 ■ Periungual dermatofibroma. There is a flesh-colored, semispherical nodule of the posterior nail fold.

DIFFERENTIAL DIAGNOSIS. Myxoid cyst, keloid, recurring digital fibrous tumor of childhood, Bowen's disease, eccrine poroma, exostosis, fibrosarcoma, pyogenic granuloma, and verruca vulgaris may be considered. High-resolution MRI may differentiate a myxoid cyst from an early evolving matrix fibroma. Histopathological confirmation is mandatory.

TREATMENT. Simple surgical excision is the treatment of choice. Tumors of the matrix and ventral nail fold are excised after reflection of the proximal nail fold. Nail bed tumors need nail plate avulsion before removal.

VASCULAR TUMORS

Benign

Glomus Tumor

ETIOLOGY. Glomus tumors are benign hamartomatous proliferations of the glomus body.

PATHOLOGY. The encapsulated tumors contain numerous vascular lumina lined by endothelial cells and many layers of glomus cells.

DIAGNOSIS. Glomus tumors are rare, accounting for 1% to 4% of tumors of the hand; three fourths of glomus tumors occur on the hand.[17] The subungual location is the most common, but the tumors may appear in the pulp or in the lateral or proximal folds.[17] A solitary tumor is the rule, but multiple localizations have been described.[17] The diagnosis usually is made in the fifth decade. Pain and temperature sensitivity are the hallmarks of glomus tumors. Pain radiates proximally and is exacerbated by cold, trauma, or pinpoint pressure. Subungual tumors may appear as bluish or red macules visible through the nail plate, longitudinal red chromonychias, or distal fissures (Fig. 11–13).[17] Tumefaction or localized destruction of the nail plate may be caused by long-standing lesions. Tumors of the periungual tissues are invisible or rarely present as a localized subcutaneous tumefaction. Radiographs may show an erosion of the distal phalanx resulting from prolonged pressure. MRI is the imaging method of choice. T1-weighted images (Fig. 11–14) show an ovoid, isointense lesion homogeneously enhanced with gadolinium injection; T2-weighted images show a hyperintense lesion.[18]

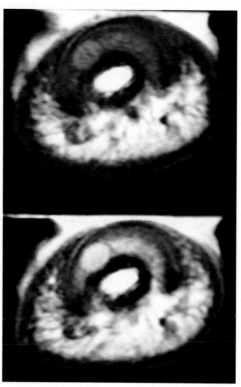

FIGURE 11–14 ■ Glomus tumor. T1-weighted images from high-resolution magnetic resonance imaging studies show an isointense subungual lesion that is homogeneously enhanced with gadolinium injection.

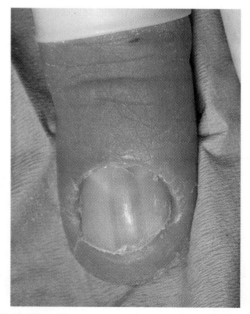

FIGURE 11–13 ■ Glomus tumor. There is a longitudinal red chromonychia associated with pain and temperature sensitivity.

DIFFERENTIAL DIAGNOSIS. Histopathological examination is mandatory to differentiate glomus tumors from other subungual tumors of the nail apparatus.

TREATMENT. Surgical excision is recommended. High-resolution MRI and the pain elicited by pinpoint pressure help to localize the tumor precisely.

Pyogenic Granuloma

ETIOLOGY. Pyogenic granuloma (PG) is a reactive process that occurs after dermal injury. Trauma, ingrown toenail, and retinoid treatment are the most common causes of PG of the nail apparatus.

PATHOLOGY. Early PG fulfills criteria for granulation tissue. Mature lesions are indistinguishable from a capillary hemangioma: there is endothelial proliferation with capillary lumina, covered by a flattened epithelium. Fibrosis is present at later stages.

DIAGNOSIS. Periungual PG usually manifests as a fleshy, ulcerated, sessile papulonodule, often surrounded by an epidermal collarette. Location in the lateral nail fold of the great toe is usually associated with an ingrowing toenail.

Nail bed PG manifests as a reddish macular discoloration seen throughout the nail plate and associated with onycholysis. Nail plate section is mandatory to visualize, biopsy, and treat the lesion.

DIFFERENTIAL DIAGNOSIS. Amelanotic malignant melanoma, ulcerated SCC, and other ulcerated tumors may be considered. Hyponychial PG located on the toe may be secondary to subungual exostosis, to be ruled out by radiographic examination. Pseudo-PG and cavernous hemangioma are possible diagnoses. Histopathological examination is always mandatory.

TREATMENT. Any provocative cause should be relieved (e.g., ingrown nail, retinoid). Shave or punch excision or electrodissection followed by slight electrodessication of the base is curative. Carbon dioxide laser treatment may be used.

BONE, ARTICULATION, AND TENDON TUMORS

Benign

Subungual Exostosis

ETIOLOGY. Subungual exostosis is a benign osteocartilaginous outgrowth. Trauma and genetic predisposition are possible etiological factors. Though there is still some debate, osteochondroma is probably the same tumor.

PATHOLOGY. The lesion is made of mature trabecular bone covered by a cartilage cap.

DIAGNOSIS. Subungual exostosis, one of the most common tumors of the toes, is rare on the digits. Young adults are most often affected. A history of trauma is frequent. The hallux is the usual location; lesser toes are more rarely involved. Typically, the lesion presents as a dorsomedial, flesh-colored, hard, painful tumefaction (Fig. 11–15). It emerges from the hyponychium, elevates the nail plate, or may appear in the nail sulcus. Centrodorsal lesions may appear as red macular discolorations of the nail bed associated with onycholysis, and

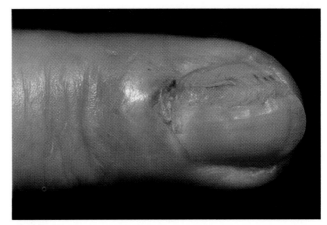

FIGURE 11–16 ■ Typical myxoid cyst.

nail avulsion may reveal a PG-like outgrowth. Digital x-ray examination usually is sufficient to confirm the diagnosis. It shows a sessile or pedunculated expansion of trabecular bone covered with radiolucent cartilage. Biopsy of the lesion is easy and diagnostic.

DIFFERENTIAL DIAGNOSIS. Enchondroma, pyogenic granuloma, verruca vulgaris, onychoclavus, acral periungual fibrokeratoma, subungual dermatofibroma, SCC, and amelanotic malignant melanoma may be considered.

TREATMENT. Nail avulsion and nail bed incision are necessary to expose the tumor, which is then cut at its base with a chisel and curetted from the distal phalanx.

Myxoid Cyst

ETIOLOGY. Myxoid cysts are the most common hand tumors. It seems that they represent a reactive process caused by degenerative osteoarthritis, although this is a debated issue.

PATHOLOGY. The jellylike fluid is composed of mucin and stains pale blue with hematoxylin-eosin.

DIAGNOSIS. Myxoid cysts mostly occur in middle-aged

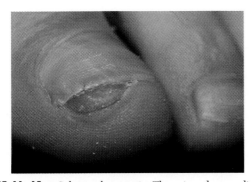

FIGURE 11–15 ■ Subungual exostosis. There is a dorsomedial, hard tumefaction that elevates the nail plate.

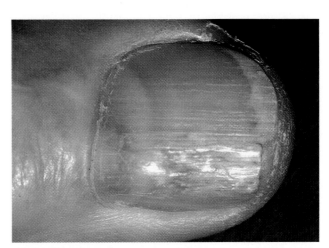

FIGURE 11–17 ■ Subungual myxoid cyst with tumefaction of the lunular area associated with nail plate dystrophy.

patients. These lesions usually are located between the distal interphalangeal crease and the cuticle. In this location, they manifest as dome-shaped, skin-colored or translucent nodules. Distal lesions may be crusted (Fig. 11–16). Inflammatory bouts may cause rapid expansion of the cyst. Secondary infectious arthritis is rare. Nail dystrophy is secondary to matrix compression. A longitudinal, irregular nail groove is frequently observed. Cyst puncturing allows evacuation of the viscous fluid. Subungual myxoid cysts are rarer and difficult to diagnose. They manifest as a tumefaction or a macular dyschromia visible through the nail plate, which may be altered (Fig. 11–17). High-resolution MRI usually permits the diagnosis.

DIFFERENTIAL DIAGNOSIS. Periungual myxoid cysts may be confused with subungual fibromas before their exteriorization. Subungual myxoid cyst mimics any subungual tumor.

TREATMENT. Periungual lesions are best treated by radical surgery to avoid recurrences. Excision of the cyst and curettage of any osteophyte surrounding the joint is the method of choice.

■ ■ ■

TUMORS OF THE PILOSEBACEOUS UNIT

ELKE-INGRID GRUSSENDORF-CONEN

Tumors of the pilosebaceous unit comprise a heterogeneous group of cutaneous cysts, plaques, and nodules. They are relatively rare, and their gross morphological appearance is commonly not characteristic. The clinical history is that of one or more slowly growing cutaneous or subcutaneous nodules. The great majority of these tumors are not diagnosed as such until after excision and histological study.

Depending on the degree of differentiation of the constituent cells and the final development toward which they are directed (hair, sebaceous gland, apocrine gland), these tumors are classified into several groups (Table 11–3). Hyperplasias are composed of mature structures, whereas adenomas show less differentiation, and benign epitheliomas less still.

Carcinomas are rare but nevertheless do occur. The majority of skin appendage tumors are locally invasive but do not metastasize. One of the exceptions to this rule is sebaceous gland carcinomas (discussed later).

It is not possible to state confidently in every case which particular part of an appendage, or even which cutaneous appendage, a tumor is differentiating from or toward. Immunohistochemical and moleculochemical methods and ultrastructural examination must be used in addition to special stains in conventionally processed material to try to assign as many of these appendage tumors as possible.[19, 20] Currently there is considerable interest in the use of monoclonal antibodies to keratins of various molecular weights, to epithelial membrane antigen (EMA), and to carcinoembryonic antigen (CEA). Both EMA and CEA are positive in sweat gland lesions but negative in hair follicle tumors, a difference that is of value in distinguishing between the two, and also occasionally in distinguishing malignant skin appendage tumors from metastatic lesions from other body sites.[21]

The complex structure and the multicentric appearance of some of these neoplasms and malformations may be explained by the assumption that they derive from pluripotent follicular stem cells, located in the bulge region of the hair follicle.[22, 23] A large number of tumors are reported, arising from the different appendage structures depending on the exact type of cell and its situation within the dermis. For complete and detailed pathological descriptions, see the bibliography of key articles in this field. Only those cysts and tumors that have a clinical aspect of common interest or are

TABLE 11-3 ■ Classification of Tumors of the Pilosebaceous Unit (Including Nevi and Cysts)

Type of Differentiation	Hair	Sebaceous	Apocrine
Complete (hyperplasias, harmatomas)	Hair nevus Becker's nevus	Sebaceous nevus	
Distinct but incomplete (adenomas)	Trichofolliculoma	Sebaceous adenoma	Apocrine cystadenoma Syringocystadenoma papilliferum
Rudimentary (epitheliomas)	Trichoepithelioma Pilomatricoma Trichilemmal tumor Trichilemmal cyst	Sebaceous epithelioma Steatocystoma multiplex (Sebaceous carcinoma)	Cylindroma

highly associated with internal disease (i.e., part of a syndrome) are described here.

In most cases, surgical removal is the best treatment.

Tumors with Hair Differentiation

HAIR NEVUS
(Synonym: hair follicle nevus)

A hair nevus, or hair follicle nevus, is simply an excessive concentration of normal hair follicles. It may appear in infancy and consists of a small nodule on the face.

Histologically, there are numerous small, well-differentiated hair follicles, occasionally accompanied by a few tiny sebaceous glands.

BECKER'S NEVUS
(Synonym: pigmented hairy epidermal nevus)

Becker's nevus is an uncommon organoid lesion with male predominance. Initially manifesting as a light- to dark-brown, enlarging macular lesion, it appears usually in the second decade and subsequently shows hypertrichosis (Fig. 11–18). Frequently the chest, shoulder, or upper arm is involved. Of importance is the occasional association with anomalies such as breast hypoplasia and spina bifida.

Histologically, hyperpigmentation of the basal cell layer and melanophages but no nevus cells are observed. The hairs are mature and appear normal.

TRICHOFOLLICULOMA

This tumor occurs in adults as a solitary, small, dome-shaped nodule, usually on the face but sometimes on the neck or scalp. There may exist a central pore with a wisp of wool like white hairs protruding from it.

Histologically, the tumors are variable in appearance. Some are dominated by cellular hair bulb–like structures, others form mature hairs, and all have a characteristic cellular stroma.

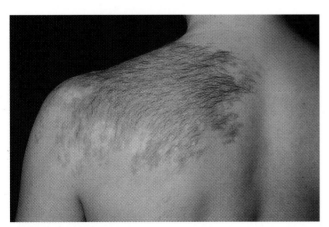

FIGURE 11–18 ■ Becker's nevus.

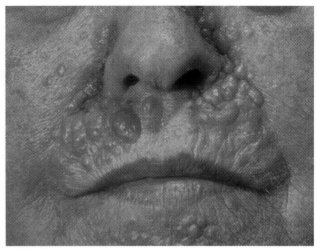

FIGURE 11–19 ■ Epithelioma adenoides cysticum.

TRICHOEPITHELIOMA
(Synonyms: epithelioma adenoides cysticum, Brooke's tumor, benign cystic epithelioma)

Clinically the tumor can be divided into two types, in which the lesions are either single or multiple and symmetrically distributed (Fig. 11–19). Multiple trichoepithelioma is transmitted as an autosomal dominant trait. The first lesions appear in childhood and gradually increase in number. They are small, rounded, and rather translucent nodules located mainly on the face but occasionally also on the scalp, neck, and upper trunk.

Histologically, the well-circumscribed lesions consist of small, dark cells, often with a degree of peripheral palisading surrounding a central area of eosinophilic amorphous material. At times, differentiation to rudimentary hair roots is apparent in some areas. The epithelial elements are enclosed by a well-developed fibrous stroma. There is no sharp boundary between trichoepithelioma and basalioma.

PILOMATRICOMA
(Synonym: calcifying epithelioma of Malherbe)

Pilomatricoma is a relatively uncommon tumor with differentiation toward hair cells, particularly hair cortex cells. It may arise at any age, but the lesion is more common in the young. It occurs predominantly on the face and scalp, usually as a solitary dermal nodule, 0.3 to 3.0 cm in diameter, which grows slowly. The consistency may vary from smooth or firm to stony-hard.

Histologically, the tumor is seen deep in the dermis surrounded by a condensed pseudocapsule of fibrous tissue. Irregularly shaped islands show two main types of epithelial cells, basophilic cells and shadow cells. The basophilic cells have deeply basophilic nuclei and scanty cytoplasm. The more mature cells, located toward the center of the tumor islands, show a gradual loss of their nuclei and finally appear as faint eosinophilic shadow cells. The central areas often calcify and occasionally

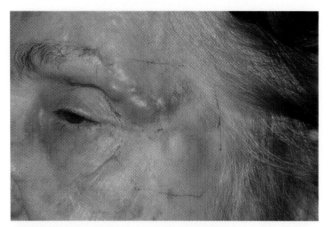

FIGURE 11-20 ■ Proliferating trichilemmal tumor.

ossify. The stroma reaction, which closely follows the epithelial foldings, usually contains inflammatory and foreign-body giant cells in the vicinity of the shadow cells.

PILAR TUMOR OF THE SCALP
(Synonyms: proliferating trichilemmal tumor, hair matrix tumor, proliferating epidermoid cyst)

This usually solitary tumor occurs almost exclusively on the scalp of elderly women and starts as a subcutaneous nodule like a wen (Fig. 11–20). The tumor grows into a large, elevated, lobulated mass that may undergo ulceration.

Histologically, pilar tumors of the scalp consist of variably sized lobules composed of squamous epithelium undergoing abrupt change into amorphous keratin, as seen in the cavity of trichilemmal cysts.

MULTIPLE TRICHILEMMOMAS
(Synonyms: Cowden's syndrome, multiple harmatoma syndrome)

Multiple trichilemmomas are diagnostic of Cowden's (multiple harmatoma) syndrome. This is an autosomal dominant, rare condition manifesting variable expressivity. The trichilemmomas consist of nonspecific, flesh-colored, pink or brown papules located mainly around the mouth, nose, and ears. Their importance lies in the fact that they precede the development of breast cancer in women with Cowden's disease. The diagnosis of tricholemmomas should therefore stimulate the search for other evidence of Cowden's syndrome, including the characteristic cobblestoned appearance of the oral epithelium and multiple skin tags.

Histologically, multiple small, clear cells are seen with surrounding palisading cells. Keratinization is usually minimal, superficial, and epidermoid.

TRICHILEMMAL CYST
(Synonyms: pilar cyst, sebaceous cyst, pilosebaceous cyst, hair cyst)

Trichilemmal cysts occur exclusively on the scalp and have the same clinical appearance as atheromas (Fig. 11–21). They appear as firm, smooth, yellow-walled nodules and are easy to enucleate. Frequently, they occur as multiple lesions and may be inherited as an autosomal dominant trait. Women are seven times more frequently affected than men.

Histologically, the wall consists of epithelial cells that possess no clearly visible intercellular bridge and do not seem to keratinize (Fig. 11–22).

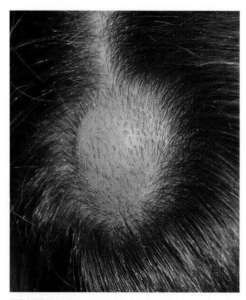

FIGURE 11-21 ■ Trichilemmal cyst.

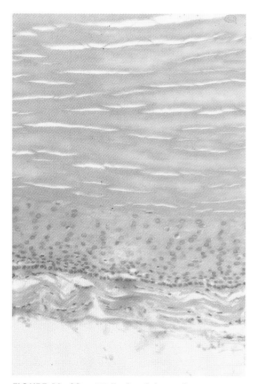

FIGURE 11-22 ■ Wall of trichilemmal cyst.

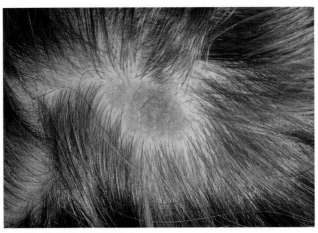

FIGURE 11–23 ■ Sebaceous nevus.

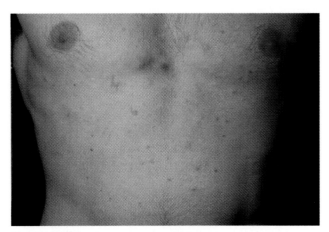

FIGURE 11–24 ■ Steatocystoma multiplex.

Tumors with Sebaceous Differentiation

SEBACEOUS NEVUS

The sebaceous nevus usually arises on the scalp or face, forming a conglomeration of gray or yellow nodules (Fig. 11–23). The lesions are present at birth or appear early in life. In adulthood several other tumors may develop in a sebaceous nevus, such as syringocystadenoma papilliferum or basal cell carcinoma. Occasionally sebaceous nevus may be associated with cerebral abnormalities, including epilepsy and mental retardation.

Histologically, large groups of sebaceous gland lobules occur within the dermis, with normal appearance. The development of the hair follicle, however, is incomplete. Also, apocrine sweat gland abnormalities may be found in the same region.

SEBACEOUS ADENOMA

The rare sebaceous adenoma occurs as a rounded, flesh-colored nodule approximately 0.5 to 1 cm in diameter, usually located on the face and neck of an older person. In some cases the occurrence of sebaceous adenomas leads to the diagnosis of Torre-Muir syndrome, which includes both multiple sebaceous tumors and multiple visceral carcinomas.

Histologically, the well-circumscribed tumor shows an increased number of sebaceous gland lobules that are irregular in size and shape and incompletely differentiated. The proportions of immature, transitional, and mature sebaceous cells may vary widely from one area to another.

STEATOCYSTOMA MULTIPLEX
(Synonym: sebocystomatosis)

This condition, inherited in an autosomal dominant manner, manifests in adolescence. Although sternal areas are infected most in boys (Fig. 11–24) and the

axillae and groin in girls, the multiple lesions may spread over most of the upper trunk and face. The early small, dome-shaped nodules are rather translucent, changing to a yellowish color with age.

Histologically, corrugated cyst wall lining spaces are revealed. The cyst wall consists of several layers of large, often vacuolated cells (Fig. 11–25). Groups of sebaceous glands or ducts may be imbedded in the wall. Frequently, invaginations resembling hair follicles are present in the wall, and in some instances there are true hair shafts.

SEBACEOUS CARCINOMA

Sebaceous carcinoma is rare and of two types: an aggressive periocular variant and a relatively nonaggressive extraocular form. The extraocular tumors arise most often on the head and neck. The tumor manifests as an ulcerated or nonulcerated nodulocystic lesion resembling a basal cell carcinoma (Fig. 11–26). The mean age at presentation is 54 years.

Histologically, sebaceous carcinoma shows irregularly dispersed lobules of cells with foamy cytoplasm, having

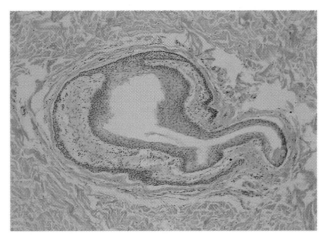

FIGURE 11–25 ■ Wall of a cyst in steatocystoma multiplex.

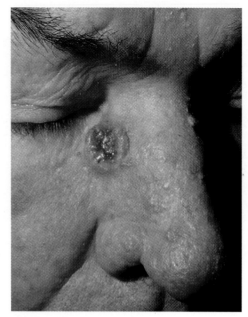

FIGURE 11–26 ■ Sebaceous carcinoma.

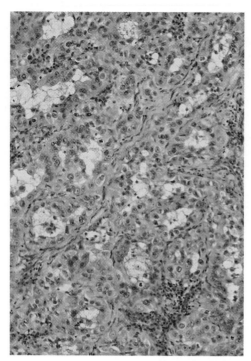

FIGURE 11–27 ■ Histological picture of sebaceous carcinoma.

in addition large numbers of mitotic figures and atypical mitoses (Fig. 11–27). Special staining for lipids is usually positive.

Tumors with Apocrine Differentiation

APOCRINE CYSTADENOMA
(Synonym: hidrocystoma)

Hidrocystomas frequently occur on the face, often in periocular sites, as small, dome-shaped, translucent papules showing a bluish color (Fig. 11–28).

Histologically, there may be several cystic spaces lined by columnar cells showing decapitation secretion and resting on flattened myoepithelial cells. Papillary projections of epithelium may extend into a central cavity.

SYRINGOCYSTADENOMA PAPILLIFERUM

The tumor occurs most commonly on the scalp or face and has been thought to represent an apocrine gland adenoma, although some cases show organoid structures of the eccrine sweat gland. It may be present at birth, or it may arise early in life as a hairless plaque that at puberty becomes larger, nodular, and often verrucous. Some of these tumors have a central umbilication, where a small fistula may discharge some fluid. Occasionally, syringocystadenoma arises within a sebaceous nevus at or after puberty.

Histologically, the lesions consist of papillary structures with a cystic invagination. The papillary structures are lined with a double layer of columnar epithelial cells that show decapitation secretion. The stroma consists of vascular connective tissue containing a dense inflammatory infiltrate in which plasma cells predominate.

CYLINDROMAS
(Synonyms: turban tumors, Spiegler's tumors)

Cylindromas usually appear as multiple nodules on the scalp (Fig. 11–29). The disease is inherited as an autosomal dominant trait, but women are affected about

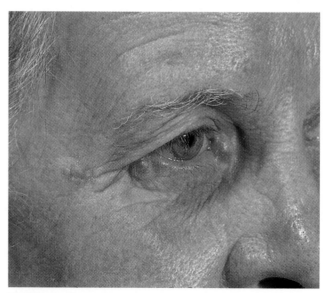

FIGURE 11–28 ■ Hidrocystoma.

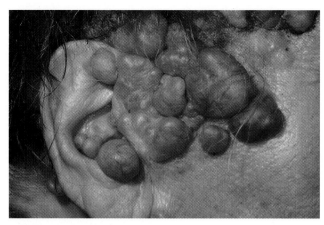

FIGURE 11-29 ■ Cylindromas.

twice as frequently as men. Onset may be in childhood or adolescence but is usually in early adult life. The rate of growth is slow and self-limited. New tumors arise over years. Solitary lesions without familial history may occur in adult life either on the scalp or on the face.

Histologically, cylindromas are composed of multilayered epithelial cell islands surrounded by a dense hyaline membrane. The centrally placed cells have a pale-staining cytoplasm with vesicular nuclei, and these are surrounded by smaller cells with darkly staining oval nuclei. These smaller cells tend to form a palisade where they abut the hyaline membrane.

REFERENCES

1. Cohen PR, Scher RK: Geriatric nail disorders: diagnosis and treatment. J Am Acad Dermatol 26:521–531, 1992.
2. Baran R, Dawber RPR (eds): Disease of the Nails and Their Management. Oxford, Blackwell Scientific Publications, 1994.
3. Baran R, Kint A: Onychomatrixoma: filamentous tufted tumour in the matrix of a funnel-shaped nail. A new entity (report of three cases). Br J Dermatol 126:510–515, 1992.
4. Baran R, Perrin C: Localized multinucleate distal subungual keratosis. Br J Dermatol 133:77–82, 1995.
5. Cobb MW: Human papillomavirus infection. J Am Acad Dermatol 22:547–566, 1990.
6. Drake LA, Ceilley RI, Cornelison RL, et al: Guide line of care for warts: human papillomavirus. J Am Acad Dermatol 32:98–103, 1995.
7. Sau P, McMarlin SL, Sperling LC, Katz R: Bowen's disease of the nail bed and periungual area: a clinicopathologic analysis of seven cases. Arch Dermatol 130:204–209, 1994.
8. Moy R: Significance of human papillomavirus induced squamous cell carcinoma to dermatologists. Arch Dermatol 130:235–237, 1994.
9. Baran R, Kechijian P: Longitudinal melanonychia (melanonychia striata): diagnosis and management. J Am Acad Dermatol 21: 1165–1175, 1989.
10. Tosti A, Baran R, Piraccini BM, Cameli N, Fanti PA: Nail matrix nevi: a clinical and histopathologic study of twenty-two patients. J Am Acad Dermatol 34:765–771, 1996.
11. Park KG, Blessing K, Kernohan NM: Surgical aspects of subungual malignant melanomas: The Scottish Melanoma Group. Ann Surg 216:692–695, 1992.
12. Finley R III, Driscoll DL, Blumenson LE, Karakousis CP: Subungual melanoma: an eighteen-year review. Surgery 116:96–100, 1994.
13. Kato T, Suetake T, Sugiyama Y, Tabata N, Tagami H: Epidemiology and prognosis of subungual melanoma in 34 Japanese patients. Br J Dermatol 134:383–387, 1996.
14. Blessing K, Kernohan NM, Park KG: Subungual malignant melanoma: clinicopathological features of 100 cases. Histopathology 19: 425–429, 1991.
15. Baran R, Kechijian P: Hutchinson's sign: a reappraisal. J Am Acad Dermatol 34:87–90, 1996.
16. Baran R, Perrin C, Baudet J, Requena L: Clinical and histological patterns of dermatofibromas of the nail apparatus. Clin Exp Dermatol 19:31–35, 1994.
17. Glicenstein J, Ohana J, Leclercq C (eds): Tumeurs de la Main. Berlin, Springer Verlag, 1988, p 185.
18. Drape JL, Idy-Peretti I, Goettmann S, et al: Subungual glomus tumors: evaluation with MR imaging. Radiology 195:507–515, 1995.
19. de Viragh PA, Szeimie RM, Eckert F: Apocrine cystadenoma, apocrine hidrocystoma, and eccrine hidrocystoma: three distinct tumors defined by expression of keratins and human milk fat globulin 1. J Cutan Pathol 24:249–255, 1997.
20. Wick MR, Cooper PH, Swanson PE, et al: Microcystic adnexal carcinoma: an immunohistochemical comparison with other cutaneous appendage tumors. Arch Dermatol 126:189–194, 1990.
21. MacKie RM: Skin Cancer, 2nd ed. London, Martin Dunitz, 1996.
22. Lavker RM, Miller S, Wilson C, Cotsarelis G, Wie Z-G, Yang J-S: Hair follicle stem cells: their location, role in hair cycle, and involvement in skin tumor formation. J Invest Dermatol 101(Suppl):16S–26S, 1993.
23. Mehregan AH: The origin of the adnexal tumors of the skin: a viewpoint. J Cutan Pathol 12:459–467, 1985.

BIBLIOGRAPHY

Headington JT: Tumors of the hair follicle: a review. Am J Pathol 85: 480–514, 1976.
Prioleau PG, Santa Cruz DJ: Sebaceous gland neoplasia. J Cutan Pathol 11:396–414, 1984.
Warkel RL: Selected apocrine neoplasms. J Cutan Pathol 11:437–449, 1984.

Pigment Disorders of the Hair and Nails

DESMOND J. TOBIN

EVA M. J. PETERS

KARIN U. SCHALLREUTER

Etiology

Pigmentation disorders of the hair and nail can be of either melanocytic or nonmelanocytic origin.

HAIR

Acquired hypomelanoses are of two types, endogenous induction and exogenous induction. The former group includes age-associated melanocyte loss (e.g., senile canities) and circumscribed poliosis (e.g., alopecia areata, vitiligo). The latter group includes disorders caused by drugs or chemicals (e.g., chloroquine), by nutritional factors (e.g., vitamin B_{12} or iron deficiency), or by endocrine factors (e.g., Cushing's syndrome). Genetic hypomelanoses include albinism, circumscribed poliosis (e.g., piebaldism, Waardenburg's syndrome), and endocrine types (e.g., homocystinuria, sometimes in phenylketonuria).

NAILS

Acquired hypermelanoses of the nail caused by endogenous induction include localized melanocyte activation and nail matrix nevi. Exogenous induction of nail hyper/hypopigmentation may be physical (e.g., subungual hematoma, radiation), neoplastic (e.g., subungual melanoma), toxic or nutritional (e.g., vitamin B_{12} or folic acid deficiency), drug or chemical (e.g., chloroquine), inflammatory (e.g., secondary to lichen planus), endocrine (e.g., Addison's disease), or infectious (e.g., fungal, bacterial, viral). Genetic hypermelanoses involve congenital nevi of the nail.

Clinical Features

HAIR

The clinical features of hair pigmentation disorders can range from hypopigmentation to complete loss of pigment. These changes involve variable areas and changes in texture.

Canities

Graying has a variable course in different body sites. On the head it is first observed in the beard or temples,

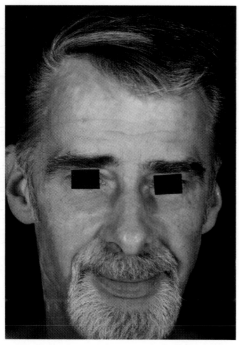

FIGURE 12-1 ■ Senile canities of the beard and of the scalp hair in a 54-year-old man. Note that the majority of the hair in the beard and temples is gray, whereas the rest of the scalp and eyebrow hair still show the original color.

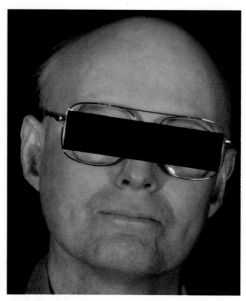

FIGURE 12-2 ■ Progeria in a 34-year-old man. Besides androgenetic alopecia, the remaining hair is completely white. (Courtesy of Dr. H. Mensing, Department of Dermatology, University of Hamburg, Hamburg, Germany.)

followed by crown, occiput, and finally eyebrows (Fig. 12–1). Each follicle is autonomous, experiencing its own graying process. Graying hair may have an increased growth rate, from 0.3 to 1.2 mm per day, in association with altered texture such as larger caliber, stand-on-end trait, or increased medullation.[1] Rarely, spontaneous remission occurs in early stages.[2]

The most common alteration in hair pigmentation is senile canities, involving gradual, age-related loss of hair color. This is observed beginning at 30 to 40 years of age and appears earlier in Caucasians than in blacks. Premature graying occurs before the second decade of life in Caucasians, and before the third decade in blacks.

Pathological early graying is less common. It is observed in vitiligo and in rare syndromes including progeria and pangeria, Böök's syndrome, dystrophia myotonica, Rothmund-Thomson syndrome, and cri du chat syndrome (Fig. 12–2). Canities symptomatica (sometimes associated with rapid graying) has been described after acute fever and together with hyperthyroidism, pernicious anemia, malnutrition, and malignant tumors. Canities subita ("overnight" graying or whitening) is a rare form of alopecia areata observed after severe emotional stress. After diffuse loss of pigmented hair, the remaining white hair is fully revealed, unobscured by pigmented hair shafts.

Exogenous Alteration of Hair Color

Reversible hair pigmentation change can be associated with drug or chemical exposure; blond or red-haired persons are most often affected. Nutritional deficiencies (e.g., kwashiorkor) and iron and vitamin B_{12} deficiencies can turn black hair reddish and brown hair blond.

Circumscribed Poliosis

Poliosis is defined as an inherited or acquired loss of pigment from a group of closely-positioned hair follicles, resulting in a patch of white or hypopigmented hair. Piebaldism, an autosomal dominant genetic disorder, is characterized by a white forelock associated with a diamond-shaped area of depigmentation on the forehead in up to 90% of cases (Fig. 12–3). Waardenburg's syndrome (types I through III) can manifest with sensorineural deafness, partial or total heterochromia iridis, dystopia canthorum, and eyebrow hyperplasia with syno-

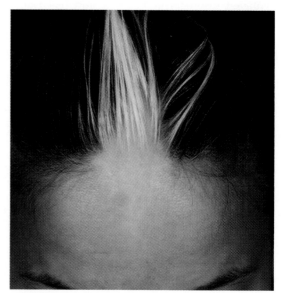

FIGURE 12-3 ■ Piebaldism in a 23-year-old woman, showing white forelock associated with diamond-shaped depigmentation on the forehead.

phrys, piebaldism features, and premature graying. Depigmented areas of the skin at birth are stable thereafter, unlike vitiligo. Clinically, these areas often show hyperpigmented macules of different sizes.

Rare cases of poliosis have been described with Tietze's, Vogt-Koyanagi-Harada, Alezzandrini's, Griscelli, Prader-Willi, and Apert's syndromes; von Recklinghausen's neurofibromatosis; and tuberous sclerosis (Pringle's disease). However, white hair can grow from any depigmented macule. Poliosis is observed with variable frequency in alopecia areata, where spontaneous or induced regrowth of hair is commonly white, regaining the original color with time (Fig. 12–4). Acquired poliosis is in most cases associated with vitiligo. Under Wood's light, the depigmentation of the scalp is demonstrated by the characteristic fluorescence of the pterins, confirming a diagnosis of vitiligo.

Genetic Hypomelanosis

Albinism consists of a group of autosomal recessive diseases that exhibit the congenital reduction or absence of melanin in skin, hair, and eyes. Patients with oculocutaneous albinism have nystagmus, photophobia, and decreased visual acuity. Like the skin color, the hair color can be affected to various degrees, ranging from complete white to red, brown, and dark (Fig. 12–5). The rare Chédiak-Higashi syndrome is additionally characterized by neuropathies, recurrent bacterial infections, and the production of silver-gray or light-blond hair on the scalp. Ectodermal dysplasias are another cause of fine, sparse, brittle hair, for example, in Christ-Siemens-Touraine syndrome (Fig. 12–6). This X-linked syndrome is associated with high intermittent fever in infancy, anodontia or hypodontia, bulbous pear-shaped nose, anhydrosis or hypohydrosis, and skeletal anomalies. The syn-

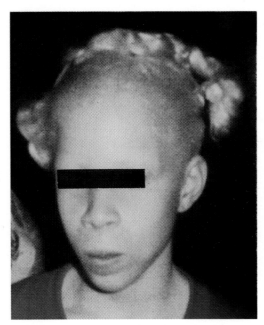

FIGURE 12–5 ■ Hermansky-Pudlak syndrome (occulocutaneous albinism) in a 12-year-old Puerto Rican girl, showing white hair and hypopigmented skin.

drome manifests in two forms, a major one in male patients and a minor one in females.

NAILS

The features associated with the clinical presentation of nail pigmentation disorders include depigmentation, hypopigmentation, or hyperpigmentation; changes in tex-

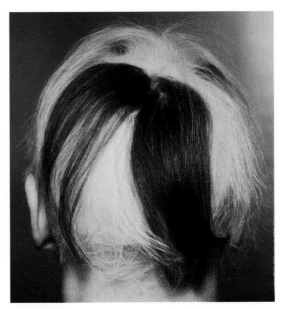

FIGURE 12–4 ■ Alopecia areata in a 38-year-old woman, showing white hair regrowth. (Courtesy of Dr. David A. Fenton, St. Thomas' Hospital, London, England.)

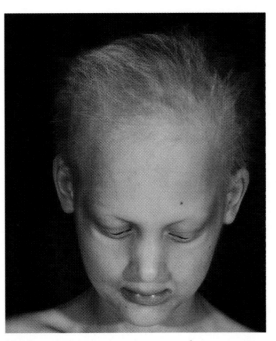

FIGURE 12–6 ■ Christ-Siemens-Touraine syndrome in an 8-year-old girl. Note the sparse, brittle, very fine, hypopigmented hair, the complete alopecia of the eyelashes and brows, and the pear-shaped nose.

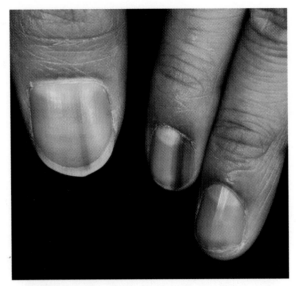

FIGURE 12–7 ■ Longitudinal melanonychia of the nails.

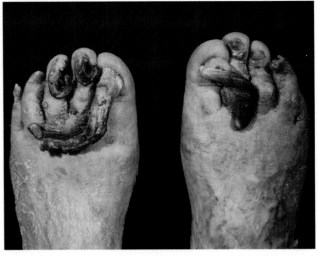

FIGURE 12–8 ■ Extensive "exogenous pigment" and nail deformation caused by neglect or trauma.

ture; variable distribution; and variable palpability. Most commonly they manifest clinically as pigmentary striations of the nail plate, showing considerable racial differences. This longitudinal melanonychia is uncommon in Caucasians, affects 10% to 20% of Japanese and Hispanics, and is frequently observed in aging African-Americans. The hyperpigmented streaks vary in width from 2 to 4 mm. They can be singular or multiple in one person, with colors ranging from brown to black (Fig. 12–7). An associated subcuticular or periungual location of pigment is often described as pseudo-Hutchinson's sign and is visible underneath the transparent cuticle.

Melanocytic Longitudinal Melanonychia

Focal activation of melanocytes may result from melanocyte hyperplasia, yielding a single dark band or nail matrix nevus with variable bands common on fingernails, particularly the thumb. Striae can also be caused by repeated trauma to the nail matrix, such as nail and cuticle biting. Toe trauma associated with ill-fitting footwear or foot deformities can also induce melanonychia at the friction sites (Fig. 12–8). Traumatic melanonychias are sometimes difficult to distinguish from malignancies such as malignant melanoma or Bowen's disease. Radiation, drugs, inflammatory skin diseases (e.g., lichen planus, psoriasis), endocrine disorders (e.g., Addison's disease, Cushing's syndrome, acromegaly), hyperthyroidism, and hormonal changes (e.g., pregnancy, adrenalectomy) can affect the pigmentation of the nails.

Nonmelanocytic Longitudinal Melanonychia

Nutritional deficiencies can result in bluish longitudinal melanonychia, for example in patients with megaloblastic anemia due to vitamin B_{12} deficiency (pernicious anemia) or folic acid deficiency. Melanonychia can also be seen with fungal, bacterial, or viral infections. Some

bacterial spores can produce green-black chromogens (e.g., *Pseudomonas aeruginosa*). Some fungi produce Fontana-Mason–positive pigment (e.g., *Trichophyton rubrum*) or other brownish pigments (e.g., *Aspergillus niger, Alternaria tenuis*). Nonmelanocytic melanonychia has also been observed in patients with the acquired immunodeficiency syndrome (AIDS).

Pathology

HAIR

Hair color is produced by a subpopulation of melanocytes located in the hair bulb which, unlike epidermal melanocytes, exhibit noncontinuous melanogenesis tightly coupled to the hair growth cycle.[3] Hair color depends on (a) the chemical nature of the melanins and the ratio of eumelanin to phaeomelanin, and (b) the number of melanocytes, their activity, and their interaction with precortical keratinocytes. Individual hairs can exhibit a gradual loss of pigment along the hair shaft. Similarly, in rare cases of spontaneous remission of canities in single hairs, the return of pigment is also gradual (Fig. 12–9). These processes are controlled at the gene level or are the result of endogenous or exogenous factors.[3, 4]

Endogenously Induced Hypopigmentation

Pathological changes in senile or premature canities include reduction, abnormality, or loss of hair bulb melanocytes. Differentiated melanocytes are retained in normal numbers in graying hair, as identified by dopa or TRP-1 positivity, but appear to be absent in fully white hair bulbs. However, reliance on differentiated melanocyte markers may miss the presence of undifferentiated cells. Melanocyte degeneration may occur and may

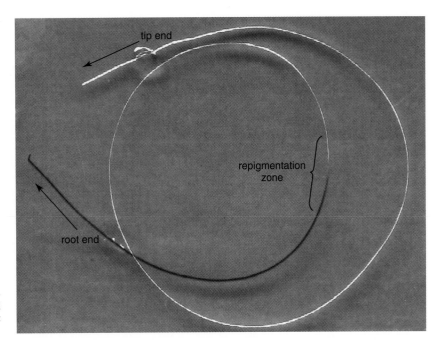

FIGURE 12-9 ■ Spontaneous remission of canities in a single hair shaft. Note that the proximal (bulbar) end is deeply pigmented and the cut distal end is white.

manifest histologically as a spectrum of changes ranging from vacuolation and melanin incontinence to deletion via apoptosis.[5, 6] Similar changes have been reported in alopecia areata, both in the targeted pigmented hair and in regrowing white hair[6] (Figs. 12–10 and 12–11).

Exogenously Induced Hypopigmentation

Drugs and other chemicals can interfere with the melanin pathway and lead to reversible hair hypopigmentation. Chloroquine binds to pheomelanin intermediates and therefore affects primarily blond and red hair.[7] Nutritional deficiency (e.g., kwashiorkor) or metabolic disorders can also lead to pigment dilution, which is reversible on correction of the deficit.

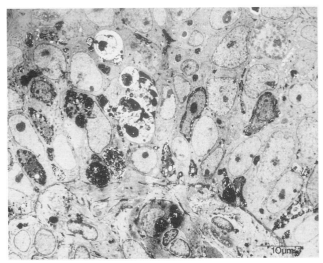

FIGURE 12-10 ■ Hair bulb melanocyte degeneration and melanin incontinence in acute alopecia areata.

Genetic Disorders

Clinical features of the different types of oculocutaneous albinism are based on the extent of skin and hair hypopigmentation. Melanogenesis is completely blocked in tyrosinase-negative albinism, whereas some melanin can be produced in tyrosine-positive albinism (e.g., Hermansky-Pudlak syndrome, Fig. 12–12). Other melanosomal defects occur in the Chédiak-Higashi and Griscelli syndromes, in which melanosome transfer to keratinocytes is affected. Piebaldism is associated with impaired melanocyte maturation and migration in affected hair bulbs.[8] Focal mutations or deletions in the *KIT* gene encoding the receptor for stem cell factor, which is critical for melanocyte proliferation and migration during development, have been identified. Molecular studies of Waardenburg (type I) syndrome also reveal mutations or deletions in the *KIT* gene, whereas the *MITF* (microphthalmia transcription factor) gene is deleted in Waardenburg type II syndrome. Reduced eumelanogenesis and melanocyte loss are observed in Prader-Willi and Angelman's syndromes, in which deletions in the *P* (pink-eyed dilution) gene have been identified (Fig. 12–13).

NAIL

The pathology of nail pigmentation disorders is still in its infancy. Increased numbers of normal or atypical melanocytes do not seem to be the cause of most nail hyperpigmentations. Physiologically, matrix melanocytes are not very productive, but melanin synthesis and dendricity can be upregulated by a variety of stimuli. Melanocyte "hyperplasia" has been reinterpreted to indicate aggregation of differentiated melanocytes to more than 6.5 cells per millimeter of basal membrane.[9] Only complete excision can identify in situ melanoma.

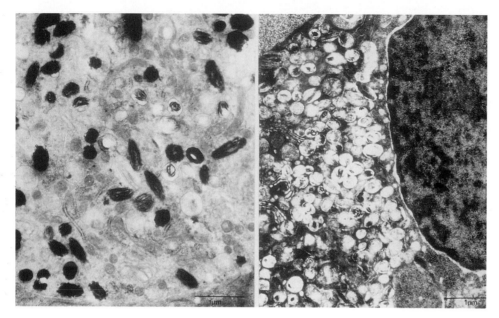

FIGURE   12–11 ■ Melanocyte morphology in a normal adult (*left*) and in a patient with acute alopecia areata (*right*). Note the negligible melanin deposition in swollen, disrupted melanosomes in alopecia areata, compared with the organized melanization in the normal cell.

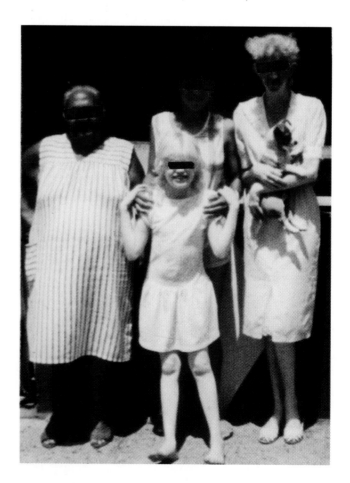

FIGURE 12–12 ■ Hermansky-Pudlak syndrome in a Puerto Rican family: in left, heterozygote mother (skin type VI); *middle back,* heterozygote daughter (skin type IV); *front,* homozygote granddaughter (no pigmentation of hair and skin) standing in front of heterozygote mother; and *far right,* homozygote daughter (no pigmentation of hair and skin).

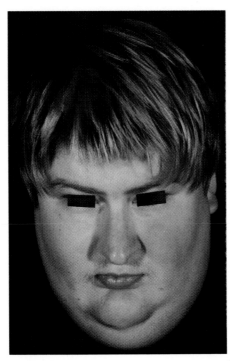

FIGURE 12–13 ■ Prader-Willi syndrome in a 24-year-old patient showing fair hair and hypopigmented skin (height, 156 cm; weight, 185 kg).

Focal Melanocyte Activation

Nail matrix nevi are usually identified by focal, melanin-laden, or poorly pigmented melanocyte accumulation at the dermoepidermal junction. Friction-induced melanonychia is associated with matrix hyperplasia in addition to increased activity of melanocytes in the basal layer and the nail plate. Acral lentiginous melanoma appears first in the basal epithelium and thereafter infiltrates the dermis, whereas superficial spreading melanoma can in-

volve the entire epidermis (Fig. 12–14). Radial growth yields wider bands compared with other types of melanocytic melanonychias and may involve the proximal nail fold epithelium (Hutchinson's sign).

Nonmelanocytic Melanonychias

Pigmentation caused by topical agents (exogenous) corresponds to the shape of the proximal nail fold. By contrast, pigmentation resulting from systemic causes (endogenous) affects the nail matrix and corresponds to the lunula pattern. Nail colonization by bacteria and fungi can be identified by scrapings, potassium hydroxide preparation, histological examination, or culture (Fig. 12–15).

▌Diagnosis

HAIR

Diagnosis of pigmentation disorders is based on the patient's history and physical examination. A very few diseases present universal depigmentation of hair and are then further distinguishable by the degree of hypomelanosis. Circumscribed hypomelanosis (i.e., poliosis) can be associated with various disorders and requires further clinical investigation (Fig. 12–16). Histological classification of hypomelanosis relies on light and electron microscopy, which yield information on melanocyte number and size, melanosome morphology, and melanization.

Canities

Senile canities is age related and therefore is easily distinguished from other forms. Loss of pigment is not abrupt, and single hairs may display gradual pigment loss

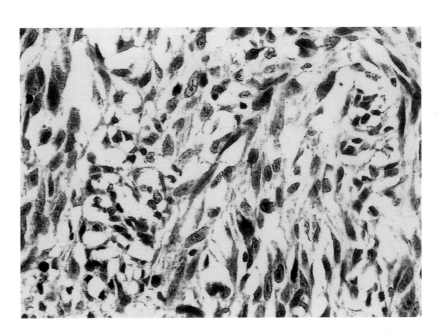

FIGURE 12–14 ■ Histological section of acrolentiginous melanoma with nests of irregularly shaped melanocytes in the dermis.

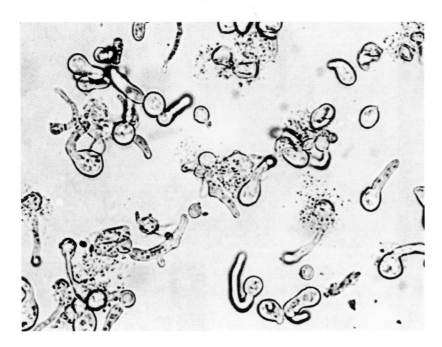

FIGURE 12–15 ■ Culture of *Trichophyton rubrum* isolated from a nail.

from dark to white. Epidermal depigmentation is not observed despite similar age-related reduction in interfollicular melanocyte numbers.

Vitiligo

In this disorder, circumscribed poliosis often occurs in hair of the scalp, pubis, eyelashes, and eyebrows or white hair in depigmented skin (i.e., leukotrichia) (Fig. 12–17). Leukotrichia with leukoderma may be present (Fig. 12–18). Spontaneous or induced repigmentation of epidermis and hair follicles is rare and may derive from infundibular hair follicle melanocytes. However, the long-standing consensus that melanocytes are completely absent in lesional skin has been challenged by our ob-

servations that small numbers of amelanotic melanocytes can persist in amelanotic epidermis (unpublished results). Canities praecox (early graying) of the hair can be inherited or acquired. It is often associated with vitiligo but can also be associated with endocrine disorders and malnutrition (Table 12–1).

Albinism

Oculocutaneous albinism can cause hypopigmentation of the skin and hair together with impaired vision and nystagmus. To distinguish between tyrosinase-positive and tyrosinase-negative albinism, further diagnosis includes examination of hair bulb tyrosinase activity, pigment formation on incubation with tyrosine and dopa, and possibly electron microscopy studies.

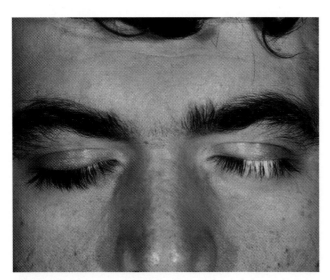

FIGURE 12–16 ■ Circumscribed poliosis of the eyelashes without any involvement of the skin in a patient with vitiligo.

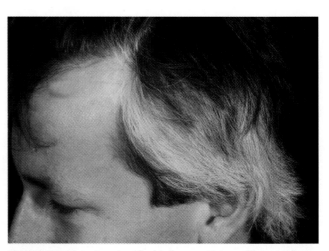

FIGURE 12–17 ■ Circumscribed poliosis in 32-year-old man with vitiligo. Note that the hypopigmented hair is located close to hair of normal color at the temple.

TABLE 12-1 ■ Premature Graying (Canities Praecox)

Cause	Diagnostic Clues
Hereditary premature canities	Appears gradually, single hairs displaying pigment loss from dark to white
Vitiligo	Single or grouped gray hairs before the age of 25 yr (canities praecox), white hair on depigmented skin (leukotrichia), acquired and progressive, unstable (spontaneous or induced repigmentation)
Hyperthyroidism	Elevated thyroid hormone, proptosis, acropathy, pretibial myxedema, onycholysis (Plummer's nail)
Progeria	"Little old man" appearance, retarded growth evident from second year, early death from artherosclerosis
Pangeria (Werner's syndrome)	Growth ceases early in second decade; from second to third decade tense, skinny adherent skin, mottled pigmentation, peripheral telangiectasia, obese trunk, bird-like facies
Waardenburg's syndrome	Piebaldism with white forelock, sharp and discrete bordered hypomelanotic macules, dystopia canthorum, hearing deficit, heterochromia iridis, positive family history
Woolf's syndrome (albinism-deafness syndrome)	Extreme piebaldism with deafness, no other associated features
Fisch's syndrome	Deafness, partial heterochromia iridis
Böök's syndrome	Peripheral vitiligo, café au lait macules, multiple lentigines, premolar aplasia, hyperhidrosis
Vitamin B_{12} or folic acid deficiency	Megaloblastic anemia, pernicious anemia
Fanconi's syndrome	Diffuse hypopigmentation from birth, café au lait macules and achromic lesions, pancytopenia, vitamin D–resistant rickets
Homocystinuria	Defective methionine metabolism, dolichostenomelia, ectopic lens, chest and spinal deformity, mental retardation; fine, sparse, brittle hair

Piebaldism

Piebaldism is associated with sharp and discrete bordered hypomelanotic patches encompassing hyperpigmented macules. Characteristic is the white forelock and presence of a diamond-shaped leukoderma of the central forehead and the ventral midline. Further clinical examination (e.g., audiometry, vision, positive family history) and genetic analysis must be included to rule out Waardenburg's syndrome (Fig. 12–19).

NAIL

Melanonychias present a considerable difficulty in diagnostic medicine, in large part because of the need to differentiate numerous clinically grouped disorders from life-threatening subungual melanoma. Appropriate biopsy or complete excision is required for fail-safe diag-

nosis and treatment, even if it is associated with significant aesthetic and functional consequences. Some authors dispute the definition of melanocyte hyperplasia of nail matrix melanocytes. However, it can be helpful for diagnosis of longitudinal melanonychia to determine the melanocyte number. Histological examination indicates active, dopa-positive melanocytes exceeding ap-

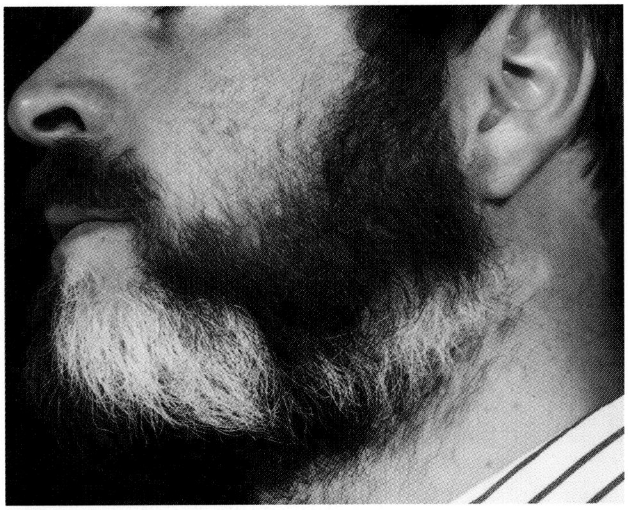

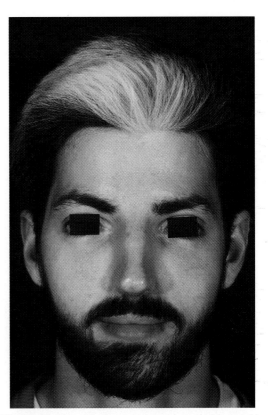

FIGURE 12-19 ■ Waardenburg's syndrome in a 30-year-old man, showing the characteristic white forelock, wide inner canthi, and graying of the beard.

FIGURE 12-18 ■ Circumscribed poliosis in 26-year-old man with vitiligo. Note hypopigmentation of both the hair and underlying skin.

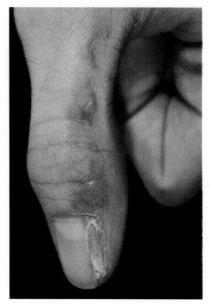

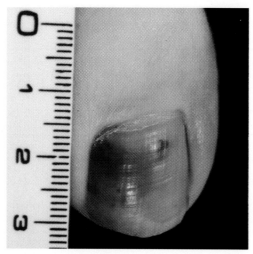

FIGURE 12–22 ■ Subungual hematoma of the toenail after physical trauma. Note the normal outgrowth of the proximal nail.

FIGURE 12–20 ■ Linear dermal nevus extending into the nail.

proximately 6.5 per millimeter of basal membrane.[9] Furthermore, pigmentation abnormalities can suggest general disease (even specific diagnoses) and may be useful for analysis and as indicators of treatment side effects.

Melanocytic Melanonychia

Longitudinal brown or black single or multiple bands in Caucasians present a serious diagnostic challenge because of the intrinsic inactivity of matrix melanocytes. Without histological examination it is often impossible to differentiate among local melanocyte activation, hyper-

plasia, matrix nevus, subungual hemorrhage, and matrix melanoma. Histochemically, the upregulation of tyrosinase activity in melanocytes in the matrix epithelium can be seen by dopa staining without cell atypia or alteration in cell number. Intensely or poorly pigmented melanonychia caused by congenital or acquired matrix nevi occur primarily in children and young adults (Fig. 12–20). They can be readily recognized histologically and may be associated with a pseudo-Hutchinson's sign. Melanoma should always be considered after an uncertain history of nail trauma, particularly in middle-aged and elderly African-American, Japanese or Hispanic persons. Melanoma-associated melanonychia can be wide, range from light brown to black in color, have sharp to blurred borders, and may show partial to complete nail plate dystrophy with Hutchinson's sign (Fig 12–21).

Nonmelanocytic Melanonychia

Many melanonychias are observed in conditions with no primary melanocyte involvement, such as hematoma (Fig. 12–22), tuberous sclerosis (Fig. 12–23), and Hailey-Hailey disease (Fig. 12–24). In the case of fungal or chromogenic bacterial infections, scrapings, microscopic examination, or positive cultures of the microorganisms aid diagnosis (Fig. 12–25). Melanonychia in AIDS patients can be associated with hyperpigmentation of mucous membranes, soles, and palms or can be observed in these patients after treatment with zidovudine. Endocrine melanonychia is associated with cutaneous and mucosal hyperpigmentation and is seen in patients with Addison's disease.

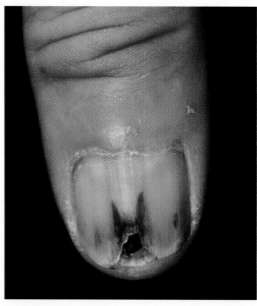

FIGURE 12–21 ■ Acrolentiginous melanoma arising from the nail bed associated with partial destruction of the nail.

Differential Diagnosis

Premature graying (see Table 12–1), hypomelanosis (Table 12–2), poliosis of the hair (Table 12–3), and melanonychia striata longitudinalis (Table 12–4) may be

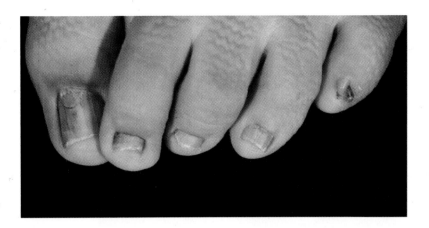

FIGURE 12-23 ■ Koenen's tumor on the little toe in an 8-year-old patient with tuberous sclerosis.

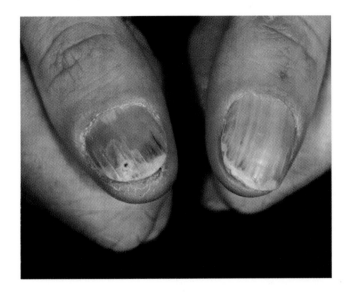

FIGURE 12-24 ■ Onycholysis and splitting of the nail in association with splinter hemorrhages in benign familial pemphigus (Hailey-Hailey disease).

TABLE 12-2 ■ Hypomelanosis (Diffuse Loss or Decrease of Pigment)

Cause	Diagnostic Clues
Vitiligo	Hypomelanosis or complete pigment loss, bluish fluorescence with Wood's light, acquired and progressive, unstable (spontaneous or induced repigmentation)
Copper deficiency (e.g., Menke's kinky hair syndrome)	Marked lightening of hair, anemia, distended blood vessels (due to defective elastin formation)
Malabsorption syndrome	Hyperpigmented skin and hair, poor and brittle nail and hair; dry, itching skin
Kwashiorkor	Protein malnutrition, loss of color intensity rather than graying
Hyperthyroidism	Elevated thyroid hormone, proptosis, acropathy, pretibial myxedema, onycholysis (Plummer's nail)
Oculocutaneous albinism (tyrosinase positive or negative)	Impaired vision nystagmus, absent or defective hair bulb tyrosinase activity
Hermansky-Pudlak syndrome (tyrosinase positive)	Autosomal recessive, tyrosinase-positive oculocutaneous albinism, creamy white skin, freckles, bleeding diathesis, ceroid storage disease affecting lungs and gut, family history
Chédiak-Higashi syndrome	Recurrent infections, giant melanin granules, neurological findings
Christ-Siemens-Touraine syndrome	X-linked, intermittent fever in infancy, anodontia or hypodontia, skeletal anomalies, major (male) and minor (female) form
Griscelli syndrome	Mutated myosin-Va gene, silver-gray hair, recurrent systemic and cutaneous pyogenic infections
Prader-Willi syndrome	Deletions of 15q11-12 region (pink-eyed dilution gene), light hair, marked hypotonia, hyporeflexia, cryptorchidism, hypoplastic penis/labia, acromicria, short stature, mental retardation, obesity, diabetes mellitus
Angelman's syndrome	Deletions of the 15q11-12 region (pink-eyed dilution gene), light hair, mental retardation, gait abnormalities, seizures
Phenylketonuria	Autosomal recessive disorder of phenylalanine metabolism, often blond hair, blue eyes, mental retardation
Homocystinuria	Defective methionine metabolism, dolichostenomelia, ectopic lens, chest and spinal deformity, mental retardation

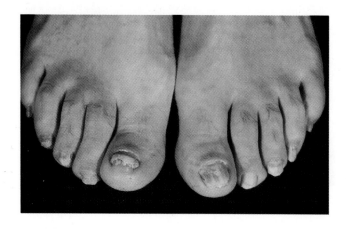

FIGURE 12–25 ■ Fungal onycholysis of the toenails. Note the brittle nails and yellow color caused by *Trichophyton rubrum*.

TABLE 12-3 ■ Poliosis (Circumscribed Loss or Decrease of Pigment)

Cause	Diagnostic Clues
Vitiligo	Acquired and progressive, unstable (spontaneous or induced repigmentation) (see Figs. 12–17, and 12–18)
Alopecia areata	Circumscribed hair loss pattern with regrowing hair initially white
Leukoderma acquisitum centrifugum	Associated with perilesional hypomelanotic halo and melanoma or nevus cell nevus
Piebaldism	Focal mutations in *KIT* gene, manifests at birth, stable course, positive family history, no other associated findings
Waardenburg's syndrome	Mutated or deleted *KIT* (type 1) or *MITF* (type 2) gene, white forelock, sharp and discrete bordered hypomelanotic patches, leukoderma of the ventral midline and the distal extremities, dystopia canthorum, positive family history, hearing deficit, heterochromia iridis (see Fig. 12–19)
Vogt-Koyanagi-Harada syndrome	Bilateral vitiligo-like depigmentation and ocular/auditory abnormalities
Alezzandrini's syndrome	Unilateral/ipsilateral vitiligo-like depigmentation and ocular/auditory abnormalities
Tuberous sclerosis (Pringle's disease)	Lanceolate white macules (ash leaf–like) and sometimes seizures since birth, Koenen's tumors

TABLE 12-4 ■ Melanonychia Striata Longitudinalis

Cause	Diagnostic Clues
Nevi	Stable, chronic, accumulation of nevus cells in epidermis and/or dermis, no other associated features (see Fig. 12–20)
Incontinentia pigmenti	Linear rows of blisters on skin following Blaschko lines; ocular, central nervous system, and dental defects; family history
Melanoma in situ	Large melanocytes with large nuclei, atypical chromatin patterns, intact basal membrane, no other associated features
Malignant melanoma	Periungual hyperpigmentation, pigmented streak or other pigmented lesion of the nail, spindle-shaped cells in nodular areas, penetration of the basal membrane (see Fig. 12–21)
Subungual hematoma	Previous trauma history, positive benzidine staining of hemoglobin deposits in histological sections (see Fig. 12–22)
Iron chromonychia	Exposure to elemental iron, resolves after water purification
Systemic photochemotherapy	Occurs after treatment, characteristic location
Minocycline-induced hyperpigmentation	Longitudinal pigmented streak of the nail associated with periungual hyperpigmentation
Familial dysplastic nevus syndrome	Family history, multiple nevi
Tuberous sclerosis (Pringle's disease)	Lanceolate white (ash leaf–like) macules and seizures since birth, Koenen tumors, family history (see Fig. 12–23)
Familial benign pemphigus (Hailey-Hailey)	Recurrent eruption of small vesicles on an erythematous base in intertriginous areas, extensive loss of intercellular bridges in suprabasal epidermis (see Fig. 12–24)
Onychomycosis/microbial chromonychia	Subungual hyperkeratosis, dystrophic nail unit, often starting from the free edge, potassium hydroxide examination, fungal cultures (see Fig. 12–25)

hallmarks of a wide variety of diseases. However, most pigmentation disorders can be distinguished on the basis of patient history, morphology, and histological and laboratory findings.

Treatment

HAIR

Treatment and management of hair color changes ranging from hypo/hypermelanosis to complete pigment loss requires first a thorough workup of diagnosis and differential diagnosis in order to identify the underlying condition. For most hair color changes only symptomatic treatment is possible, limited to artificial coloring. However, many patients benefit from diagnosis and treatment of the underlying condition.

Canities

There is no mechanism by which hair color lost with aging can be naturally recovered. Treatment by coloring may be of some benefit, particularly in the cases of canities praecox. Repigmentation of canities has been sporadically reported in the literature after radiation therapy for unrelated cancer. Spontaneous repigmentation of the hair has been observed in early stages of canities[2] (see Fig. 12–9). Large oral doses of p-aminobenzoic acid can lead to darkening of gray hair, although the color is lost after cessation of treatment. Recovery of hair color has been reported in association with correction of nutritional, metabolic, and endocrine defects, such as cobalamin and intramuscular cyanocobalamin treatment in pernicious anemia and vitamin B_{12} deficiency, respectively. Increased hair pigmentation and growth has been seen after topical use of latanoprost for glaucoma.

Alopecia Areata

Current treatments for alopecia areata are still unsatisfactory. Hair regrowth has been observed after treatment with corticosteroids taken systematically or applied intralesionally, or after contact dermatitis–inducing topical irritants, oral zinc and so on. Regrowing hair is commonly hypomelanotic but usually recovers its original color with time. No further treatment is required.

Vitiligo

Current treatment options for loss of hair color due to vitiligo are very limited and less than successful. Limited efficacy is achieved with psoralens and ultraviolet radiation and with topical or intralesional corticosteroids. Leukotrichia may repigment by autologous grafting of cultured normal melanocytes. We have observed, in rare instances, spontaneous repigmentation of white body hair resulting from vitiligo (unpublished results).

Neoplasm

Hypomelanosis of hair associated with nevus cell nevus may spontaneously resolve, and usually no treatment is required. Surgical intervention is mandatory for any malignant neoplasm.

Piebaldism

Grafting with normally pigmented skin and/or autologous cultured normal melanocytes has been attempted with moderate success.

Congenital Hereditary Hypomelanosis

Hair coloring is the only option in albinism. In phenylketonuria, the removal or limiting of dietary phenylalanine may increase hair pigmentation, but it is not able to reverse mental retardation, once present. Although Vogt-Koyanagi-Harada syndrome is self-limited, treatment for the depigmentation is as for vitiligo.

NAIL

The most important step in the treatment of hyperpigmentations of the nail is to differentiate benign from malignant disorders.

Malignancies

Longitudinal melanonychias rarely undergo spontaneous remission. Biopsy of the nail matrix and the nail bed in persistent lesions is indicated, especially in Caucasians, to rule out subungual melanoma. Histological evidence of melanocytic atypia should indicate complete excision of the lesion.[10, 11] In uncertain cases, removal of nail matrix nevi is also justified.

Exogenously Induced Pigmentation

Removal of causative agents aids melanonychias caused by drug eruptions. Color changes of the nail caused by fungi or bacteria can be treated with antimycotics or antibiotics, respectively. *Trichophyton rubrum* (Fig. 12–25), for example, produces a diffusible black pigment and can be successfully treated with itraconazole, whereas discoloration caused by colonization of the subungual space with *Candida humicola* can be treated with ketoconazole.

REFERENCES

1. Nagl W: Different growth rates of pigmented and white hair in the beard. Br J Dermatol 132:94, 1995.
2. Tobin DJ, Cargnello JA: Partial reversal of canities in a 23 year old normal Chinese male. Arch Dermatol 129:789, 1993.
3. Slominski A, Paus R: Melanogenesis is coupled to murine anagen: towards new concepts for the role of melanocytes and the regulation of melanogenesis in hair growth. J Invest Dermatol 101:90S, 1993.
4. Dawber RPR, Gummer CL: The color of hair. In: Dawber RPR (ed): Diseases of the Hair and Scalp, 3rd ed. London, Blackwell Scientific, 1998, pp 97–417.

5. Tobin DJ, Fenton DA, Kendall MD: Ultrastructural observations on hair-bulb melanocytes and melanosomes in alopecia areata. J Invest Dermatol 94:803, 1990.

6. Messenger AG, Bleehen SS: Alopecia areata: light and electron microscopic pathology of the regrowing white hair. Br J Dermatol 110:155, 1984.

7. Sam WM Jr, Epstein JH: The affinity of melanin for chloroquine. J Invest Dermotol 45:482, 1965.

8. Murphy M, Reid K, Williams DE, Lyman SD, Barlett PF: Steel factor is required for maintenance, but not differentiation, of melanocyte precursors in the neural crest. Dev Biol 153:396, 1992.

9. Tosti A, Piraccini BM, Baran R: The melanocyte system of the nails and its disorders. In: Nordlund JJ, Boissy RE, Hearing VJ, King RA, Ortonne J-P (eds): The Pigmentary System. New York, Oxford University Press, 1998, pp 937–942.

10. Daniel CR, Osment LS: Nail pigmentation abnormalities: their importance and proper examination. Cutis 25:595, 1980.

11. Zaias N: Pigmentation. In: Zaias N (ed): The Nail in Health and Disease, 2nd ed. Norwalk: Appleton & Lange, 1990, pp 187–251.

BIBLIOGRAPHY

Baran R, Dawber RPR: Diseases of the nails and their management, 2nd ed. Oxford, Blackwell Scientific, 1994.

Fitzpatrick TB, Eisen AZ, Wolff K, Freedberg IW, Austen HF: Dermatology in General Medicine, 4th ed. New York, McGraw Hill, 1993.

Ortonne J-P, Mosher DB, Fitzpatrick TB: Topics in Dermatology: Vitiligo and Other Hypomelanoses of the Hair and Skin. New York, Plenum, 1983.

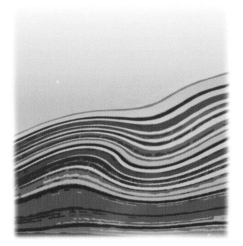

Treatments

Cosmetic and Ethnic Issues

...

HAIR COSMETIC ISSUES

CHRISTOPHER L. GUMMER

The ends of the hair fibers from normal shoulder-length (20 cm) hair are at least 1½ years old. During this period they could have been subjected to more than 500 washes and several thousand comb or brush strokes, in addition to bleaching, perming, or heat treatments. Simply considering the hair on a patient's head as a uniform mass misses a unique clinical history that may span several years. A head of hair is a collection of fibers varying from completely normal new growth to aged, treated, and damaged older growth (Fig. 13–1). Because hair grows at approximately 1 cm/mo, it is possible to establish a timeline of both systemic and extraneous events that affect the quality and quantity of hair on the head. For the same reason, when a patient presents with a cosmetic problem, *all* previous treatments must be considered as potentially causative or complementary. A single perm treatment near the scalp changes hair properties and fiber longevity for the total length and duration of the style. Consequently, a permanent wave conducted close to the scalp in a 30-cm hair style may take 30 months to grow out.

Hair Care Practices

Normal hair care practices present no problems if they are conducted with care and skill. This is evidenced by the fact that chemically treated hair can attain great length and still be in excellent condition. However, any cosmetic practice, if conducted carelessly and without adequate thought to hair condition and product choice, can result in significant hair fiber damage with potentially catastrophic results.

The overall aim of a hair care regimen is to exploit to the maximum the potential of the hair. Hair is, however, a finite tissue that is at its best when just emerging from the skin, where the hair cuticle is perfectly formed and provides maximum protection. From that point on, the hair progressively breaks down. The speed at which this breakdown occurs is under personal control. The careful choice of cosmetic products, shampoos, conditioners, and so forth allows the individual to maintain and often augment hair qualities.

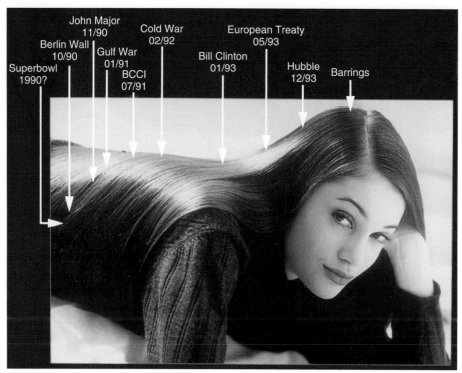

FIGURE 13–1 ■ Growing at 1 cm/mo, hair contains a unique history reflecting both physiological changes and cosmetic practices over a long period. (Courtesy of Proctor and Gamble Co.)

Sudden changes in hair quality are invariably attributed to the product used last. However, "sudden onset" (an acute event) is different from "sudden awareness," when a series of events reaches a level at which their cumulative effect suddenly becomes noticeable. Chemical damage to hair may become fully obvious to a person only after more serious events such as hair breakage or tangling occur. Almost all problems can be traced back to either previous "aggressive" treatments or the way the hair is handled.

HAIR LOSS

Hair loss is often attributed to shampoos, especially with the use of a new product. It is well established that shampoos have no effect on hair loss.[1] The simple act of changing products leads to new expectations and focuses a person's attention on the hair. At this point two events are likely to occur. First, loss of hair during the washing process may be observed. Approximately 50 hairs (or more) may be lost, normally unnoticed, at each wash. Although this is normal, it may suddenly appear excessive, especially when dark hair contrasts with light-colored showers and sink basins. Rarely, there may be some slight increase in the number of hairs lost coinciding with a change to a new product. This results from the individual's putting more "work" into the wash due to different lathering, rinsing, or conditioning properties imparted by the product. Early telogen hairs are pulled prematurely from the follicle. These are easily charac-

terized under light microscopy (Fig. 13–2) as having a small, pointed tail to the telogen bulb. Within a few washes, hair fall returns to normal.

Second, new attention to the hair often highlights other underlying hair disorders, especially androgenetic alopecia, although hair loss caused by postpartum effluvium, anemia, or other problems may also be attributed to shampoos. Indeed, it is surprising how many mothers are not told of the effects of childbirth and breastfeeding on hair loss.

As a rule, hair care products do not cause hair loss. The only notable exceptions involve the *improper use* of chemical treatments such as perms and relaxers, which could cause follicular scarring and subsequent permanent hair loss.

When patients present with hair loss it is vital to establish whether the hair is being lost from the follicle or simply breaking off very close to the scalp. Follicular hair loss almost certainly has a systemic cause that is vital to diagnose, whereas hair breakage close to the scalp may implicate an unusual or excessive cosmetic practice (e.g., traction alopecia, overbleaching).

Matting

Catastrophic tangling, or bird's nest hair, is a rare occurrence.[2] However, tangling and matting of the hair ends occurs frequently, especially on chemically treated hair (Fig. 13–3). Remarkably, many women consider this a known and "accepted" problem of chemical treatments.

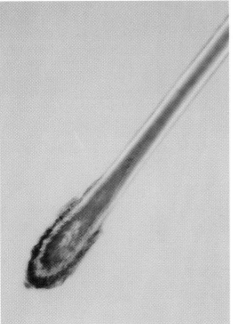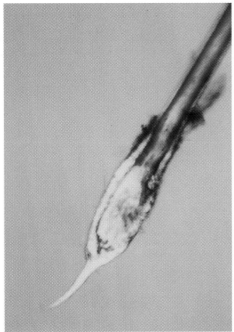

FIGURE 13-2 ■ Changes in hair care practices may cause early telogen hairs to be removed. A hair with a small epithelial tail (*right*) is compared with a normal telogen hair (*left*).

To tangle, hair must be of sufficient length and the ends of the fibers must be brought into a position to interact with the rest of the hair mass. In a long style, not all hairs will have reached the full style length. On a scalp of 100,000 hairs with up to 10% in telogen at any time, as many as 10,000 hair tips will be somewhere between the scalp and the end of the hair style. Consequently, hundreds if not thousands of "ends" will be hidden in the hair mass. It is easy to tangle normal long hair by simply piling it on top of the head and massaging during the shampoo process. At this point water increases the friction of keratin and increases surface roughness. Normally parallel fibers, lower in friction from root to tip, are randomly turned around. The re-sultant fiber disarray tangles easily. This event is often experienced by young children having their hair washed, when the parent stands over the child and lifts the hair on top of the head to achieve easy shampooing.

Tangling of the hair is easily avoided, at all ages, by keeping the hair as straight as possible during washing. Hair should always be washed with a milking, rubbing action. This keeps the hair in almost perfect parallel arrays. The copious use of a conditioner, applied with a similar milking action, ensures virtually tangle-free hair and greatly aids the combing out of any small residual tangles.

Chemically treated hair is particularly prone to tangling and matting (see Fig. 13–3). Perms and bleaches cause lifting of the cuticle scale edges, increased roughness, and increased hydrophilicity, allowing more rapid weathering of the fiber. Broken hairs, caused by rapid weathering, may also be present. These fibers, typically with "brush-break" ends, are high in friction and roughness and particularly interactive in the hair mass. The increased frictional properties, combined with incorrect washing, can result in catastrophic tangling, or bird's nest hair. The hair forms a solid mass of interlocking loops with no knots (Fig. 13–4). Onset is sudden and distressing and occurs during washing. Any action or manipulation of the hair, especially while it is wet, only exacerbates the problem. Pulling one loop simply tightens another, and the hair rarely can be untangled. Even if the mass is untangled, the damaged fibers are still present and are still prone to tangling. Removal of the tangled mass and damaged hair is recommended. It should be noted that the chemical treatment leading to this problem may not have been recent. Previous treatments that are close to growing out are more likely to cause tangling because the hair ends are at their most damaged and are likely to tangle when brought into contact with the hair mass.

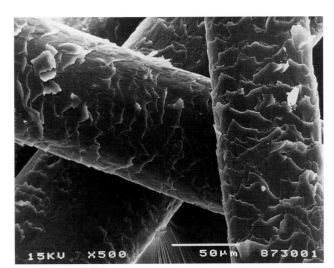

FIGURE 13-3 ■ Hair matting usually is preceded by chemical treatments that increase surface roughness, cuticle lifting, and fiber-fiber interactions.

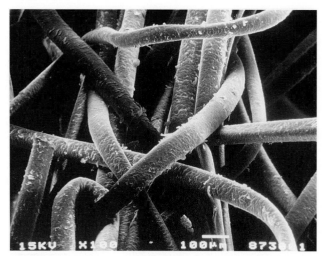

FIGURE 13–4 ■ Bird's nest hair or severe matting typically involves chemically treated hair. The hair forms masses of interlocking loops that cannot be untangled. Knots are not present.

Bubble Hair

Bubble hair is characterized by the formation of large bubblelike structures within the hair cortex[2, 3] (Fig. 13–5). The hair is brittle and dry and breaks easily at the site of the bubbles. The patient usually presents complaining of sudden hair loss or hair breakage, attributing the problem to a new hair care product.

Hair styling often involves the use of heated appliances such as rollers, curling irons, or hair dryers. Curling irons (tongs) operate at temperatures greater than 100°C (the boiling point of water). It is not unusual to see curling tongs covered with brown lines caused by melted hair. Scalp burns are also common. The formation of bubbles is caused by the application of heated

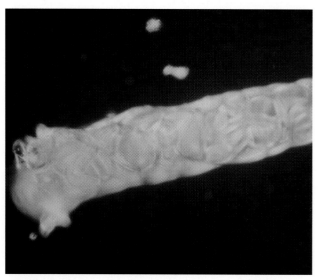

FIGURE 13–5 ■ Bubble hair is caused by local heating of damp hair, which undermines the structure of the fiber, leading to breakage.

appliances to damp hair. (At normal appliance temperatures, bubbles do not form in *dry* hair.) The heat softens the keratin. At the same time, water inside the hair is turned to steam, which both hydrolyzes keratin and expands rapidly. Unable to escape, the expanding steam forms large bubbles inside the hair. These undermine the mechanical integrity of the hair, causing breakage. Although the patient may be a regular user of a heated styling implement, a small interruption during the procedure, such as answering the telephone, may allow the tongs to get too hot. Rushing to style the hair while it is still too wet or use of a faulty, overheating appliance may be all that is required to cause bubble hair.

Diagnosis is confirmed by the presence of numerous bubbles at the broken ends of the fibers, although most of these may be lost if the hair has been cut to regain an acceptable style before the patient presents to the clinician. Chronic damage produces bubbles throughout the hair and numerous broken hairs of different lengths, indicating several heating events. Acute damage may manifest as numerous hairs all broken at the same length, as if the hair had been cut. The distribution of bubbles across the head also depends on the type of appliance used. Any damaged ends remaining will rapidly degrade to "split ends."

Bubble hair may also be caused by the application of hydrogen peroxide to bleach or highlight the hair. The breakdown of H_2O_2 to form oxygen is catalyzed by various metals. Once started, this reaction is self-catalyzing. Metals such as iron and copper, absorbed into the fibers from tap water, can catalyze the rapid breakdown of hydrogen peroxide. The hair is seen to steam or smoke, and there is accompanying rapid heat formation. The event is rare and normally is seen only in salons. Failure to act quickly results in serious damage to the hair, with breakage close to the scalp.

Chemical Treatments

Chemical treatments include permanent waving, bleaching, highlighting, and relaxing. Usually the permanent wave is not considered to be permanent for the life of the hair; that is, after 6 months another perm may be applied even though the hair still shows a permanent record of the effects of the previous treatment. Therefore, further investigation usually is unnecessary. The cuticle typically shows increased lifting, separation, or both. Amino acid analysis reveals a reduction in cystine. Increased cysteic acid levels (normal, 0.5 mol per 100 mol) are typical after both perms and bleaches. Electron microscopy and amino acid analysis are warranted only to establish the severity of the damage.

Although the chemistry varies, all chemical treatments work from the outside in and must penetrate via the cuticle into the hair cortex to achieve the desired result. Perms and relaxers need to achieve disulfide bond cleavage in the cortex. Similarly, melanin, the target for bleaches, exists only in the cortex. Overall, the need for deep penetration into the fiber is the reason these treatments can be so damaging. All treatments result in

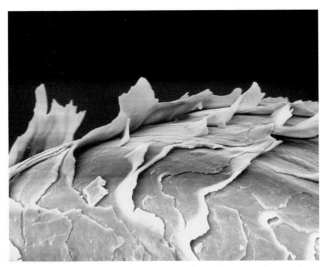

FIGURE 13-6 ■ Tortuous curves and tight styles cause the cuticle to lift and be broken off by simple combing.

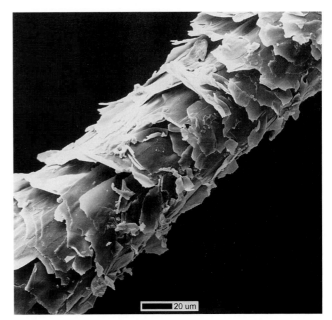

FIGURE 13-8 ■ Overbleaching causes severe cuticle damage through oxidative cleavage of disulfide bonds and removal of structural lipids from the cuticle cell membranes.

cleavage of disulfide bonds, the greatest concentration occurring in the cuticle. Consequently, although the treatment needs to penetrate through the cuticle, it is partially consumed en route to the cortex. Therefore, higher concentrations or increased application times are required. In achieving the desired end result, the cuticle is noticeably damaged.

All chemical treatments cause significant changes in the amount of extractable bound lipids. Removal of covalently bound surface lipids causes the fiber to become more hydrophilic and reduces adhesion between cuticle cells, particularly when the fiber is bent into new shapes (Fig. 13-6). Also, both permeability and swelling are greatly increased, the latter aided by an increased number of cysteic acid residues. Once damaged, the cuticle

weathers rapidly, resulting in complete breakdown of the fiber (Figs. 13-7 through 13-10). Patients often complain that their hair does not grow past a certain length. In fact, the hair will grow much longer; the problem is the poor cosmetic state of the hair, which results in premature breakage. In these cases, the quality of the hair dictates the style. All chemical treatments should be conducted by skilled stylists. Processes such as perming use the same chemicals as used in depilatory preparations (i.e., thioglycolates). There is, therefore, a

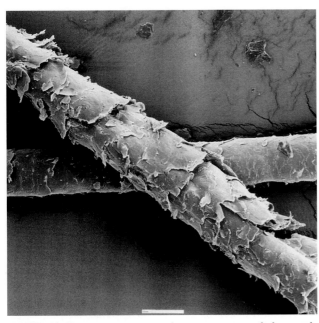

FIGURE 13-7 ■ Overperming results in separation of the cuticle from itself and from the cortex.

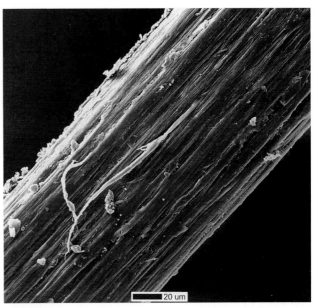

FIGURE 13-9 ■ Excessive chemical treatment (perms and bleaches) combined with normal combing can remove all of the cuticle, exposing the cortex to rapid weathering.

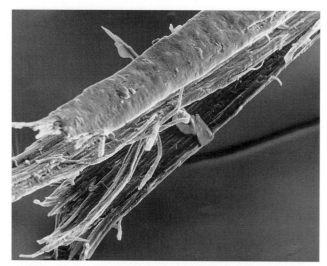

FIGURE 13–10 ■ Split ends occur on all fibers if they are left to grow long enough. Chemical treatments cause the hair to break down quickly unless it is treated with extra care.

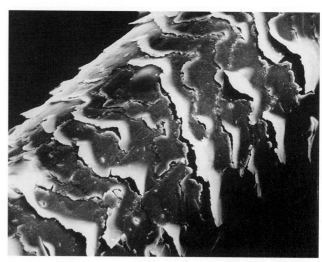

FIGURE 13–11 ■ Stretching of relaxed or chemically treated hair, especially when it is wet, leads to rupture and lifting of individual cuticle cells.

fine balance between achieving a perfect perm and removing all of the hair!

During the treatment process one of the most damaging events to the fiber is intense fiber swelling. This is caused not only by the active ingredients but by rinsing with plain water between applications of active solutions. During perming, bleaching, and relaxing, disulfide bonds are cleaved to allow manipulation of the fiber shape. The diffusion of active agents into the fiber results in proportionally high ionic concentrations inside the fiber. When the hair is rinsed with water, it attempts to establish an equilibrium by rapid penetration into the weaker fiber, resulting in massive swelling. Hair swells approximately 15% in water alone, but when thioglycolate is rinsed from a fiber, swelling may reach 200%. In addition, chemically treated hair is particularly prone to stretching in the wet state owing to the failure of the permanent wave process to re-form all of the disulfide bonds. Although they may be present in stretched normal hair, transverse cracks and fissures readily appear in treated hair (Fig. 13–11).

Trichorrhexis nodosa is a typical finding in hair that receives either regular chemical treatments or general overstyling. Focal explosions of the cortex (Fig. 13–12) are visible with the naked eye and can be considered diagnostic. Treatment takes the form of a quality haircut to remove as much of the damaged hair as possible, advice on suitable hair care practices, and liberal use of conditioner when handling the remaining hair until the problem has completely grown out.

During any chemical treatment, and especially with relaxers, handling of the hair should be kept to a minimum. All treatments significantly weaken the tensile strength of the fiber.[4] This is most important while the treatment is taking place. Even low forces can cause breakage (a normal hair breaks at approximately 100 g). The relaxing process is particularly damaging to the hair. Two chemical approaches are taken: lye (NaOH) and

no-lye guanidine hydroxide relaxers. Both have similar effects, and it is the process as much as the aggressive chemistry that can cause much of the fiber damage. Relaxing is often started at the roots first. Therefore, any subsequent manipulation while the rest of the fiber is relaxed pulls on the already weakened roots, where the chemical process is at its most advanced. This leads to breakage close to the scalp. However, it is the geometric form of African-American hair that poses the greatest problem. The hair has a characteristic crimp; to achieve perfectly straight hair, this crimp needs to be unwound during the relaxing process. Because this is

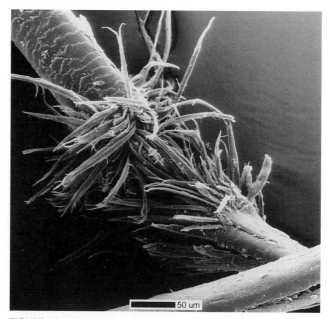

FIGURE 13–12 ■ Trichorrhexis nodosa, a typical feature of hair that has been chemically or physically overtreated.

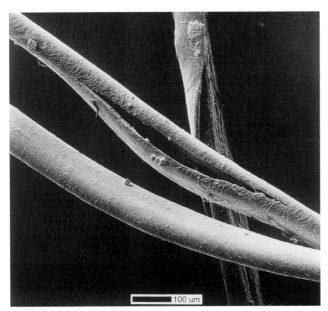

FIGURE 13–13 ■ Longitudinal splits are common in African-American hair types but are rarely found in Caucasian hair types.

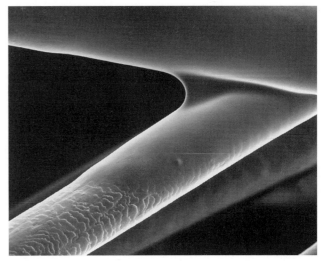

FIGURE 13–15 ■ A typical hair spray bond or "weld" joining two hair fibers.

not possible for every fiber, the hairs are relaxed and simply pulled straight, resulting in stretched and wavy fibers. Each hair is left under huge mechanical stresses, the word "relaxer" being something of a misnomer.

Whereas trichorrhexis nodosa is typical of excessive chemical and physical treatments in Caucasian hair types, longitudinal splits in the fiber (Figs. 13–13 and 13–14) are typical of overtreated African-American hair and can usually be considered diagnostic of an inappropriate hair care regimen.

Temporary Styling

A number of products are designed to place and hold the hair into a temporary style, including hair sprays, gels, and mousses. All of these products are based on a carrier solvent and fixative resin. They are either alcohol or water based (Figs. 13–15 through 13–18).

It is often said (incorrectly) that styling products "build up" on the hair, but this is a result of a person's hair care habits rather than the product. For most users, normal shampooing removes all of the styling resin. Typical shampoo frequency is more than four times per week. However, a small percentage of users apply styling products two or three times per day and have a shampoo frequency of only once per week. Conse-

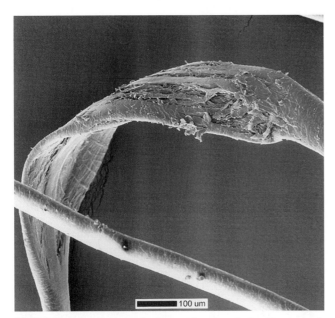

FIGURE 13–14 ■ Relaxing the fiber with sodium hydroxide can result in longitudinal splits and compression from styling implements. Although "relaxed," the hair is put under great mechanical stress.

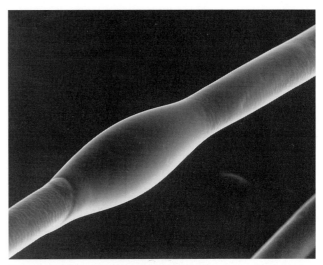

FIGURE 13–16 ■ Small droplets of hair spray remain discrete when another hair is not available to form a bond.

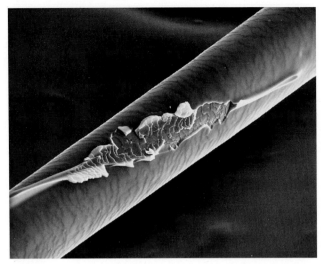

FIGURE 13–17 ■ A replica of the cuticle remains in the styling resin after the adjacent hair has been removed. Normal shampooing removes the remainder of the resin.

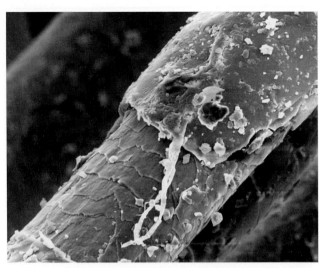

FIGURE 13–19 ■ Infrequent washing together with heavy use of styling products leads to entrapment of extraneous debris.

quently, environmental dirt, sebaceous secretions, and squames are held in place by successive styling product applications, making the overall soil component on the hair difficult to remove with a single shampoo (Figs. 13–19 and 13–20). Also, any attempts to comb out the problem will cause hairs to break. As with most hair problems, it is important to educate the patient about the effects of daily habits on the condition and quality of the hair.

Treatments and Solutions

Hair care products, especially shampoos and conditioners, are used by a very wide range of individuals with virtually no adverse events. Consequently, when a pa-

tient presents with a hair or scalp problem it is unlikely that such products are the cause. On the other hand, chemical treatments such as perms or bleaches, by the nature of their chemistry and mode of action, may well be implicated, especially if they are used incorrectly.

The hair is a unique body tissue that provides a continuous record of events occurring in the follicle and around the fiber for up to 7 years. Therefore, it is possible to read the record of the hair to aid in a successful diagnosis. The patient must first understand that hair stays on the head for a considerable time, generally longer than their own memory of hair treatment events. Furthermore, any adverse treatment of the fiber (e.g., chemical treatments, heated appliances) will cause it to break down faster, even under the normal cosmetic regimen. Finally, the fiber is at its best when it emerges from the follicle; after that, it undergoes a

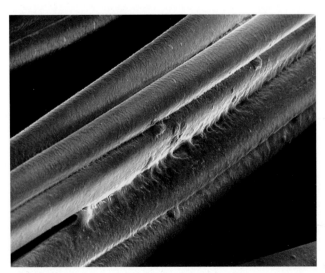

FIGURE 13–18 ■ Styling gels and mousses group fibers together via seam "welds" to hold the hair in place.

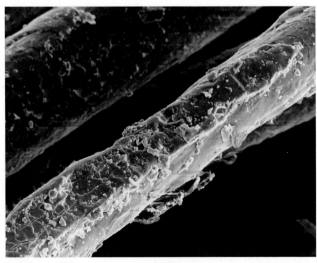

FIGURE 13–20 ■ Repeated styling product application without regular washing results in heavy polymer deposition and the accumulation of skin cells and sebum.

progressive breakdown (weathering), resulting in a split end. Consequently, protection and prevention are essential.

There are perhaps three rules to managing hair:

- When washing, never pile the hair on top of the head. This avoids bringing damaged fiber ends into contact with the hair mass, which would cause matting.
- Always use a conditioner. Conditioning eases wet detangling and prevents dry flyaway, both of which are areas of high mechanical damage from combs.
- Always comb the hair from the bottom first. Combing from the root first compounds tangles and knots. The longer the hair, the more important to start from the bottom.

Each of these rules needs to be adjusted according to the style and condition of the hair. For example, chemically treated hair should be cut regularly to remove damaged ends. Washing should be less frequent and should involve shampoos and conditioners formulated for treated hair. Conditioners should be used in excess rather than sparingly. Combing should be done gently, with a wide-tooth comb, and all other treatments should be reduced, especially subsequent chemical treatments.

Because hair grows from the roots and not the tip, any serious damage, although distressing, will eventually grow out. Patients respond well to acknowledgment that their hair condition is real and is being treated successfully with commercially available products, and very few present again.

■ ■ ■

NAIL COSMETIC ISSUES

ZOE D. DRAELOS

Nail Manicure

CLINICAL FEATURES

Dermatological side effects of a poorly performed manicure include onychoschizia accompanied by paronychia.

DIAGNOSIS

Improper nail filing leads to onychoschizia (Fig. 13–21), whereas disruption of the cuticle predisposes to paronychial bacterial, fungal, or viral infection (Fig. 13–22).

TREATMENT

Professional grooming of the nails for both men and women is known as a manicure. The manicure is designed to cut the nails, according to current fashion standards, while improving their cosmetic appearance. The procedures followed for a manicure (grooming of the fingernails) and a pedicure (grooming of the toenails) are essentially the same. The nails are first soaked in a soap solution to remove any debris and to soften the nail plate before cutting. Softening of the nail is important to prevent cracking, splitting, and horizontal layering (onychoschizia), which may occur when trying to cut a brittle nail plate.

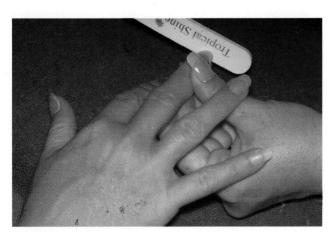

FIGURE 13–21 ■ It is important to direct the file perpendicularly to the nail plate to prevent onychoschizia.

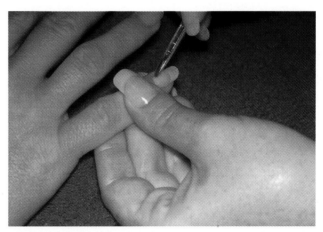

FIGURE 13–22 ■ Disruption of the cuticle predisposes to paronychia and onychodystrophy.

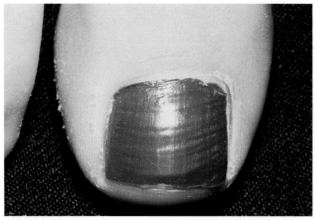

FIGURE 13–23 ■ Deep red nail polish can temporarily stain the nail plate.

Current fashion dictates that the nails should be trimmed to a delicate arc at the middle of the fingertip and filed to remove any corners at the medial and lateral nail. Although this shape is esthetically pleasing and serves to create the illusion of long, slender fingers and toes, it predisposes to nail plate fracture, hangnails, and ingrown nails. Ideally, the nail should be trimmed with as slight a curve as possible, and the corners of the nail should be left untouched. This is particularly important when trimming the toenails, because they frequently ingrow due to pressure from ill-fitting shoes or trauma encountered during exercise. Recurrent ingrown toenails are best prevented by leaving the nail corners longer than the center of the toenail to create a concave shape.

Ideally, the nail should not be cut but should be frequently filed to avoid cracking as a result of shearing forces created by scissors or clippers. However, if cutting is necessary, the nails should be trimmed with a sharp scissors or nail clipper after softening. The cutting implement should be held perfectly perpendicular to the nail surface to avoid layering of the nail plate, which predisposes to onychoschizia. Any remaining sharp edges should be filed with a diamond-dust file.[5]

Under no circumstances should the cuticle be re-moved or traumatized because this may precipitate the formation of paronychia, onychomycosis, or onychodystrophy. Unfortunately, the cuticle is considered to be unattractive by most manicure artists because it complicates the even application of nail polish. Most of the problems arising from a professional manicure are related to manipulation of the cuticle.

The last step in the manicure is grooming of the surface of the nail plate. Sometimes this is as simple as buffing the nail plate to a shine with creams containing finely ground pumice, talc, kaolin, or precipitated chalk as an abrasive, with wax added to increase nail shine.[6] Sometimes a white pencil, known as nail white, is stroked beneath the nail plate free edge to brighten the nail.

Nail Polish

CLINICAL FEATURES

Nail polish can cause staining of the nail plate or simulate the appearance of onychodystrophy.

DIAGNOSIS

Nail polishes, especially of the deep red color, can cause a yellowish staining of the nail plate that wears away in approximately 2 weeks (Fig. 13–23). Nail polish that is touched before drying can become uneven, creating the appearance of an abnormal nail plate (Fig. 13–24). The astute dermatologist must recognize temporary cosmetic-induced nail problems.

TREATMENT

Nail polish consists basically of pigments suspended in a volatile solvent to which film-formers have been added. The ingredients are listed in Table 13–1.[7]

Nitrocellulose is the most commonly employed primary film-forming agent in nail lacquer. It produces a shiny, tough, nontoxic film that adheres well to the nail

TABLE 13-1 ■ Composition of Nail Polish

Classification	Examples
Primary film-former	Nitrocellulose, methacrylate polymers, vinyl polymers
Secondary film-forming resin	Formaldehyde, p-toluene sulfonamide, polyamide, acrylate, alkyl and vinyl resins
Plasticizers	Dibutyl phthalate, dioctyl phthalate, tricresyl phosphate, camphor
Solvents and diluents	Acetates, ketones, toluene, xylene, alcohols
Colorants	Organic D&C pigments, inorganic pigments
Specialty fillers	Quanine fish scale or titanium dioxide-coated mica flakes or bismuth oxychloride for iridescence
Suspending agents	Stearalkonium hectorite

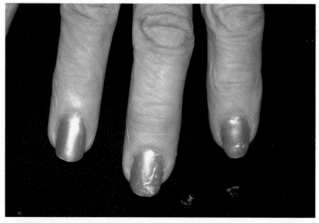

FIGURE 13–24 ■ Touching the nail polish before drying is completed can simulate the appearance of onychodystrophy.

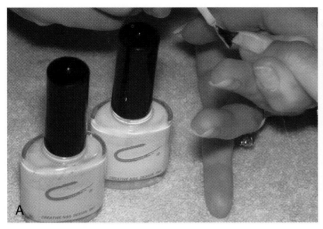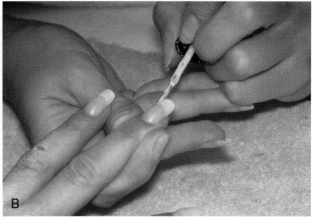

FIGURE 13-25 ■ The French manicure involves painting a pink polish over the nail plate (A) and a white polish over the nail free edge (B).

plate. The film is somewhat permeable to oxygen, allowing gas exchange between the atmosphere and the nail plate, of importance to ensure nail plate health. Resins and plasticizers are then added to increase the flexibility of the film, minimizing chipping and peeling.

The most popular resin used to enhance the nitrocellulose film is toluene-sulfonamide-formaldehyde. However, it is the source of allergic contact dermatitis in some nail enamels. Hypoallergenic nail enamels employ polyester resin or cellulose acetate butyrate, but sensitivity is still possible.[8] Plasticizers, such as dibutyl phthalate, are also used to keep the product soft and pliable. All of these ingredients are dissolved in a solvent, such as *N*-butyl acetate or ethyl acetate, with toluene and isopropyl alcohol added as diluents.

Variety in nail polish color can be achieved through the addition of coloring agents, such as organic colors selected from a list of certified colors approved by the U.S. Food and Drug Administration. Inorganic colors and pigments may also be used, but they must conform to standards for low heavy metal content.[9] These colors can be suspended within the lacquer with suspending agents such as stearalkonium hectorite to produce colors ranging from white to pink, purple, brown, orange, blue, and green. If the pigments are dissolved rather than

suspended in the polish, nail staining is more likely. The pigments most likely to cause staining are D & C Reds Nos. 6, 7, 34, and 5 Lake.

Other specialty additives are used to create variety. Guanine, fish scale, bismuth oxychloride, or titanium dioxide–coated mica can be added to enhance light reflection and give a frosted appearance. Chopped aluminum, silver, or gold can be added for a metallic shine. Nylon or rayon fibers can be added for nail strengthening purposes.

French Nail Manicure

CLINICAL FEATURES

An abnormal nail can be concealed by the artistic application of nail polish to simulate the nail bed and accompanying free edge.

DIAGNOSIS

A French nail manicure is a method of applying a pink nail polish to the nail bed (Fig. 13–25A) and a white

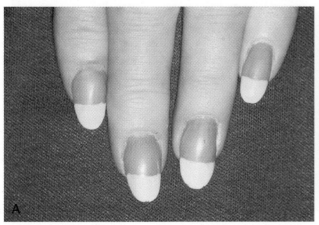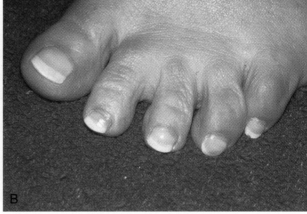

FIGURE 13-26 ■ Completed French manicure (A) and pedicure (B).

TABLE 13-2 ■ Nail Grooming Products

Nail Cosmetic	Main Ingredients	Function	Adverse Reactions
Nail polish	Nitrocellulose, toluene-sulfonamide resin, plasticizers, solvents, and colorants	To add color and shine to nail plates	Allergic contact dermatitis to toluene-sulfonamide resin, nail plate staining
Nail hardener	Formaldehyde, acetates, acrylics, or other resins	To increase nail strength and prevent breakage	Allergic contact dermatitis to formaldehyde
Nail enamel remover	Acetone, alcohol, ethyl acetate, or butyl acetate	To remove nail polish	Irritant contact dermatitis
Cuticle remover	Sodium or potassium hydroxide	To destroy keratin that forms excess cuticular tissue on nail plate	Irritant contact dermatitis
Nail white	White pigments	To whiten free nail edge	Practically none
Nail buffing cream	Pumice, talc, or kaolin	To smooth ridges in nails	Practically none
Nail moisturizer	Occlusives, humectants, lactic acid	To increase water content of nails	Practically none

nail polish to the free nail edge (Fig. 13–25B) to simulate normal fingernails (Fig. 13–26A) or toenails (Fig. 13–26B). Dermatologists should ask patients to remove all nail polish before evaluating the health of the nail bed.

TREATMENT

The discussion of nail polish presented previously also pertains to the products used in a French nail manicure. A summary of other nail grooming products, including their main ingredients, function, and possible adverse reactions, is provided in Table 13–2.

Nail Adornments

CLINICAL FEATURES

A source of nickel contact allergy is nickel-containing nail adornments.

DIAGNOSIS

Nickel may be present in artificial nail plates (Fig. 13–27A) and in nail jewels or ribbons (Fig. 13–27B).

TREATMENT

A variety of adornments can be applied to the fingernails immediately before drying of the nail lacquer, which adheres the decoration to the nail plate. Allergic contact dermatitis may be caused by the adornments, rather than the nail polish, in some nickel-sensitive patients, so gold or nickel-free jewels should be selected.

Artificial Nail Tips

CLINICAL FEATURES

A piece of plastic can be glued to the nail tip, simulating an elongated natural nail plate (Fig. 13–28).

DIAGNOSIS

The use of artificial nail tips can create several nail problems. Occlusion of the natural nail, which inhibits oxygen transfer, results in a thinned nail plate that many times cannot support its own weight after the plastic tip is removed. Patients may not be aware of the condition of the natural nail plate, which is usually visible beneath the plastic tip (Fig. 13–29A). Traumatic removal of the

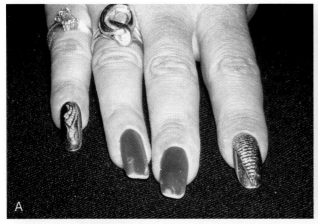
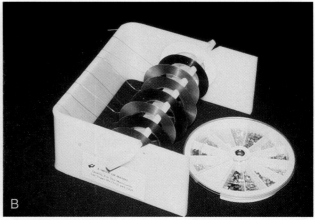

FIGURE 13–27 ■ Nickel-containing artificial nails (A) or jewels and ribbons (B) used to adorn the nail can be a source of allergic contact dermatitis in the nickel-sensitive patient.

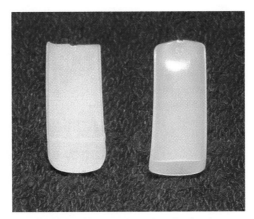

FIGURE 13–28 ■ Preformed artificial nail tips.

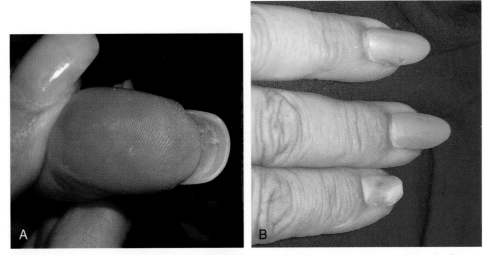

FIGURE 13–29 ■ Problems associated with artificial nails include thinning of the natural nail plate, seen beneath the prosthesis (*A*), and onycholysis resulting from traumatic removal of artificial nails (*B*).

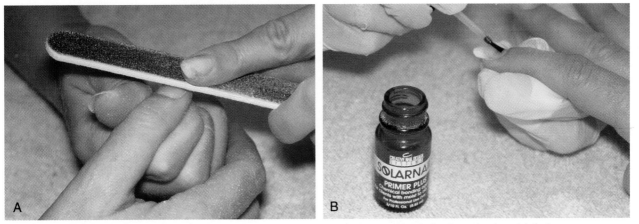

FIGURE 13–30 ■ The natural nail plate is roughened (*A*) and painted with decolorized iodine (*B*) before application of the artificial nail.

plastic tip may also result in onycholysis and nail pitting[10] (Fig. 13–29B).

TREATMENT

The use of artificial nail tips involves preparation of the nail bed by roughening of the surface with a nail file to increase adhesion (Fig. 13–30A) and application of decolorized iodine to prevent fungal growth between the preformed plastic tip and the natural nail plate (Fig. 13–30B). A plastic tip is then glued, typically with a methacrylate-based adhesive, to the natural nail plate (Fig. 13–31A). The methacrylate adhesive is a possible cause of allergic contact dermatitis in some patients. An alternative nail adhesive made from ethyl 2-cyanoacry-

late provides better adhesion but can cause onycholysis.[11]

The artificial nail tip is then trimmed to the desired length (Fig. 13–31B), and a formable acrylic is applied over the remaining exposed natural nail plate (Fig. 13–31C). A drill is then used to grind the undersurface of the nail smooth (Fig. 13–31D), and the prosthesis is completed (Fig. 13–31E).

Artificial Nail Sculptures

CLINICAL FEATURES

Artificial nail sculptures coat the entire nail plate with a methacrylate-based polymer (Table 13–3).

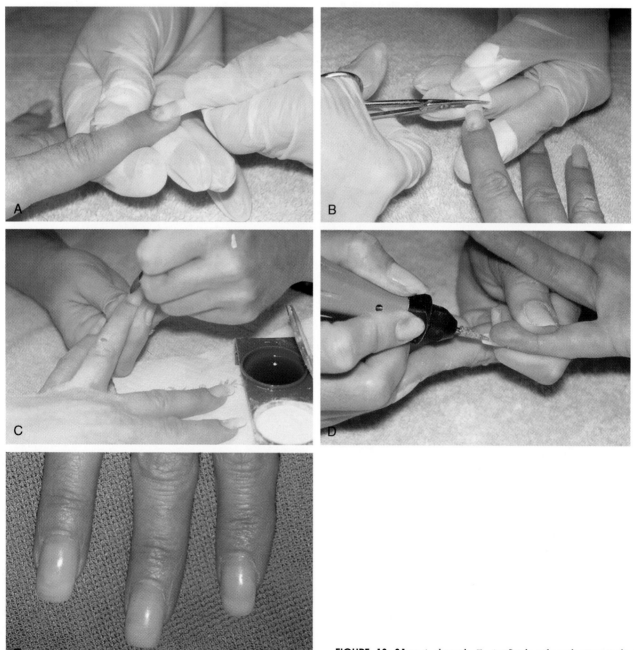

FIGURE 13–31 ■ *A* through *E*, Artificial nail application technique.

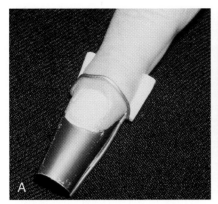 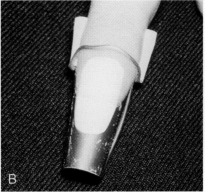 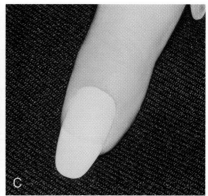

FIGURE 13–32 ■ *A through C, Sculptured nail application technique.*

DIAGNOSIS

Artificial nail sculptures can result in the same problems as artificial nail tips. However, the sculptures use no preformed pieces but rather custom fit the entire nail from a formable acrylic.

TREATMENT

Either the entire nail plate or a portion of the nail plate can be covered with a formable acrylic. The acrylic uses liquid ethyl or isobutyl methacrylate as the monomer to be mixed with the powdered polymethyl methacrylate polymer (see Fig. 13–31C). The product is allowed to polymerize in the presence of a benzoyl peroxide accelerator, and a formable acrylic is made that hardens in 7 to 9 minutes.[12] Usually, hydroquinone, monomethyl ether of hydroquinone, or pyrogallol is added to slow polymerization.[13] If the entire nail is to be sculptured, a form is placed beneath the nail (Fig. 13–32A) and the acrylic is applied to the template (Fig. 13–32B) to com-

plete the nail elongation process (Fig. 13–32C). Fabric, such as linen, can be imbedded in the acrylic before curing to add strength to the elongated nail (Fig. 15–33).

Many patients are not aware that finished nail sculptures require more care than natural fingernails. With continued wear of the sculpture, the acrylic loosens from the natural nail, especially around the edges. These loose edges must be clipped and new acrylic applied approximately every 3 weeks to prevent development of an environment for infection. The sculpture grows out with the natural nail plate, and more polymer must be added proximally, depending on the nail growth rate. This procedure is known as "filling." If necessary, the sculptured nails can be removed by soaking in acetone.

Allergic contact dermatitis remains an issue, even though methyl methacrylate is no longer used. The isobutyl, ethyl, and tetrahydrofurfuryl methacrylates are still strong sensitizers,[14, 15] but it should be emphasized that only the liquid monomer, not the polymerized, cured acrylic, is sensitizing.[16] Therefore, a careful operator who avoids skin contact with the uncured acrylic can avoid sensitizing the patient. Patch testing should be performed for persons with suspected sensitization, us-

TABLE 13-3 ■ Artificial Nail Sculpture Application Technique

1. All nail polish and oils are removed from the nail.
2. The nail is roughened with a coarse emery board, pumice stone, or grinding drill to create an optimal surface for sculpted nail adhesion.
3. An antifungal, antibacterial liquid, such as decolorized iodine, is applied to the entire nail plate to minimize onychomycosis and paronychia.
4. The loose edges of the cuticle are either trimmed, removed, or pushed back, depending on the operator.
5. A preformed plastic tip is glued to the distal edge of the natural nail plate, if tips are to be used. If no tips are to be used, a flexible template is placed beneath the natural nail plate on which the elongated sculpted nail will be built.
6. The acrylic is mixed and applied with a paintbrush to cover the natural nail plate proximal to the preformed tip. Or, if the nail is to be completely made from the formable acrylic, it is placed over the entire natural nail plate and extended onto the template to the desired nail length.
7. The final artificial nail is sanded to a high shine.
8. Nail polish, jewels, decals, and decorative metal strips may be added.

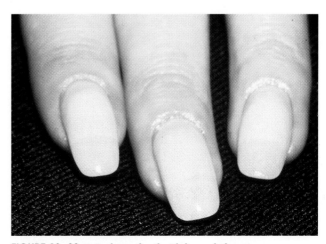

FIGURE 13–33 ■ Sculptured nail with linen cloth wrap.

ing methyl methacrylate monomer, 10% in olive oil, and methacrylate acid esters, 1% and 5% in olive oil and petrolatum.[17]

REFERENCES

1. Kullavanijiya P, Gritiyarangsan P, Bisalbutra P, Kulthanan R, Cardin CW: Absence of effects of dimethicone and non-dimethicone containing shampoos on daily hair loss rates. J Soc Cosmet Chem 43:195–206, 1992.
2. Gummer CL: Bubble hair: a cosmetic abnormality caused by brief, focal heating of damp hair. Br J Dermatol 131:901–903, 1994.
3. Detweiller SP, Carson JL, Woosley JT, et al: Bubble hair: case caused by an overheating hair dryer and reproducibility in normal hair with heat. J Am Acad Dermatol 30:54–60, 1994.
4. Robbins CR: Chemical and Physical Behaviour of Human Hair. New York, Springer Verlag, 1998.
5. Engasser PG, Matsunaga J: Nail cosmetics. In: Scher RK, Daniel CR (eds): Nails: Therapy, Diagnosis, Surgery. Philadelphia, WB Saunders, 1990, pp 214–215.
6. Cohen PR, Scher RK: Nail changes in the elderly. J Geriatric Dermatol 1:45–53, 1993.
7. Wing HJ: Nail preparations. In: de Navarre MG (ed): The Chemistry and Manufacture of Cosmetics. Wheaton, IL, Allured Publishing Corporation, 1988, pp 983–1005.
8. Schlossman ML: Nail-enamel resins. Cosmetic Technology 1:53, 1979.
9. Schlossman ML: Nail polish colorants. Cosmetic Toil 95:31, 1980.
10. Lazar P: Reactions to nail hardeners. Arch Dermatol 94:446–448, 1966.
11. Baran R: Pathology induced by the application of cosmetics to the nails. In: Frost P, Horwitz SN (eds): Cosmetics for the Dermatologist. Philadelphia, CV Mosby, 1982, p 182.
12. Barnett JM, Scher RK, Taylor SC: Nail cosmetics. Dermatol Clin 9:9–17, 1991.
13. Viola LJ: Fingernail elongators and accessory nail preparations. In: Balsam MS, Sagarin E (eds): Cosmetics, Science and Technology, 2nd ed. New York, Wiley-Interscience, 1972, pp 543–552.
14. Marks JG, Bishop ME, Willis WF: Allergic contact dermatitis to sculptured nails. Arch Dermatol 115:100, 1979.
15. Fisher AA: Cross reactions between methyl methacrylate monomer and acrylic monomers presently used in acrylic nail preparations. Contact Dermatitis 6:345–347, 1980.
16. Fisher AA, Franks A, Glick H: Allergic sensitization of the skin and nails to acrylic plastic nails. J Allergy 28:84, 1957.
17. Baran R, Dawber RPR: The nail and cosmetics. In: Samman PD, Fenton DA (eds): The Nails in Disease, 4th ed. Chicago, Yearbook Publishers, 1986, p 129.

BIBLIOGRAPHY

Gummer CL, Dawber RPR: Diseases of the Hair and Scalp, 3rd ed. London, Blackwell Scientific, 1997, chap. 15.
Olsen EA: Disorders of Hair Growth: Diagnosis and Treatment. New York, McGraw-Hill, 1994, chaps. 16, 17.

Surgical Treatments

ECKART HANEKE

Diagnostic Procedures

Although nail disorders may be difficult to diagnose clinically, biopsies are far too rarely performed. There are several biopsy techniques that yield good specimens for histopathology if the correct biopsy site is chosen.[1, 2]

NAIL PLATE BIOPSIES

The simplest way to biopsy a nail plate is to clip a part of its free portion; commonly the most proximal area of the onycholytic nail should be included. This technique is often sufficient to make the diagnosis of an onychomycosis or to determine the nature of a pigment. The nail clipping requires no formalin fixation. Periodic acid–Schiff stain is recommended for identification of fungi, argentaffin reaction for melanin, and peroxidase reaction for blood. (Subungual hematomas remain Prussian blue negative.)

Discoloration of the nail plate over the nail bed and matrix can be diagnosed by punching out a little disc of the plate. In case of proximal subungual onychomycosis, there is usually no plate–nail bed adherence, so the nail disc may be punched out without local anesthesia. It is wise to soak the digit in warm water for about 10 minutes beforehand to render the nail plate softer and the punching easier. This technique is also useful for the differential diagnosis of subungual hemorrhage and melanin pigmentation.[1, 3]

NAIL BIOPSIES

Depending on the pathological process suspected, a biopsy of the nail bed, matrix, or nail fold may be indicated (Fig. 14–1). These biopsies are best carried out under ring block anesthesia at the base of the digit.

Nail bed biopsies may be performed with a punch or a scalpel. Again, the plate should be softened with a warm bath. A 4- to 6-mm hole may be punched into the plate, and a 3- to 4-mm punch is taken from the nail bed. The punch is run down to the bone, and the tissue is carefully dissected from the bone without crushing it with pincers. A fine injection needle, bent to a fine hook, may be used to gently elevate the tissue cylinder, which is cut from its deep anchoring with curved iris scissors. A 3- to 4-mm defect in the nail bed needs no suture. If a scalpel biopsy is preferred, a 6-mm hole is cut or punched into the nail plate to allow a narrow fusiform biopsy to be cut. All incisions in the nail bed are carried out in a longitudinal direction, respecting the unique, longitudinally arranged rete ridges of the nail bed. The defect may be sutured with 6-0 polyglactin after the adjacent nail bed is dissected from the underlying bone.

Matrix biopsies are useful in the diagnosis of longitudinally striated lesions. Either a punch or a scalpel may be used. Punch defects smaller than 3 mm in diameter need no suture. Depending on the location of the pathology, it may be necessary to reflect the proximal nail fold. This is done after carefully freeing the undersurface of the proximal nail fold from the underlying nail plate using a septum elevator, the curved tip of which is directed to the plate. The punch is run through the soft plate and matrix down to the bone, and the entire specimen is transferred to the fixative. Lesions wider than 3 mm require a fusiform excision that, in contrast to the nail bed, is always oriented transversally to avoid a split nail from a longitudinal scar in the matrix. The distal margin of the biopsy should run parallel to the lunula

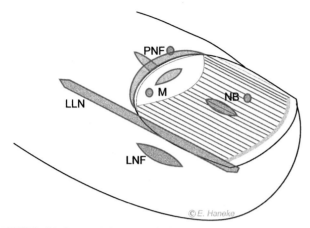

FIGURE 14-1 ■ Nail biopsies of the nail apparatus. LLN, lateral longitudinal nail biopsy; LNF, narrow longitudinal biopsy of the lateral nail fold; M, transverse fusiform or small punch biopsies of the nail matrix; NB, longitudinal and punch biopsies of the nail bed; PNF, punch, narrow wedge, and crescentic biopsies of the proximal nail fold.

border. Careful undermining usually allows a reduced size of the biopsy defect, but care should be taken because the matrix tissue is very friable. Finally, the proximal nail fold is resutured, and antibiotic tulle gras and a thick padded dressing are applied.

Lateral longitudinal nail biopsies including the whole length of the nail organ with proximal nail fold, matrix, nail bed, plate, and hyponychium provide maximal information. Because of the growth characteristics of the nail, a longitudinal biopsy reflects the many months that it takes for the nail to grow out. A linear incision is carried out from the distal dorsal crease of the distal interphalangeal joint all along through the nail down to the bone to the hyponychium, and a second incision is performed 2 mm lateral to the first, running along the lateral nail sulcus. The lateral nail wall is left intact.[1, 3]

BIOPSY OF THE NAIL FOLDS

The proximal nail fold may exhibit characteristic alterations confirming a particular disease (e.g., connective tissue disease). Usually, a 2-mm punch is used to take a small piece from the fold, leaving its free margin intact. No suture is necessary. A narrow wedge excision with its longitudinal axis perpendicular to the border of the nail fold or a crescent of tissue 2 to 3 mm wide and parallel to the free margin of the proximal nail fold may be taken (see Fig. 14–1). A shave excision can yield an excellent specimen for the diagnosis of superficial lesions such as actinic keratoses or blisters.

A narrow, fusiform excision is adequate for biopsy of the lateral nail fold (see Fig. 14–1).

Specific Procedures

NAIL AVULSION

Nail avulsion is performed far too often and appears to be the only nail surgery procedure done by many gen-

eral practitioners, surgeons, and dermatologists. Nail avulsions are often done as a substitute for diagnosis and even as a treatment per se. However, because the avulsed nail is never the origin of the disorder but the consequence of a diseased matrix, nail bed, or periungual tissue, these must be the target of subsequent therapy.

Whenever possible, atraumatic chemical avulsion using a 40% urea or 50% potassium iodate paste should be considered, and nail avulsion should be restricted to the diseased portion or the area of altered nail bed and matrix (i.e., partial nail avulsion). For partial plate removal, a septum elevator with its curved tip directed upward is gently inserted under the nail and advanced a few millimeters more proximal than the diseased area; it is then brought laterally while being moved back and forth. The detached plate area is cut with sturdy curved scissors. Nail bed hyperkeratoses may be cautiously curetted or atraumatically removed using 20% to 40% urea or 10% to 20% salicylic acid ointment.

Total nail avulsion may be performed in a similar way. The septum elevator is placed under the nail and pushed proximally, keeping its curved end up to the plate, to detach the plate from nail bed and matrix with back-and-forth motions. The elevator is then rotated 180 degrees and inserted, with the tip showing down to the plate, under the proximal nail fold to free the nail plate, which can then be taken out with a forceps (Fig. 14–2). The technique of using a sturdy hemostat that is run under the lateral margin of the plate and proximal nail fold, grasping the plate firmly and tearing it out with a turning of the hemostat, is extremely traumatizing and should be abandoned.

The proximal approach is less damaging to the nail apparatus. The proximal nail fold is freed from the plate, and the elevator is then turned 150 to 180 degrees to get under the most proximal portion of the nail plate. This is then gently separated from the matrix and the nail bed, again using back-and-forth motions from one side of the nail to the other. This technique is much less traumatizing because the keratin filaments form a continuous line slowly ascending from basal matrix cells into the nail plate[1] (see Fig. 14–2).

After avulsion, the vulnerable matrix and nail bed are treated with an antibiotic or antifungal ointment. After completion of re-epithelialization, the specific treatment must be started and continued until a normal nail has regrown.

MATRICECTOMY

Certain nail conditions such as onychogryphosis and severe post-traumatic nail dystrophy are not amenable to either conservative or surgical treatment. To permanently free the patient from pain, a complete matricectomy may be necessary.

In onychogryphosis and onychauxis, the nail is thickened and does not adhere to the nail bed, but there is usually a hard hyperkeratosis just distal to the nail bed–matrix transition, so that considerable force would be necessary to perform a distal nail avulsion. In contrast, the adherence to the proximal nail fold is weak and the

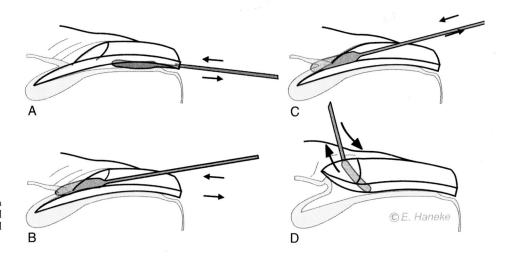

FIGURE 14–2 ■ Nail avulsion techniques. *A* and *B*, Distal nail avulsion. *C* and *D*, Proximal nail avulsion.

nail pocket is shallow, so that the dystrophic nail can easily be removed by the proximal approach. A tourniquet is applied to achieve a bloodless field, and liquefied phenol (90% phenol) is vigorously rubbed into the matrix epithelium for 2 to 3 minutes. Special attention is paid to the treatment of the lateral matrix horns to avoid the development of nail spicules. Because phenol treatment results in the formation of an eschar from coagulated protein, "neutralization" with alcohol is unnecessary. Further, after the tourniquet is released, blood inactivates any phenol. The procedure is completed with a padded dressing, using plenty of antimicrobial ointment. The dressing is changed in an antiseptic bath (e.g., povidone-iodine soap solution) daily until oozing stops completely.

Surgical matricectomy is an alternative to complete matrix phenolization, but it demands much greater surgical skills and causes more morbidity immediately postoperatively. The entire matrix field must be resected, incising all around the matrix. This can be difficult because the lateral matrix horns often reach far back proximally and volarly. Especially in the great toe, the matrix may cover almost half of the circumference of the base of the distal phalanx. Further, in the center of the proximal tip of the matrix, the distance between the matrix epithelium and the bone with its tendon insertion is less than 1 mm. The proximal nail fold is incised on both sides to be reflected and to demonstrate the extent of the matrix and its lateral horns. An incision is carried out just distal to the lunula border down to the bone to allow the matrix to be dissected from the bone. The use of blunt-tipped curved scissors helps to prevent injury to the extensor tendon insertion. Particular attention must be paid to dissecting all of the lateral matrix horns. The undersurface of the proximal nail fold is de-epithelialized and turned back to cover about 60% of the defect, the rest of which heals by secondary intention.

If an artificial nail is to be applied laterally, a nail pocket may be created. The proximal nail fold is incised horizontally from its proximal origin about halfway, and the proximal lower portion is pulled distally, sutured at both sides to the lateral wall of the defect, and fixed to the bone with fibrin glue. This shallow new nail pocket

is kept open by insertion of a soft, flexible sheet of silicone that is removed only after healing and re-epithelization of the remaining surgical defect. Although this operation is fairly radical, it is not rare to observe nail spicules emerging from the former lateral matrix horns some months later.

NAIL ABLATION

Nail ablation may be necessary for severely painful nail dystrophy and some nail tumors. The surgical technique is similar to that described previously, but the incision is carried all around the entire nail organ, thus including all nail walls, hyponychium, nail bed, and matrix. The defect may be closed with a free full-thickness skin graft, a reversed dermal graft, or a cross-digit flap (Fig. 14–3).

LATERAL HYPERTROPHIC NAIL LIP

The great toenail of neonates and infants may be covered a one-third extent by a grossly hypertrophic nail fold, usually of the medial aspect of the toe. Surgery is rarely necessary when the hypertrophic nail lip is gently but consistently massaged from a medial to a lateral-

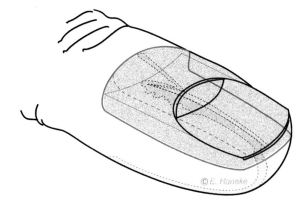

FIGURE 14–3 ■ Surgical matrix excision and nail ablation. Distal phalanx with the nail and sagittal section through the nail *(dotted lines)*; red line represents incisions, shaded area marks excised tissue.

plantar direction. If this is not sufficient, the portion of the nail fold overlying the nail plate may simply be cut. A hard hypertrophic lateral nail fold may develop from long-standing ingrown toenail when the chronic granulation tissue becomes fibrotic to eventually form a dense mass. A fusiform excision from the lateral aspect of the toe under the hypertrophied lateral nail fold pulls it down and releases the margin of the nail plate.

CONGENITAL MALALIGNMENT

Congenital malalignment is a relatively common condition.[1, 4] Neonates and infants have one, or more often both, great toenails thickened, discolored, and transversally overcurved. The long axis of the nail deviates laterally from the axis of the terminal phalanx. In addition, the phalanx may be short and bulbous, with the nail growing slightly upward. This condition may resolve spontaneously, or it may lead to permanent nail dystrophy, epidermization of the nail bed with lack of nail bed–nail plate attachment, and repeated nail loss. It is thought that the deviation of the nail axis causes unphysiological stress to the matrix with frequently repeated disruption of nail formation, leading to the oystershell-like appearance of the plate. There is no sign or symptom indicating the future course. Permanent nail dystrophy may develop, or the nail may reattach to the nail bed and grow normally despite the malalignment, and even in the most obvious deviation from the correct axis the nail may grow normally from birth. Clinical experience has shown that nail dystrophy after the age of 2 years carries a high risk of being irreparable. Surgical correction is therefore recommended before that age.

Usually with the patient under general anesthesia, an incision is carried around and approximately 3 mm under the entire nail organ, and a second incision is performed to allow excision of a crescentic wedge of tissue. This wedge is widest in its distal-medial part. The nail bed and matrix are dissected from the terminal phalanx bone and rotated into their correct axis. A small Burrow's triangle may have to be excised at the medial pole of the wedge. The defect is sutured with 5-0 monofil, nonabsorbable sutures left in place for 10 to 14 days. Healing is usually uneventful, and there appears to be little postoperative pain. It takes usually more than 6 months before normal nail growth is observed. Twice-daily application of 20% azelaic acid cream appears to be beneficial.

When the great toe is bulbous, the wedge to be excised may have to be wider, and a small layer of the cartilaginous dorsal distal end of the phalanx must also be removed.

Nail malalignment is a constant feature of pincer toenails and very common in foot malformations.

INGROWN TOENAILS

Nails may grow into the periungual tissue at any age.[1, 5]

Neonatal Ingrown Toenails

In neonates, the nails may not yet have overgrown the tip of the digits and may grow into the distal nail wall and distal portion of the lateral nail walls. Treatment is essentially nonsurgical.

Infantile Ingrown Toenails

Infantile ingrown toenails are usually caused by either nail malalignment or hypertrophic lips (see previous discussion).

Juvenile Ingrown Toenails

Ingrown toenails in adolescents are common. Usually the patients are tall and have hyperhidrosis of the feet. Their nails are wide and transversally overcurved, cutting into the lateral nail sulci. They are often cut at their distal corners, but sharp nail spicules remain at the lateral margins. These grow into the periungual tissue, giving rise to painful inflammation that tends to get secondarily infected. There are many treatment recommendations, ranging from purely conservative to grossly inadequate radical surgery. In general, the treatment should respect the pathogenesis and avoid any mutilation.

Conservative therapy consists of placing a gutter over the lateral margin to allow the nail to grow out without digging into the distal portion of the lateral nail groove. This procedure usually requires anesthesia. However, the factors that caused the nail to grow in are still present, and recurrences are therefore rather the rule than an exception.

The logical treatment of a condition that is caused by a discrepancy between too wide a nail and too narrow a nail bed is narrowing of the nail plate (Fig. 14–4). This is best done under a proximal ring block of the toe. The lateral margins of the nail plate are freed from the proximal nail fold and the nail bed and are cut with

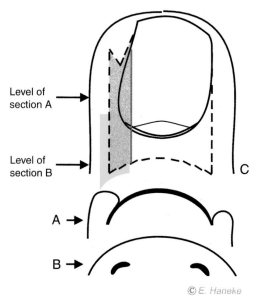

© E. Haneke

FIGURE 14–4 ■ Juvenile ingrown toenail. *A,* The nail plate is overcurved, digging deep into the lateral groove. *B,* The lateral matrix horns are reaching far proximally. *C,* Surgical treatment. The red line represents the section of the nail plate; the yellow area is either dissected or cauterized with liquified phenol. The shaded area shows the lateral strip to be avulsed.

straight, sturdy scissors. To permanently narrow the nail plate, the lateral matrix horn is either cauterized or dissected. For cauterization, liquefied phenol (90% phenol) is used. A tourniquet is applied to preclude any bleeding, and the lateral matrix horn is cleaned and dried. A cotton-tipped applicator is dipped into liquefied phenol and then vigorously rubbed into the matrix for 2 to 3 minutes. Excess granulation tissue may also gently be touched with the phenol to speed its involution. Liquefied phenol cauterizes the matrix epithelium, forming a barrier against further phenol penetration, so there is no risk of phenol cardiotoxicity, nephrotoxicity, or delayed and protracted action. Phenol has, in addition, an antiseptic and local anesthetic effect. Postoperative morbidity and pain are considerably reduced. A padded dressing with antiseptic tulle gras is applied and changed daily after a bath containing povidone-iodine soap solution until healing, which takes 3 to 6 weeks. Recurrences are very rare provided the phenol was rubbed in long enough.

The lateral matrix horns may be removed surgically. After avulsion of the lateral ingrown nail strips, an incision is made in the proximal nail fold from the junction of the proximal and lateral nail folds in a proximal plantar direction to open the lateral portion of the nail pocket and allow the lateral matrix horns to be visualized. They are then meticulously dissected and excised. Care must be taken not to leave any matrix remnants behind; they would give rise to a matrix cyst or nail spicules. Small antibiotic tablets are placed into the wound cavity, and the section of the proximal nail fold is closed with a Steri-Strip or a 5-0 skin suture. A thick padded dressing that allows blood to be absorbed is applied for 24 hours and changed after a disinfecting foot bath. Further changes of dressing depend on the degree of infection and amount of granulation tissue. Healing is usually complete after 10 to 14 days. Raising the feet above the horizontal line reduces postoperative pain.

In my experience, complete nail avulsion some weeks before surgery of the ingrown toenail is not necessary with this technique. Nail avulsion causes a distal nail wall, interfering with nail growth. Wedge excisions, often taking a large portion of the lateral nail wall and a strip of the nail bed and nail plate, are inadequate methods. They reduce the width of the nail bed, take the lateral nail groove away, and narrow the toe. However, they do not consider the true shape of the lateral matrix horn, which reaches far proximally and plantarly so that the matrix often covers more than 40% of the circumference of the toe's base. For the common type of lateral ingrowing, a horizontal, crescent-shaped wedge excision also is not adequate.[5]

In the case of a distal nail wall preventing the nail from growing over it, a crescentic wedge excision is indicated. An excision is carried out around the distal half of the toe, 3 mm under the hyponychium. A second incision is carried out, beginning and ending at the same points but taking a width of about 4 mm at the tip of the toe. The distal nail wall is mobilized just proximal to the hyponychium and pulled down by suturing it to the plantar wound margin. If there is also distal-lateral ingrowing, the crescentic wedge should take more tissue

beneath the lateral nail grooves. Healing of this operation wound takes 2 to 3 weeks.[1]

ADULT-TYPE INGROWN NAIL

In adults, usually those older than 50 years of age, a gradual transverse overcurvature and thickening of the nail plate may develop. This can lead to painful pressure on the lateral nail grooves that may be aggravated by hyperkeratosis of the grooves (onychophosis). Padding of the lateral nail groove with a whisp of cotton wool and thinning of the nail plate by grinding it down to make it more pliable may help in some cases. A definitive cure is achieved with the use of selective lateral matrix horn cautery or dissection.

PINCER NAIL

This condition is characterized by a transversally overcurved nail that pinches the nail bed. The overcurvature usually increases distally. Pain often is not closely related to the degree of nail bed constriction. However, pain may be so excruciating that even a bedsheet cannot be tolerated.

The various types of pincer nails must be differentiated.[6] The symmetrical form appears to be a hereditary trait. The hallux nails are most severely involved and show a lateral deviation; the lesser toes, when affected, are medially deviated. The overcurvature increases distally. X-ray films invariably show a widening of the base of the distal phalanx, often with hooklike osteophytes. The wide base decreases the normal transverse curvature of the nail proximally, which in turn increases the curvature distally. The widening of the base is more pronounced on its medial aspect, thus pushing the nail to the lateral side. Corresponding changes can be seen in the lesser toes.

Acquired forms are usually asymmetrical and may be caused by foot deformation, degenerative osteoarthritis of the distal interphalangeal joints with formation of Heberden's nodes, or chronic skin diseases, particularly (arthropathic) psoriasis.

Conservative treatment using orthonyx braces is commonly unsuccessful because the underlying bone alteration is not considered. It takes many months with several sessions to adapt the braces to get a flatter nail, but it will soon overcurve again.

Surgical treatment is aimed at releasing the decurving force on the proximal nail plate portion, spreading and flattening the nail bed, and removing the distal dorsal osteophyte developing from the traction of the heaped-up nail plate on the nail bed, which is firmly bound to the bone (Fig. 14–5). Because the base of the distal phalanx cannot be narrowed without damaging the ligaments, the nail plate must be narrowed permanently. This is done as described for the treatment of ingrown toenails. Depending on the degree of overcurvature, the nail plate may be partially, or more rarely completely, avulsed. A median sagittal incision is then carried out along the height of the pinched nail bed, which is carefully dissected from the bone. The distal dorsal osteophyte is removed with a rongeur or a nail clipper, and

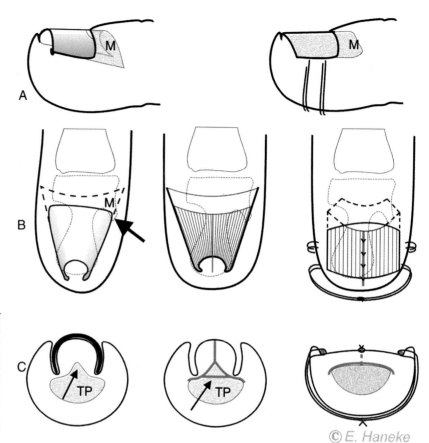

FIGURE 14–5 ■ Pathogenesis and treatment of pincer nail. *A,* Lateral view of pincer nail in the preoperative state *(left)* and the postoperative state *(right). B,* Dorsal view in the preoperative state *(left),* with an outline of the incision *(middle),* and in the postoperative state *(right). C,* Transverse section through the distal phalanx in the preoperative state *(left),* with an outline of the incision *(middle),* and in the postoperative state *(right).* M, matrix; *thick arrow,* medial osteophyte; *thin arrow,* distal dorsal traction osteophyte (TP).

© E. Haneke

the nail bed is gently pressed onto the bone and sutured with 6-0 polyglactin. Reversed tie-over sutures are made from one lateral nail fold to the other after placement of fine rubber tubes into the lateral grooves to prevent the sutures from cutting through the lateral nail fold. These stitches are removed after 18 to 20 days.

Selective matrix horn resection is also the treatment of choice for most acquired forms of pincer nails.

SUBUNGUAL HEMATOMA

Subungual hematoma is a common event that occurs after a single heavy, usually painful, trauma or after repeated microtrauma that often remains unnoticed. A painful subungual hematoma may be treated by drilling a hole into the nail plate and evacuating the blood. The pain usually stops immediately. If more than 50% of the nail bed and matrix are occupied by the hematoma, laceration of the soft tissue and a bone fracture are probable. A radiographic study is mandatory. Any dislocation of bone fragments should be corrected, and the matrix and nail bed should be cleaned and sutured to avoid subsequent nail dystrophy.

▌ Infections

FUNGAL NAIL INFECTIONS

Onychomycoses are the most common nail diseases and the most difficult to treat of all dermatomycoses. As already pointed out, nail avulsion must never be the first-line treatment; in fact, it is no therapy per se. The removal of the nail plate overlying the diseased portion of the nail bed enables a topical treatment to be carried out. Even partial nail avulsion should be performed as atraumatically as possible, preferably using 40% urea paste under occlusion. This also softens the subungual hyperkeratosis that contains the majority of fungi, so that it can be painlessly scraped off.

CHRONIC PARONYCHIA

Long-standing inflammation of the proximal nail fold, whatever its cause, leads to a thickening with loss of the cuticle and attachment of the eponychium to the nail plate. This gives rise to a slit-like space under the proximal nail fold, where foreign material may be entrapped. When conservative treatment fails despite removal of foreign bodies and successful eradication of any infectious cause, a crescentic excision of the proximal nail fold is often helpful (Fig 14–6). Using a no. 15 scalpel angled at 45 to 60 degrees, a 3-mm strip of tissue is removed to form a new proximal nail fold. Re-epithelialization takes place within 8 to 12 days. With the creation of an acute angle at the free margin of the proximal nail fold a new cuticle can be formed, sealing the nail pocket.[1, 7]

WHITLOW

This superficial bacterial infection is usually caused by *Staphylococcus aureus* and develops after a minor pene-

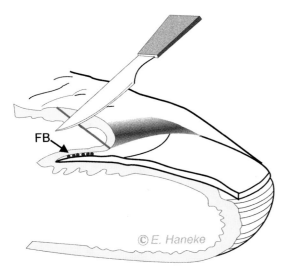

FIGURE 14–6 ■ Surgical treatment of chronic paronychia. FB, foreign body.

trating injury. A blister forms that is at first clear but soon becomes putrid and may extend around the proximal half of the nail ("run-around"). The blister roof is removed, and the digit is soaked with disinfective compresses two or three times a day. Systemic antibiotics are not routinely needed.

(SUBUNGUAL) FELON

A felon is a deep bacterial infection of the periungual and subungual tissue, usually caused by *S. aureus*. When it drains under the nail, pus is accumulated between the matrix and plate because the attachment is less firm to the matrix than to the nail bed. This may permanently damage the matrix, especially in children. If a subungual felon does not respond to antibiotic treatment within 24 to 48 hours, a partial proximal nail plate removal is indicated. A piece of gauze impregnated with antibiotic ointment is then placed under the proximal nail fold to allow the pus to drain.[1]

Tumors and Pseudotumors

WARTS

Viral warts are the most common tumors of the nail region. They are predominantly located around the nail but may be found under the proximal nail fold, in the nail grooves, and under the nail plate. They are notoriously resistant to most conservative treatment regimens. I prefer to apply saturated monochloroacetic acid and cover it with salicylic plaster. Hot hand baths twice daily are important supportive measures. After 1 week, the plaster is removed, the necrotic wart material is removed, and the procedure is repeated until all warts have disappeared. For subungual warts, the overlying plate must be removed. Alternatives are bleomycin needling, carbon dioxide laser vaporization, cautious cryotherapy, and curettage.

MYXOID PSEUDOCYST

This lesion, also called *dorsal finger cyst,* is a degenerative pseudotumor. About 90% arise in the proximal nail fold of fingers. Of the many treatment modalities, I recommend cryosurgery and radical excision. Cryosurgery has a success rate of approximately 80%. One course of liquid nitrogen is applied after needling and expression of the lesion. Healing takes several weeks. For radical surgery, 0.05 to 0.1 mL of 1% methylene blue solution is injected into the distal joint and an incision is carried around the lesion, which is then meticulously dissected. A small transposition flap is raised and sutured into the defect (Fig. 14–7). The cure rate is 95%.[1, 8]

EPIDERMOID CARCINOMA

Bowen's disease and squamous cell carcinoma of the nail unit are the second most common malignant nail tumors. They often mimic warts or other benign inflammatory lesions. A biopsy or complete excision is neces-

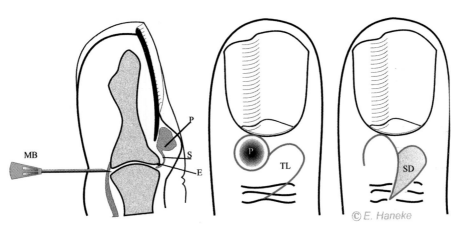

FIGURE 14–7 ■ Treatment of myxoid pseudocysts (dorsal finger cysts). E, exostosis; MB, injection of methylene blue; P, pseudocyst; S, stalk connecting pseudocyst with joint; SD, secondary defect for second intention healing; TL, transposition flap.

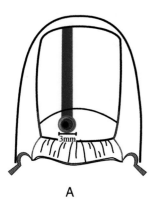 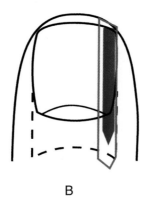 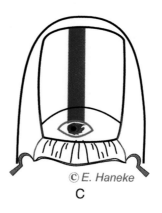

FIGURE 14–8 ■ Diagnostic biopsies in longitudinal melanonychia. *A,* Narrow band may be biopsied with a 3-mm punch. *B,* Pigment streak in the lateral position may be removed using the lateral longitudinal nail biopsy technique. *C,* Central melanonychia wider than 3 mm requires fusiform excision.

sary for such lesions when they occur in persons older than 40 years of age. Mohs' micrographic surgery is the treatment of choice to save as much tissue as possible and ensure the highest cure rate.[9] Defects in the lateral nail region can often be repaired using a nail flap, either by the method of Schernberg and Amiel[10] or with a bridge flap.[11]

LONGITUDINAL MELANONYCHIA AND UNGUAL MELANOMA

About 70% of nail melanomas begin with a pigmentation that appears as a longitudinal brown streak. Any streak wider than 5 mm occurring in an adult is highly suggestive of malignant melanoma. Streaks in lateral position can be removed by the technique used for the lateral longitudinal nail biopsy (Fig. 14–8). Pigmented bands located in the central third of the nail if less than 3 mm wide require a punch biopsy of the melanocyte focus in the matrix. Those wider than 3 mm should be removed by a transverse fusiform excision; suture of the defect should avoid cutting through the fragile matrix. Wide bands require a nail flap, but this often leaves a split nail.[1, 12]

The patient's age, intensity of pigmentation, and width of the melanonychia are not reliable signs, and a biopsy is recommended in all cases of acquired pigmented nail streaks in persons with fair complexion. Histopathology of early melanoma can be difficult, and step and serial sections are necessary.

Simple Reconstructive Surgery

SPLIT NAIL

The most common cause of nail splits is longitudinal scars of the matrix resulting from trauma or a scarring dermatosis. Split nail repair requires excision of the sterile matrix portion and suture without any step formation in matrix and nail bed (Fig. 14–9). The matrix and nail bed scar is excised, and the corresponding nail plate with 1 to 2 mm additional nail is removed. Matrix and nail bed are sutured with 6-0 absorbable stitches, and the nail plate is then approximated using 4-0 skin sutures. This brings matrix and nail bed closer together

and relieves the fine sutures. The success rate is approximately 50%.[3]

RECONSTRUCTION OF THE LATERAL NAIL FOLD

Lateral longitudinal nail biopsies and other excisions of the lateral nail fold may cause loss of the lateral nail fold. A simple modification of the suture can reconstruct the nail fold (Fig. 14–10). A backstitch suture beginning in the middle of the lateral aspect of the digit, carried

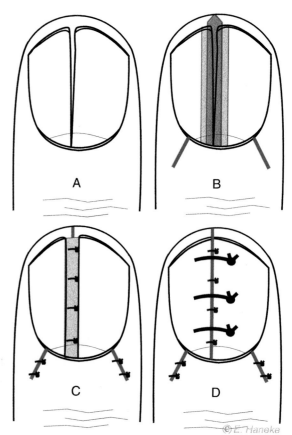

FIGURE 14–9 ■ Split nail correction. *A,* The proximal nail fold is incised to permit reflection. *B,* A small strip of the nail is removed. *C,* The nail bed and the proximal nail folds are sutured with 6-0 absorbable material. *D,* The nail plate is sutured with 3-0 material.

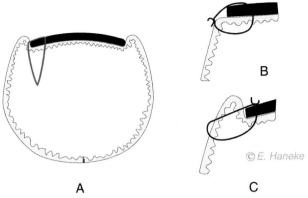

FIGURE 14–10 ■ Reconstruction of the lateral nail fold. *A,* Outline of the lateral nail biopsy. *B,* Suture without backstitch makes the lateral nail fold disappear. *C,* Backstitch suture elevates the lateral aspect of the digit and creates a new lateral nail fold.

through the nail bed and plate, and running back through the lateral side dorsally raises the skin and creates a new lateral nail fold.[13]

RACKET NAIL CORRECTION

The racket nail deformity is caused by premature ossification of the epiphysis of the terminal phalanx so that the longitudinal growth stops but the base still grows wider. Characteristically, there are no pronounced lateral nail folds. Correction of this condition requires two longitudinal nail biopsies, one on each side of the nail, with reconstruction of the lateral nail folds as outlined previously[1, 14] (Fig.14–11).

RECONSTRUCTION OF THE PROXIMAL NAIL FOLD

Loss of the proximal nail fold can lead to nail dystrophy, longitudinal striations, lusterlessness, and discoloration. A new nail fold can be created with the use of two narrow transposition flaps from the sides of the digit or a bridge flap from the dorsal aspect of the digit. How-

ever, loss of the most proximal part of the undersurface of the proximal nail fold and matrix cannot be repaired, and therefore a completely smooth and shiny nail plate will never regrow.

Anesthesia, Preoperative and Postoperative Care, and Complications

In most cases, a proximal ring block using 2 to 3 mL of 2% lidocaine or similar local anesthetic without vasoconstrictor is sufficient. Distal infiltration anesthesia is more painful and carries a greater risk of infection.

Before the operation, a disinfective hand or foot scrub should be performed. Smoking is forbidden to the patient from the evening before until the day after surgery. Perioperative antibiotic prophylaxis may be considered. Raising the extremity above the horizontal line relieves pain, which may be intense for 24 hours; if pain persists and becomes pulsating, infection may be the cause. The dressing should use nonadherent gauze and should be thick enough to absorb shock and blood. A new dressing is often necessary after 24 hours.

Possible complications are infection, prolonged bleeding, numbness, and, rarely, sympathetic reflex dystrophy. Other complications may be disease-related.[15]

REFERENCES

1. Haneke E, Baran R: Nail surgery and traumatic abnormalities. In: Baran R, Dawber RPR (eds): Diseases of the Nails and Their Management, 2nd ed. Oxford, Blackwell, 1994, pp 345–415.
2. Salasche S: Surgery. In: Scher RK, Daniel CR III (eds): Nails: Therapy, Diagnosis, Surgery. Philadelphia, WB Saunders, 1990, pp 258–280.
3. Haneke E: Cirugía dermatológica de la región ungueal. Mongrafias de Dermatología 4:408–423, 1991.
4. Baran R, Haneke E: Etiology and treatment of nail malalignment. Dermatol Surg 24:719–721, 1998.
5. Haneke E: Surgical treatment of ingrowing toenails. Cutis 37:251–256, 1986.
6. Haneke E: Etiopathogénie et traitement de l'hypercourbure trans-

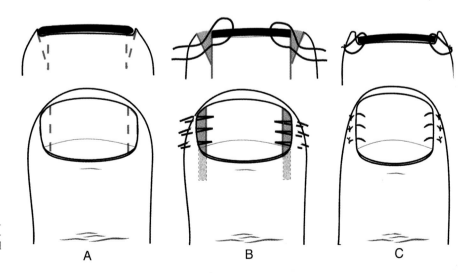

FIGURE 14–11 ■ Racket nail correction. *A,* Outline of incisions. *B,* Lateral excisions of the nail bed and matrix. *C,* End of the operation.

versale de l'ongle du gros orteil. J Méd Esthét Chir Dermatol 19:123–127, 1992.

7. Baran R, Bureau H: Surgical treatment of recalcitrant chronic paronychia of the fingers. J Dermatol Surg Oncol 7:106–107, 1981.

8. Haneke E: Operative Therapie der myxoiden Pseudozyste. In: Haneke E (ed): Fortschritte der operativen Dermatologie 4. Berlin, Springer, 1988, pp 221–227.

9. Mikhail G: Subungual epidermoid carcinoma. J Am Acad Dermatol 11:291–298, 1984.

10. Schernberg F, Amiel M: Etude anatomo-pathologique d'un lambeau unguéal complet. Ann Chir Plast Esthet 30:217–231, 1985.

11. Haneke E: Deckung von Defekten des Nagelorgans mit einem Brückenlappen. In: Konz B, Wörle B, Sander A: Ästhetische und korrektive Dermatologie. Fortschritte der operativen und

onkologischen Dermatologie, vol 14. Berlin, Blackwell, 1999, pp 82–87.

12. Baran R, Kechijian P: Longitudinal melanonychia (melanonychia striata). Diagnosis and management. J Am Acad Dermatol 21:1165–1175, 1989.

13. Haneke E: Reconstruction of the lateral nail fold after lateral longitudinal nail biopsy. In: Robins P (ed): Surgical Gems in Dermatology. New York, Journal Publishing Group, 1988, pp 91–93.

14. Haneke E: Behandlung einiger Nagelfehlbildungen. In: Wolff HH, Schmeller W (eds): Fehlbildungen, Nävi, Melanome: Fortschritte der Operativen Dermatologie, vol 2. Berlin, Springer, 1985, pp 71–77.

15. Haneke E, Baran R: Nail surgery. In: Harahap M (ed): Complications of Dermatologic Surgery: Prevention and Treatment. Berlin, Springer, 1993, pp 84–91.

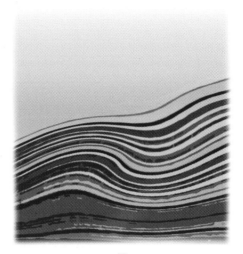

SPECIAL
ISSUES

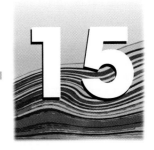

chapter

15

Adverse Effects and Drug Interactions of Medications Used to Treat Hair and Nail Disorders

H. IRVING KATZ

The purpose of this chapter is to stimulate the reader to learn more about the medications prescribed for hair and nail disorders. The systemic medications used include oral antifungals, antibiotics, hormone and hormone modulators, and psychotherapeutic agents. Examples of adverse effects and drug interactions are discussed in this chapter. The reader should refer to the most current manufacturer's product information or an in-depth reference source for details regarding a particular agent before starting treatment.

Drug-induced adverse effects and drug interactions are iatrogenic diseases. The frequency, scope, and intensity of adverse experiences are listed in the specific manufacturer's package insert and described in the literature. Pregnancy, lactation, and a documented past hypersensitivity to a specific medication are well-known warning signals. Any one of these signals is sufficient reason to rethink or not to administer a medication for a disorder affecting hair or nails. In addition, if a patient is elderly, is taking other medications, or has hepatic, renal, or cardiac impairment, avoidance or extra caution is necessary.

A drug-related adverse experience is defined as any

undesirable event that occurs in the course of treatment with an agent and is at least possibly related to the medication in question. Adverse experiences can be subdivided according to the organ system involved (e.g., cardiovascular, gastrointestinal, hepatic), their intensity (mild, moderate or severe), and whether they represent a serious threat to patients. Serious adverse experiences include those that cause cancer, are disabling, are life-threatening, are fatal, or result in a congenital anomaly.

Drug interactions are a unique type of adverse experience resulting from alterations in the way a drug is handled or acts in a patient when two or more agents are administered concurrently; the second agent may be a food, a chemical, or another drug. The altered response may be of little significance, or it may result in a clinically significant, serious adverse experience.

Drug interactions are classified as being either pharmacokinetic or pharmacodynamic.[1, 2] The term *pharmacokinetic* refers to how a patient handles a particular drug. Pharmacokinetic interactions encompass the absorption, distribution, metabolism, and elimination of therapeutic agents. Pharmacokinetic interactions ultimately affect the blood level or concentration of a particular drug. *Pharmacodynamic* interactions involve the actual physiological effects of a drug in a patient. Pharmacodynamic drug interactions entail what a drug does to a person. Competition among drugs for similar receptors or competition in a physiological system may result in either agonist or antagonist effects.

Although medications are sometimes eliminated in their native, unchanged form, most must be metabolized by one or more enzymatic catalytic processes that change a parent lipophilic, water-immiscible drug into a more water-soluble form. Such biotransformation may begin in the lumen of the gut or the gut wall, but it usually occurs primarily in the liver.[1] Some drugs are extensively (almost 100%) metabolized during their first pass through the gut or liver. Any interference with such first-pass metabolism can cause significant adverse effects. The orderly breakdown of drugs occurs during phase I and phase II metabolic processes, as summarized in the following paragraphs. Generally, the metabolites of a parent compound are less pharmacologically active than their parent form.

Phase I metabolic reactions are catalyzed by the cytochrome P450 family of heme-containing enzymes.[1, 3–5] Cytochrome P450 enzymes are subclassified into families (e.g., CYP1), subfamilies. (CYP1A). and isoenzymes (CYP1A2), conforming to progressive similarities in their amino acid makeup and substrate specificity.[3] The activity of a CYP isoenzyme may be influenced by the genetic makeup of the patient, by hepatic impairment, or by exogenous chemicals or drugs. Many of the more clinically significant and potentially serious pharmacokinetic drug interactions involve alteration of CYP isoenzymes. CYP isoenzymes have specificity for certain substrate drugs (Table 15–1). One or more CYP isoenzyme pathways may be involved in biotransformation of a specific drug. Cytochrome P450 enzymes may exert a rate-limiting effect on drug metabolism, especially if only one isoenzyme is required for such biotransformation. Understanding of cytochrome pathways is important in many potential drug interactions.

CYP isoenzymes can be either induced or inhibited by other drugs. Agents that cause CYP induction accelerate drug biotransformation and may lead to therapeutic failure as a result of decreased blood levels of the parent substrate drug. In contrast, CYP inhibition decreases drug metabolism and may cause increased blood levels of a parent substrate drug (see Table 15–1) Enzyme inhibitors generally produce decreased drug metabolism within a shorter time (hours to days) than enzyme inductors (days to weeks). CYP inhibition can cause increased blood levels of a substrate drug and resultant drug toxicity. Drug toxicity is especially relevant when a concomitant medication has a *narrow therapeutic window* or depends on complete first-pass metabolism after absorption from the gastrointestinal tract.

Phase II metabolism produces highly polar, water-soluble glucuronic acid or other conjugates that are readily eliminated. Noncytochrome enzymes catalyze these conjugation transformations.

The rest of this chapter presents an overview of certain antifungals, antibiotics, hormones or hormone modulators, and psychotherapeutics that may be used to treat hair or nail disorders. Their therapeutic benefit should be balanced by a number of other factors, including the risks for potential adverse effects or drug interactions. The listings in the table should not be considered complete. Also, note that italicized drug classes mentioned in text and tables are elaborated in Table 15–2.

Antifungals

Systemic oral antifungal agents used to treat superficial fungal infections involving hair and nail tissues include the azole/triazoles, griseofulvin and terbinafine. Use of any oral antifungal agent should be avoided, if possible, in a person with severe hepatic impairment. The more common adverse experiences with these agents include drug eruptions, headaches, gastrointestinal complaint, and transient elevations of liver enzymes. Very rare idiosyncratic hematological reactions (leukopenia) or hepatotoxic reactions may occur with some agents. Monitoring of hematological, hepatic, and renal function is generally recommended during long-term treatment with any of the oral antifungal agents listed.

AZOLE/TRIAZOLES

The azole/triazoles include fluconazole, itraconazole, and ketoconazole. They should not be given to pregnant women. Itraconazole capsules and ketoconazole are best absorbed if taken with meals and in an acid gastric milieu. The azole/triazoles inhibit the fungal CYP enzyme, lanosterol 14-demethylase, and to a variable extent inhibit human CYP3A4. Human CYP3A4 inhibition may result in increased blood levels of a number of CYP3A4 substrate drugs (see Table 15–1).[2] Therefore, potent CYP3A4 inhibitors such as itraconazole and ketoconazole (and possibly fluconazole in large doses) should not be used concurrently with certain benzodiazepines, several 3-hydroxy-3-methylglutaryl coenzyme A reductase inhibitors, or selected nonsedating antihistamines, because excessive sedation, myopathy, cardiotoxicity, or other serious adverse effects may occur[1, 2] (see Table 15–1). In addition, fluconazole can act as a CYP2C9 inhibitor[6] (see Table 15–1). Careful patient selection, close monitoring, and certain intermittent dosing schedules theoretically may eliminate or reduce the potential drug interaction risks when concurrent medications are prescribed. Examples of some azole/triazole-related drug interactions are found in Table 15–3.

GRISEOFULVIN

Griseofulvin should not be given if a patient has porphyria or liver impairment or is pregnant. The absorption of griseofulvin from the gastrointestinal tract is increased after a fat-containing meal. Griseofulvin may rarely be associated with hepatotoxic, nephrotoxic, hematotoxic, or phototoxic adverse effects. Griseofulvin is a CYP enzyme inducer and may accelerate the metabolism of drug substrates such as oral contraceptives and

TABLE 15-1 ■ Examples of Cytochrome P450 Substrates, Inducers, and Inhibitors

Isoenzyme	Substrates	Inducers	Inhibitors
CYP1A2	Caffeine[a-c] Clozapine[a-c] Imipramine[a-c] Tacrine[b, c] Theophylline[a-c] Warfarin-r[a, b]	Charcoal-broiled meats[c] Cigarette smoke[c] Phenobarbital[c]	Ciprofloxacin[c] Enoxacin[c] Erythromycin[c] Fluvoxamine[c, d]
CYP2C9/10	Ibuprofen[b, c] Phenytoin[a-c] Tolbutamide[a-c] Warfarin-s[a-c]	Carbamazepine[c] Phenobarbital[c] Rifampin[c, d]	Cimetidine[c] Fluconazole[a] Fluoxetine[c] Fluvoxamine[c] Omeprazole[c]
CYP2D6	Chlorpromazine[c] Clomipramine[a, c] Codeine[a-c] Desipramine[a-c] Dextromethorphan[a, b, d] Encainide[a-c] Flecainide[a-c] Fluoxetine[a-c] Haloperidol[b, c, e] Hydrocodone[b, c] Imipramine[a, c] Metaprolol[a-c] Paroxetine[a-c] Perphenazine[c] Propafenone[a-c] Propranolol[a-c] Risperidone[b, c] Thioridazine[c] Timolol[a-c] Venlafaxine[a, f]		Cimetidine[c, d] Fluoxetine[a, c, d] Haloperidol[c, e] Norfluoxetine[c-e] Paroxetine[a, c, e, g] Propafenone[c] Quinidine[c, e] Terbinafine[h] Thioridazine[c, e]
CYP3A4	Alfentanil[a, c, e] Alprazolam[a, c, e] Amitriptyline[a, c] Astemizole[a-c] Carbamazepine[a, c] Cisapride[a, c] Clarithromycin[a] Cyclosporine[a, e] Dapsone[a] Dexamethasone[a, e] Diazepam[a, e] Diltiazem[a, c] Disopyramide[a, e] Erythromycin[a, e] Ethinyl estradiol[a, i] Felodipine[a, f] Lidocaine[a, c, e] Loratadine[a-c] Lovastatin[c, e] Midazolam[a, c, e] Nifedipine[a, e] Pimozide[j] Quinidine[a, e] Sertraline[a-c, e] Tacrolimus[a, i] Triazolam[a, c, e] Venlafaxine (demethylvenlafaxine)[a, b] Verapamil[a, c, e]	Carbamazepine[c, e] Griseofulvin[i] Isoniazid[i] Phenobarbital[c] Phenytoin[c, e] Rifampin[c, e] Ritonavir[i]	Cimetidine[c, d] Clarithromycin[c, i] Diltiazem[c, e] Erythromycin[c, e] Fluconazole (in large doses)[c] Fluoxetine[a, c, e] Fluvoxamine[a, c, e] Grapefruit juice[c, e] Itraconazole[c, e] Ketoconazole[c, e] Ritonavir[i] Verapamil[e]

[a] Preskorn SH: Clinically relevant pharmacology of selective serotonin reuptake inhibitors. Clin Pharmacokinet 32:1–21, 1997.
[b] Ereshefsky L: Drug-drug interactions involving antidepressants: focus on venlafaxine. J Clin Psychopharmacol 16:37S–53S, 1996.
[c] Aeschlimann JR, Tyler LS: Drug interactions associated with cytochrome P-450 enzymes. J Pharmaceutical Care in Pain and Symptom Control 4:35–54, 1996.
[d] Kerremans AL: Cytochrome P450 isoenzymes: importance for the internist. Neth J Med 48:237–243, 1996.
[e] Ketter TA, Flockhart DA, Post RM, et al: The emerging role of cytochrome P450 3A in psychopharmacology. J Clin Psychopharmacol 15:387–398, 1995.
[f] Albers LJ, Reist C, Helmeste D, Vu R, Tang SW: Paroxetine shifts imipramine metabolism. Psychiatry Res 59:189–196, 1996.
[g] Paxil (paroxetine) [package insert]. Philadelphia, PA: Smith Kline Beecham Pharmaceuticals; 1997.
[h] Personal communication, V. Fischer, PhD, Novartis Pharmaceuticals, East Hanover, NJ, 1999.
[i] Singer MI, Shapiro LE, Shear NH: Cytochrome P-450 3A: interactions with dermatologic therapies. J Am Acad Dermatol 37: 765–771, 1997.
[j] Orap (pimozide) [package insert]. Sellersville, PA: Gate Pharmaceuticals; 1997.

warfarin, leading to subtherapeutic plasma levels and therapeutic failures with these agents[1, 2] (see Table 15–1). Concomitant alcohol ingestion and griseofulvin use should be avoided, because disulfiram-like reactions with tachycardia, diaphoresis, and flushing may occur.

TERBINAFINE

Terbinafine is a synthetic allylamine that inhibits the fungal enzyme squalene epoxidase.[7] Squalene epoxidase is not a CYP enzyme. Terbinafine is extensively bound to plasma proteins, metabolized in the liver by multiple CYP isoenzymes, and primarily eliminated by the renal system.[7] Terbinafine should not be given to persons with renal insufficiency or hepatic impairment. Adverse effects with terbinafine include those common to other antifungals (discussed earlier), along with infrequent (about 2%), reversible taste aberration. Currently there are no drugs that are contraindicated if terbinafine is also given.[7] However, recently terbinafine has been found to be a potent in vitro CYP2D6 inhibitor.[8] Nevertheless, the clinical relevance of this finding is unknown because only a single case report of an adverse interaction with a CYP2D6 substrate (nortriptyline) in an elderly patient who was on multiple other medications has been published.[9] Examples of other CYP2D6 substrates are found in Table 15–1. Clinical monitoring of a patient's therapeutic response is recommended if rifampin and terbinafine are given concurrently. Rifampin may cause a 50% decrease in terbinafine blood levels. Cimetidine may cause a 33% decrease in terbinafine clearance.[7]

TABLE 15-2 ■ Further Clarification and Examples for *Italicized Medications* Found in Text and Tables°

Medication Class	Selected Examples (Generic Names)†
Antidiabetics	Acetohexamide, chlorpropamide, glipizide, insulin, metformin, tolazamide, troglitazone
Antihypertensives	Angiotensin-converting enzyme inhibitors, angiotensin II receptor antagonists, amiloride, beta blockers, calcium channel blockers, clonidine, diuretics, doxazosin, guanabenz, guanethidine, hydralazine, methyldopa, reserpine, terazosin
Benzodiazepines (oxidative metabolism [O] or nonoxidative metabolism [NO])	Alprazolam (O), chlordiazepoxide (O), diazepam (O), lorazepam (NO), midazolam (O), oxazepam (NO), temazepam (NO), triazolam (O)
CNS depressants	Alcohol, barbiturates, benzodiazepines, buprenorphine, buspirone, desflurane, dezocine, droperidol, enflurane, glutethimide, haloperidol, isoflurane, ketamine, meprobamate, methoxyflurane, molindone, narcotics, propofol, sedating antihistamines
Dibenzazepine derivatives	Amoxapine, amitriptyline, carbamazepine, clomipramine, desipramine, doxepin, imipramine
Dihydropyridine calcium channel blockers	Amlodipine, felodipine, isradipine, nicardipine, nifedipine, nimodipine, nisoldipine
Diuretics	Acetazolamide, amiloride, chlorthalidone, ethacrynic acid, furosemide, spironolactone
Drugs with narrow therapeutic window	Amphotericin B, carbamazepine, cyclosporine, digoxin, insulin, methotrexate, phenytoin, tacrolimus, theophylline, warfarin
Gastric acid alkalinizers	Antacids, anticholinergics, didanosine, H₂ blockers, proton pump inhibitors such as lansoprazole or omeprazole, sucralfate
Hyperkalemics	Amiloride, angiotensin-converting enzyme inhibitors, NSAIDs, potassium chloride and other potassium supplements, spironolactone, triamterene, trimethoprim
Hypokalemics	Acetazolamide, amphotericin B, furosemide, sympathomimetics, theophylline, thiazide diuretics
Immunosuppressants	Antithymocyte globulin, anti-Rh₀(D), azathioprine, cyclosporine, muromonab-CD3, mycophenolate mofetil, tacrolimus
Monoamine oxidase inhibitors (MAOIs)	Isocarboxazid, isoniazid (partial), furazolidone (partial), pargyline, phenelzine, procarbazine (partial), tranylcypromine
Nonsteroidal antiinflammatory drugs (NSAIDs)	Diclofenac, etodolac, flurbiprofen, ibuprofen, indomethacin, ketoprofen, ketorolac, meclofenamate, mefenamic acid, nabumetone, naproxen, oxaprozin, piroxicam, sulindac, tolmetin
Oral hypoglycemics	Acetohexamide, chlorpropamide, glipizide, insulin, metforman, repaglinide, tolazamide, troglitagone
Phenothiazines	Chlorpromazine, fluphenazine, mesoridazine, methdilazine, methotrimeprazine, perphenazine, prochlorperazine, promazine, promethazine, thioproperazine, thioridazine, trifluoperazine, triflupromazine, trimeprazine
Polyvalent cations	Aluminum carbonate, aluminum hydroxide, aluminum phosphate, bismuth hydroxide, bismuth subsalicylate, calcium carbonate, calcium citrate, calcium gluconate, ferrous gluconate, ferrous sulfate, magnesium carbonate, magnesium gluconate, magnesium hydroxide, magnesium trisilicate, zinc sulfate
Psychostimulants	Amphetamine, methylphenidate, pemoline
Retinoids	Acitretin, etretinate, isotretinoin, tretinoin
Selective serotonin reuptake inhibitors	Citalopram, fluoxetine, fluvoxamine, paroxetine, sertraline
Sympathomimetics	Dextroamphetamine, dobutamine, dronabinol, ephedrine, epinephrine, fenfluramine, isometheptene, isoproterenol, mephentermine, metaproterenol, methamphetamine, methoxamine, methyldopa, methylphenidate, norepinephrine, phendimetrazine, phentermine, phenylephrine, phenylpropanolamine, pseudoephedrine
Tricyclic antidepressants	Amitryptyline, amoxapine, clomipramine, clozapine, desipramine, doxepin, imipramine, nortriptyline, protriptyline, trimipramine
Tyramine-containing foods	Aged cheeses, aged meats, aged ripened avocados, aged ripened bananas, alcoholic beverages, anchovies, bananas, beers, caviar, Chianti wines, chocolates, fava beans, liqueurs, liver preparations, pickled herring, processed spicy meats such as bologna, pepperoni, salami and sausages, raisins, sauerkraut, sherry, sour creams, soy sauce, yeast extracts, yogurts

° Not all members of the drug class are necessarily associated with the adverse effect or drug interaction. Refer to the individual manufacturer's package insert for details.
† This is not a complete list.

TABLE 15-3 ■ Examples of Azole/Triazole Drug Interactions

Interacting Drug	Potential Consequences of Interactions
Alcohol	May cause a disulfiram-like reaction with ketoconazole[a]
Dihydropyridine types of calcium channel blockers	Monitor; edema reported with itraconazole[a]
CYP3A4 enzyme inducers (see Table 15–1)	Avoid or monitor therapeutic efficacy; decreased fluconazole, itraconazole, or ketoconazole levels may occur[b]
CYP3A4 substrate drugs (see Table 15–1)	Avoid (cisapride, alprazolam, midazolam, triazolam, lovastatin, simvastatin, astemizole, terfenadine) or monitor closely (other CYP3A4 substrate drugs); serious adverse experiences may occur[c, d] (see text)
Digoxin	Monitor; increased digoxin levels may occur with itraconazole or ketoconazole[d]
Gastric acid alkalinizers	Monitor therapeutic efficacy; alkaline gastric pH can decrease itraconazole capsules or ketoconazole absorption[d]
Oral hypoglycemics	Avoid or monitor glucose levels closely; clinically significant increased hypoglycemia may occur with fluconazole[a]
Theophylline	Monitor; increased theophylline blood levels may occur with fluconazole[a]
Vincristine	Monitor; aggravation of vincristine-induced neurotoxicity may occur with itraconazole[d]
Warfarin	Monitor; increased anticoagulant effect and bleeding may occur[d]
Zidovudine	Monitor; increased zidovudine blood levels may occur with fluconazole[c]

Italicized drug classes are elaborated in Table 15–2.
[a] Katz HI, Gupta AK: Oral antifungal drug interactions. Dermatol Clin 15:535–544, 1997.
[b] Gillum JGG, Israel DS, Polk RE: Pharmacokinetic drug interactions with antimicrobial agents [review]. Clin Pharmacokinet 25: 450–482, 1993.
[c] Katz HI: Corticosteroids. In: Katz HI (ed): Guide to Adverse Treatment Interactions for Skin, Hair and Nail Disorders. Philadelphia, Lippincott-Raven Publishers, 1998, pp 51–54.
[d] Sporanox (itraconazole) [package insert]. Titusville, NJ: Janssen Pharmaceutica; 1997.

Antibiotics

The cephalosporin, fluoroquinolone, macrolide, penicillin (penicillinase-resistant), and tetracycline antibiotics may be used to treat uncomplicated skin and soft tissue infections caused by susceptible staphylococcal or streptococcal microorganisms. General types of antibiotic adverse experiences include gastrointestinal distress (nausea, vomiting, or diarrhea, including the rare occurrence of pseudomembranous colitis); hypersensitivity reactions (a variety of drug eruptions, anaphylaxis); and hematological, hepatic, and renal toxicity.[1, 10–12] The concurrent administration of antibiotics and oral contraceptives is controversial. There are isolated case reports of oral contraceptive failures with concurrent use of tetracycline or penicillin-type (ampicillin) antibiotics.[1, 13] Theoretically, broad-spectrum antibiotics could eradicate certain colonic bacteria that are vital to the enterohepatic recirculation of ethinyl estradiol in a small number of women who depend on this extra boost of hormone for proper ovulation. If ethinyl estradiol enterohepatic recirculation is interrupted, then theoretically oral contraceptive pill failure may occur in this small group of women. The individual manufacturer's package insert or product monograph should be consulted for more details.

CEPHALOSPORIN ANTIBIOTICS

Cephalosporins are grouped into generations according to their general antimicrobial profiles.[1, 10, 14] The first-generation cephalosporins are active primarily against gram-positive, methicillin-sensitive staphylococcal and streptococcal organisms. The first-generation oral cephalosporins include cefadroxil, cephalexin, and cephradine. Parenteral first-generation cephalosporins include cepha-

lothin, cefazolin, and cephradine. The higher-generation cephalosporins, such as cefaclor, cefuroxime axetil, cefamandole, cefprozil, and cefpodoxime proxetil, are generally more active against gram-negative microbes and less active against gram-positive microbes. Cephalosporins should not be given to a person who is allergic to penicillins or other cephalosporins, because cross-sensitivity–type reactions may occur. Renal impairment may compromise some cephalosporin elimination. Most cephalosporins are absorbed well; however, absorption of cefuroxime axetil or cefpodoxime proxetil may be less than optimal with an alkaline gastric pH; therefore, use of antacids or cimetidine decreases bioavailability.[1, 14] The adverse experiences with cephalosporins are similar to those with other antibiotics, already discussed. Antibacterial antagonism may occur if cephalosporins are given concurrently with penicillins.[1, 10, 12, 15] Later generations of cephalosporins containing a methylthiotetrazole side chain, such as cefamandole, cefotetan, cefoperazone, or moxalactam, may cause a disulfiram-like reaction with alcohol or possible bleeding if given with warfarin.

FLUOROQUINOLONE ANTIBIOTICS

Fluoroquinolone antibiotics include ciprofloxacin, enoxacin, lomefloxacin, norfloxacin, and ofloxacin.[1, 11, 15] Fluoroquinolones should not be given to patients with tendonitis or tendon rupture associated with the administration of any quinolone antibiotic. Some fluoroquinolones may cause hypersensitivity reactions (including anaphylaxis), central nervous system (CNS) stimulation (anxiety, insomnia), disorientation, mental confusion, phototoxicity, or eye abnormalities, or they may lower the threshold for seizures.[11] Simultaneous administration of *polyvalent cations* should be avoided, because decreased fluoroquinolone antibiotic absorption may result.[1, 11, 15] Certain fluoroquinolone antibiotics, to variable extents, may inhibit CYP1A2 substrate metabolism. Therefore, metabolism of caffeine and theophylline may be decreased, leading to increased levels, especially with concurrent administration of ciprofloxacin or enoxacin. Caution should be exercised if fluoroquinolones are given with *nonsteroidal antiinflammatory drugs* or other drugs that lower the threshold for seizures. The anticoagulant effects of warfarin may be increased with concurrent use of certain fluoroquinolones.

MACROLIDE ANTIBIOTICS

Macrolide antibiotics include azithromycin, clarithromycin, and erythromycin. These agents are metabolized by the liver and eliminated primarily by the hepatobiliary route.[12, 15, 16] Hepatic impairment may decrease clearance. Erythromycin and clarithromycin are CYP3A4 or CYP1A2 inhibitors, but azithromycin does not appear to be a clinically significant CYP inhibitor (see Table 15–1). Macrolide adverse effects include abdominal cramping and discomfort as a result of prokinetic gastrointestinal activity. Macrolides may also cause hypersensitivity reactions (anaphylaxis), reversible hearing loss, hepatic dysfunction, and ventricular arrhythmias, including torsades de pointes in persons with prolonged QT intervals on electrocardiography. Examples of macrolide antibiotic drug interactions are found in Table 15–4.

PENICILLINS (PENICILLINASE-RESISTANT) ANTIBIOTICS

The penicillinase-resistant penicillins include cloxacillin, dicloxacillin, nafcillin, and oxacillin. Penicillins are organic acids like the cephalosporins and are eliminated unchanged by the kidney via tubular secretion. Some prominent adverse effects of penicillin derivatives include hypersensitivity reactions such as urticaria or anaphylaxis.[14, 17] Antibacterial antagonism may occur if aminoglycoside, cephalosporin, or tetracycline antibiotics are given concurrently with penicillins.[1, 15, 17] Large doses of penicillins may interfere with the renal elimination of methotrexate, leading to methotrexate toxicity. Probenecid, a renal tubular secretion inhibitor, can inhibit penicillin clearance and cause increased levels of the penicillin derivatives. If warfarin and nafcillin or dicloxacillin are given concurrently, prothrombin levels should be monitored, because increased warfarin dosing may be needed.

TETRACYCLINES

Tetracyclines (including minocycline and doxycycline) may be used to treat folliculitis and other inflammatory processes involving the pilosebaceous apparatus.[18, 19] The absorption of tetracycline from the gastrointestinal tract is decreased in the presence of food, divalent cations (calcium, magnesium, aluminum), resins, and antacids. Administration of tetracyclines should be avoided during the third trimester of pregnancy or in children less than 8 years of age because permanent tooth discoloration may occur. Tetracyclines can cause exaggerated sunburn reactions (photosensitivity) in some individuals when exposed to ultraviolet light. Pigmentary changes can occur with minocycline. In addition, central nervous system adverse effects such as lightheadedness and vertigo have been reported with minocycline. Pseudotumor cerebri is

TABLE 15–4 ■ Examples of Macrolide Antibiotic Drug Interactions

Interacting Drug	Potential Consequences of Interactions
Astemizole	Avoid (clarithromycin, erythromycin) or monitor (azithromycin); cardiotoxicity may occur[a-c]
Carbamazepine	Monitor; increased carbamazepine levels may occur with clarithromycin or erythromycin[a-c]
Cisapride	Avoid (clarithromycin, erythromycin) or monitor (azithromycin); cardiotoxicity may occur[a-c]
Cyclosporine	Monitor; increased cyclosporine levels may occur with clarithromycin or erythromycin[a-c]
CYP1A2 substrates (see Table 15–1)	Avoid (clarithromycin, erythromycin) or monitor (azithromycin); increased blood levels of the substrate drug may occur due to impaired metabolism[a-c]
CYP3A4 substrates (see Table 15–1)	Avoid (clarithromycin, erythromycin) or monitor (azithromycin); increased blood levels of the substrate drug may occur due to impaired metabolism[a-c]
Digoxin	Monitor digoxin levels; digoxin toxicity may occur[c]
Ergotamine	Monitor; ergotism may occur with clarithromycin or erythromycin[a, b]
Lovastatin	Avoid (clarithromycin, erythromycin) or monitor (azithromycin); myopathy (rhabdomyolysis) may occur[a, b]
Methadone	Avoid (clarithromycin, erythromycin) or monitor (azithromycin); increased methadone blood levels may occur[a-c]
Phenytoin	Monitor phenytoin levels; phenytoin toxicity may occur with clarithromycin or erythromycin[a-c]
Pimozide	Avoid; cardiotoxicity may occur[d]
Rifabutin	Monitor; increased rifabutin levels or uveitis reported with erythromycin and clarithromycin[c]
Tacrolimus	Avoid or monitor; increased tacrolimus levels may occur with clarithromycin or erythromycin[c]
Terfenadine	Avoid (clarithromycin, erythromycin) or monitor (azithromycin); cardiotoxicity may occur[a-c]
Theophylline	Monitor; increased theophylline levels or theophylline toxicity may occur with clarithromycin or erythromycin[a-c]
Triazolam	Avoid (clarithromycin, erythromycin) or monitor (azithromycin); excessive sedation may occur[a-c]
Warfarin	Monitor for increased anticoagulant effects[c]

[a] Biaxin (clarithromycin) [package insert]. North Chicago, IL: Abbott Laboratories; 1997.
[b] Zithromax (azithromycin) [package insert]. New York: NY: Pfizer Labs Division; 1997.
[c] Katz HI: Corticosteroids. In: Katz HI (ed): Guide to Adverse Treatment Interactions for Skin, Hair and Nail Disorders. Philadelphia, Lippincott-Raven Publishers, 1998, pp 51–54.
[d] Orap (pimozide) [package insert]. Sellersville, PA: Gate Pharmaceuticals; 1997.

a rare but potentially serious adverse effect associated with the use of this class of medications. Enzyme inducers such as barbiturates, carbamazepine, and phenytoin may render doxycycline therapeutically ineffective. Concurrent use of tetracycline with the general anesthetic methoxyflurane or oral *retinoids* may lead to nephrotoxicity or pseudotumor cerebri, respectively. Concurrent use of tetracyclines with warfarin may decrease prothrombin activity, necessitating a lower dose of the anticoagulant to prevent bleeding. Rare oral contraceptive failures are reported when they are used with tetracyclines.

Hormones and Hormone Modulators

Hormones and hormone modulators represent a diverse group of pharmacologically active agents that can have important endocrinological, metabolic, and antiinflammatory activities. The hormones and hormone modulators include corticosteroids, cyproterone acetate, estrogen, finasteride, flutamide, leuprolide, and spironolactone.

CORTICOSTEROIDS

The corticosteroids include methylprednisolone, prednisone, and triamcinolone. Triamcinolone may be given by intradermal injection.[20, 21] These agents should not be used in persons with systemic antifungal infections or during administration of live vaccines. Exogenous (systemic) corticosteroids can cause drug-induced adrenal insufficiency or cushingoid changes. Other adverse effects include gastrointestinal distress, glucose intolerance, hypokalemia, hypernatremia, fluid retention, psychic disturbances, osteoporosis, cataracts, and pseudotumor cerebri. Impairment of growth and development may occur in children. Corticosteroids are CYP3A4 substrates. Therefore, examples of corticosteroid drug interactions include concurrent administration of CYP3A4 inducers or inhibitors that may respectively decrease or increase corticosteroid levels in a patient[22] (see Table 15–1). Certain *diuretics* or other *hypokalemics* given with corticosteroids may cause further hypokalemia. The varied metabolic and immunosuppressant effects of the corticosteroids may interfere with the efficacy of concurrent *antidiabetics, antihypertensives, immunosuppressants,* or vaccines.

CYPROTERONE ACETATE

Cyproterone acetate is an antiandrogenic steroid that acts both directly as a target-tissue dihydrotestosterone receptor blocker and indirectly to decrease the testosterone production.[23] Cyproterone acetate may cause metabolic changes including impaired glucose tolerance, hypothalamic-pituitary-adrenal axis suppression, negative nitrogen balance, and hypercalcemia. Cyproterone acetate is readily absorbed, and most is excreted unchanged in the feces and urine. It should not be given to a patient with active liver dysfunction or renal insufficiency. Hepatotoxicity manifested by elevated liver enzymes, icterus, toxic hepatitis, hepatic failure, or a fatal outcome has been reported with the use of cyproterone acetate. Other adverse effects include fatigue, gynecomastia, reversible inhibition of spermatogenesis, gastrointestinal distress, mental depression, hypercoagulability state, and hypersensitivity reactions (drug eruptions, photosensitivity). Periodic hematological and serum chemistry analyses are recommended. Alcohol may reduce the antiandrogenic activity of cyproterone acetate. Concurrent use of estrogens such as ethinyl estradiol may increase coagulability. Antidiabetic dosing may have to be monitored because of the hyperglycemic activity of cyproterone acetate. Concurrent use of potentially hepatotoxic or renal-compromising agents should be monitored closely.

ESTROGEN

Examples of commercially available estrogens include esterified estrogens, conjugated estrogens, and those found in oral contraceptives.[24] Estrogens are CYP3A4 substrates; they are metabolized in the liver, excreted in the bile, and subject to enterohepatic recirculation into the systemic circulation. Water-soluble estrogen conjugates are eliminated by the kidney. Estrogens should not be used during pregnancy or in a person with an estrogen-dependent neoplasm, active thrombophlebitis or a thromboembolic disorder, or a history of either of the last two conditions occurring with previous use of estrogen. Adverse effects with estrogens include gastrointestinal distress, fluid retention, mastodynia, depression, liver function test abnormalities, cholestatic jaundice, vaginal candidiasis, melasma, and sexual dysfunction. Estrogens may increase the risk of endometrial carcinoma in postmenopausal women. Estrogens may impair glucose tolerance, reduce responsiveness to metyrapone testing, decrease serum folate levels, increase coagulation factors, decrease fibrinolysis, and interfere with certain thyroid function test results. Examples of estrogen drug interactions include concurrent administration of CYP3A4 inducers or inhibitors that may respectively decrease or increase the estrogen level in a patient[22, 24] (see Table 15–1). Estrogens may interfere with the efficacy of concurrent *antidiabetics, antihypertensives,* and *diuretics.* Oral contraceptive failure may occur when estrogens are given with either rifampin or griseofulvin.[1, 13] The concurrent administration of broad-spectrum antibiotics and oral contraceptives is controversial (see previous discussion).

FINASTERIDE

Finasteride (1 mg) is a competitive inhibitor of type II 5-α reductase that catalyzes the transformation of testosterone to dihydroxytestosterone in the skin and other organs.[25] It reverses the miniaturization process seen in male androgenetic alopecia. Finasteride should not be used during pregnancy. Adverse experiences are infrequent and include some type of sexual dysfunction (<3% of patients), breast tenderness, breast enlargement, and rare hypersensitivity reactions (e.g., lip swelling, drug eruptions). Finasteride may possibly lower the blood level of prostate-specific antigen. Such an iatrogenic effect theoretically may mask an increase in antigen level that might otherwise occur with prostate cancer.

FLUTAMIDE

Flutamide is an antiandrogen and antineoplastic agent used to treat advanced prostate cancer.[26] Flutamide interferes with androgen activity by blocking either testosterone cellular uptake or nuclear incorporation in the target-tissue sites. Flutamide should not be used in men with hepatic impairment, anemia, hypertension, or lupus erythematosus, because worsening of these conditions may occur. Flutamide adverse experiences include diarrhea, anorexia, gynecomastia, photosensitivity, lupus erythematosus eruptions, leukopenia, anemia, thrombocytopenia, and hepatotoxicity. Concurrent use of warfarin and flutamide should be monitored, because an increase in prothrombin time has been recorded.

LEUPROLIDE

Leuprolide is a synthetic gonadotropin-releasing hormone analogue. Leuprolide inhibits gonadotropin secretion and, after an initial period of adjustment, decreased steroidogenesis by the testes or ovaries ensues.[27] Leuprolide is used along with flutamide to treat advanced cases of prostate cancer. In addition, leuprolide is used to decrease gonadal steroidogenesis in children with central precocious puberty and in the management of endometriosis. Leuprolide should not be used during pregnancy or in women with undiagnosed vaginal bleeding. Leuprolide adverse experiences include hypersensitivity reactions (anaphylaxis, erythema multiforme), gynecomastia, hot flashes, changes in sexual drive, hepatic dysfunction, acne, seborrhea, and local reactions at the injection site.

SPIRONOLACTONE

Spironolactone is an aldosterone antagonist and potassium-sparing diuretic with antiandrogenic properties.[28] Spironolactone increases the renal excretion of sodium and water while causing retention of potassium. Hyponatremia, dehydration, and hyperkalemia are potential consequences of spironolactone therapy. Therefore, spironolactone should not be used in persons who are anuric or hyperkalemic or who have acute renal insufficiency or renal impairment. Additional spironolactone adverse experiences include gastrointestinal intolerances, gynecomastia, masculinization in females, decreased libido, and hematological toxicity. Concurrent use of hyperkalemics that might increase the potential for hyperkalemia should be avoided.[22, 28] Hypotension may occur with concurrent antihypertensive therapy. Increased levels of digoxin or lithium may occur if these drugs are used with spironolactone. The anticoagulant effect of warfarin may be decreased if it is used concurrently with spironolactone.

Psychotherapeutics

The psychotherapeutics include antianxiety, antidepressant, antipsychotic, and psychostimulant drugs. Individual agents within this therapeutic class may also have variable effects on adrenergic, dopaminergic, histaminic, or serotonergic receptors that contribute to their therapeutic and adverse experience profiles. Elderly patients and those with a seizure disorder or hepatic or renal impairment may be particularly vulnerable to an adverse experience. Selected common adverse effects that may occur during treatment with psychotherapeutic agents are presented in Table 15–5. Examples of distinctive adverse effects and drug interactions are described here for individual members of each class. Many psychotherapeutic agents, such as certain antidepressants and antipsychotics, require CYP2D6 for their metabolism. However, a small percentage of the population (<10%) are considered slow metabolizers. Slow metabolizers have reduced CYP2D6 activity, resulting in increased blood levels of substrate drugs that require this CYP isoenzyme[1, 29] (see Table 15–1). Added precautions such as closer monitoring and reduced dosing may be required. In general, concurrent ingestion of alcohol should be avoided with almost all psychotherapeutics because of possible additive psychomotor impairment. Combinations of some psychotherapeutic agents, such as monoamine oxidase inhibitors (MAOIs) and selective serotonin reuptake inhibitors (SSRIs), should be avoided.[30]

ANTIANXIETY DRUGS

The antianxiety drugs include benzodiazepines and buspirone. Benzodiazepines with short half-lives are used as hypnotics (e.g., temazepam, triazolam). Some benzodiazepines (e.g., alprazolam, diazepam, triazolam) are CYP substrates and undergo phase I metabolism.[31, 32] Others (e.g., lorazepam, oxazepam, temazepam) undergo primarily phase II metabolism. Benzodiazepine metabolites are excreted in the urine. Benzodiazepines should be avoided in persons with acute narrow-angle glaucoma. The more common adverse experiences of benzodiazepines include extension of their CNS depressive effects, such as drowsiness, lightheadedness, incoordination, memory loss, or dysarthria. Other CNS depressants may be potentiated with concurrent use of benzodiazepines. CYP inducers (see Table 15–1) such as carbamazepine, phenobarbital, phenytoin, or rifampin may increase biotransformation and lower concentrations of benzodiazepine substrates (e.g., alprazolam, diazepam, triazolam) that undergo phase I metabolism to subtherapeutic blood levels.[31, 32] In contrast, CYP inhibitors (see Table 15–1), such as clarithromycin, erythromycin, itraconazole, or ketoconazole, may increase these benzodiazepine substrates to potentially toxic blood levels.[22] Fluvoxamine and fluoxetine may also increase some benzodiazepine blood levels.[33] Benzodiazepines may increase desipramine or imipramine levels if given concurrently with either of these tricyclic antidepressants.[22] Theophylline may cause blood levels of some benzodiazepines to be decreased.

TABLE 15-5 ■ Examples of Adverse Effects That May Occur with Certain Psychotropic Medications°

System Involved or Specific Entity	Overt Manifestations of Adverse Effect
Autonomic nervous system dysfunction	Diaphoresis, dry mouth, urinary retention, blurred vision, paralytic ileus, priapism
Cardiovascular system dysfunction	Orthostatic hypotension, tachycardia, arrhythmias, prolongation of the electrocardiographic QT interval, cardiovascular collapse, sudden death
Central nervous system dysfunction	Anxiety, cognitive impairment (confusion, disorientation, delusions, hallucinations), motor impairment (dyscoordination), sedation, restlessness, seizures
Extrapyramidal symptoms	Akathisia (muscle restlessness), dysarthria, dysphagia, dystonia (muscle spasms), oculogyric crisis and/or Parkinson-like changes (tremors)
Hematological dysfunction	Anemia, leukopenia, agranulocytosis (clozapine, *phenothiazines*)
Hepatic dysfunction	Elevated liver function test results, cholestatic jaundice (*phenothiazines*), hepatitis
Neuroleptic malignant syndrome	Symptom complex consisting of altered mental status, diaphoresis, hyperpyrexia, labile cardiovascular responses including arrhythmias, muscular rigidity, myopathy, acute renal failure and/or elevated creatine phosphokinase that potentially may be fatal
Serotonin syndrome	Symptom complex that may include altered mental status with autonomic nervous system and neuromuscular dysfunction that may potentially be fatal
Tardive dyskinesia	Potentially irreversible rhythmical involuntary movements of the face, mouth, tongue and/or extremities

° Buspar (buspirone) [package insert]. 1995.
Orap (pimozide) [package insert]. Sellersville, PA: Gate Pharmaceuticals; 1997.
Prozac (fluoxetine) [package insert]. Carolina, Puerto Rico: Dista Products Company; 1997.
Reynolds RD: Serotonin syndrome cause and treatment [letter]. J Am Board Fam Pract 9:73–74, 1996.
Thorazine (chlorpromazine) [package insert]. Philadelphia, PA: Smith Kline Beecham; 1995.
Xanax (alprazolam) [package insert]. Kalamazoo, MI: Pharmacia and Upjohn, Inc; 1997.

Buspirone is a nonbenzodiazepine agent that is used to treat anxiety disorders.[34] Buspirone should not be given within at least 2 weeks of administration of an MAOI.[34, 35] Adverse experiences include excitement, nervousness, insomnia, nausea, fatigue, headache, and sexual dysfunction. Examples of buspirone drug interactions include increased CNS depression with concurrent use of CNS depressants. Increased psychiatric symptomatology and CNS toxicity have been reported with concurrent use of fluoxetine or other SSRIs. Hepatotoxicity has been reported with the combination of trazodone and buspirone.[35] Increased levels of haloperidol may occur if it is used with buspirone.

ANTIDEPRESSANTS

Antidepressants are used to treat significant depression, and some of the agents may be used by persons with obsessive-compulsive disorders. The major drugs in this group are the MAOIs, SSRIs, and tricyclic antidepressants. Each major antidepressant group is summarized separately.

Monoamine Oxidase Inhibitors

MAOIs include phenelzine and tranylcypromine. MAOIs block monoamine oxidase activity that detoxifies serotonin and norepinephrine.[35] The MAOIs have serotonergic and adrenergic activities that contribute to their efficacy and potential adverse experience profiles. MAOIs should be avoided in a person with significant cardiovascular disease (e.g., hypertension, congestive heart failure), hepatic impairment, or pheochromocytomas. Hypertensive crises, hypomania, intracranial hemorrhage, orthostatic hypotension, and seizures are illus-

trations of possible serious adverse experiences that may occur with MAOIs. Examples of MAOI drug interactions are found in Table 15–6.

Selective Serotonin Reuptake Inhibitors

SSRIs include fluoxetine, fluvoxamine, paroxetine, and sertraline. SSRIs exert increased serotoninergic activity by blocking the neuronal uptake of serotonin in the brain.[30, 36] The SSRIs should not be used with tryptophan or within at least 2 weeks (up to 5 or more weeks for fluoxetine) of exposure to MAOIs because of potential additive serotoninergic effects (ie, neuroleptic malignant syndrome) (see Table 15–5). In addition, sertraline and fluvoxamine should not be used with astemizole, cisapride, or terfenadine because of potential cardiotoxicity. The SSRIs are highly protein bound and are extensively metabolized. The SSRIs may initially cause some temporary impaired psychomotor function. The more common SSRI adverse effects include nausea, diarrhea, sedation, insomnia, agitation, palpitations, diaphoresis, dry mouth, hyponatremia, dizziness, tremor, restlessness, and seizures.[30, 36] Caution, monitoring, and dosage alteration may be necessary if certain SSRIs are prescribed with highly protein-bound drugs, serotonergic agents, lithium, digoxin, or warfarin. SSRIs given concurrently with either cimetidine or quinidine may cause increased SSRI levels. There are major pharmacokinetic differences among the SSRIs in their ability to impair CYP isoenzyme–mediated substrate drug biotransformation in a clinically significant way (see Table 15–1).[5, 30, 36] Fluoxetine, paroxetine, and possibly sertraline in large doses may interfere with the metabolism of CYP2D6 substrate drugs. Fluoxetine may also minimally inhibit CYP3A4 and CYP2C19. Norfluoxetine, a metabolite of fluoxetine, is a more potent

TABLE 15-6 ■ Examples of Monoamine Oxidase Inhibitor Drug Interactions

Interacting Drugs	Potential Consequences of Drug Interactions
Amphetamines	Avoid; increased sympathomimetic effects such as a hypertensive crisis may occur[a]
Antidiabetics	Monitor glucose levels; change in glucose tolerance may occur[b, c]
Antihypertensives	Monitor; bradycardia or hypotension may occur[b]
Bupropion	Avoid within at least 14 days; serious adverse experiences may occur[b]
Buspirone	Avoid within at least 10 days; serious cardiovascular adverse experiences such as hypertensive crisis may occur[b]
Central nervous system depressants	Avoid; increased central nervous system depression may occur[b]
Dibenzazepine derivatives	Avoid within at least 14 days; serious cardiovascular (hypertensive crisis) and central nervous system (seizures) adverse experiences, at times fatal, may occur[b]
Guanethidine	Avoid within at least 14 days; serious cardiovascular adverse experiences (hypertensive crisis) may occur[b]
L-tryptophan	Avoid within at least 14 days; serious cardiovascular adverse experiences (hypertensive crisis) may occur[b]
Levodopa	Avoid within at least 14 days; serious cardiovascular adverse experiences (hypertensive crisis) may occur[b, c]
Meperidine	Avoid within at least 14 to 21 days; serious cardiovascular (hypertensive crisis) and central nervous system (seizures) adverse experiences may occur[b, c]
Methylphenidate	Monitor; increased sympathomimetic effects such as a hypertensive crisis may occur[d]
Monoamine oxidase inhibitors	Avoid other monoamine oxidase inhibitors within at least 14 days; serious cardiovascular (hypertensive crisis) and central nervous system (seizures) adverse experiences, at times fatal, may occur[b, c, e]
Reserpine	Avoid within at least 14 days; serious cardiovascular adverse experiences (hypertensive crisis) may occur[b]
Selective serotonin reuptake inhibitors	Avoid within at least 14 days (5 weeks or more with fluoxetine); serious neuroleptic malignant syndrome-like adverse effects may occur[b, f]
Sympathomimetics	Avoid; serious cardiovascular (hypertensive crisis) adverse experiences, at times fatal, may occur[b, c]
Tricyclic antidepressants	Avoid; serious cardiovascular (hypertensive crisis) and central nervous system (seizures) adverse experiences, at times fatal, may occur[b, c, e]
Tyramine-containing foods	Avoid within at least 14 days; serious cardiovascular (hypertensive crisis) and central nervous system (seizures) adverse experiences may occur[b, g]

Italicized drug classes are elaborated in Table 15–2.
[a] Adderall (amphetamine, dextroamphetamine) [package insert]. Florence, KY: Shire Richwood Inc; 1998.
[b] Nardil (phenelzine) [package insert]. Morris Plain, NJ: Parke-Davis; 1998.
[c] Strain JJ, Caliendo G, Himelein C, Hammer JS: Part II: Drug-psychotropic drug interactions and end organ dysfunction. Clinical management recommendations. Gen Hosp Psychiatry 18:300–313, 1996.
[d] Ritalin (methylphenidate) [package insert]. East Hanover, NJ: Novartis Pharmaceutical Corporation; February 1998.
[e] Elavil (amitriptyline) [package insert]. Wilmington, DE: Zeneca Pharmaceuticals; 1998.
[f] Prozac (fluoxetine) [package insert]. Carolina, Puerto Rico: Dista Products Company; 1997.
[g] Katz HI: Corticosteroids. In: Katz HI (ed): Guide to Adverse Treatment Interactions for Skin, Hair and Nail Disorders. Philadelphia, Lippincott-Raven Publishers, 1998, pp 51–54.

CYP3A4 inhibitor. Fluvoxamine interferes with the metabolism of CYP1A2 and CYP3A4 substrate drugs. Therefore, frank avoidance or use of caution along with judicious laboratory monitoring and/or dosage alterations may be needed, especially for those *drugs with narrow therapeutic windows.*

Tricyclic Antidepressants

The *tricyclic antidepressants* include amitriptyline, clomipramine, desipramine, doxepin, and nortriptyline. These drugs may have antihistaminic, anticholinergic, serotonergic, and sympathomimetic effects.[37] Depending on the specific agent, a number of CYP isoenzymes (CYP1A2, CYP2C9, CYP2D6, and CYP3A4) may be involved in metabolism and ultimate elimination by the kidney (see Table 15–1). Tricyclic antidepressants and MAOIs should not be used within at least 14 days of each other, because serious and even fatal cardiovascular adverse experiences have occurred. The adverse effects of tricyclics include anticholinergic effects (dry mouth,

constipation, urinary retention), CNS depression, cardiovascular effects (arrhythmias, orthostatic hypotension), psychic disturbances, and rare hematological or hepatic disturbances. These adverse effects may be exacerbated by concurrent medications that interfere with a tricyclic metabolism or that have similar pharmacodynamic profiles.

ANTIPSYCHOTIC AGENTS

The antipsychotic agents include clozapine, haloperidol, pimozide, risperidone, and *phenothiazines* such as chlorpromazine or thioridazine.[29, 38–41] The antipsychotics should be avoided in persons with severe CNS depression due to any cause. In addition, clozapine should not be given to a patient with an uncontrolled seizure disorder, myelosuppression, or use of ritonavir or agents that may cause bone marrow suppression.[29] Pimozide is also contraindicated in persons with cardiac arrhythmias or congenital long QT syndrome and in those taking drugs that may prolong the QT interval, such as the macrolide antibiotics.[29] The modes of action of the antipsychotics are generally not known. However, dopamine receptor blockade in the brain may be involved. The antipsychotics may act, to a variable extent, as adrenergic, cholinergic, histaminic, or serotonergic receptor antagonists; these effects may contribute to their pharmacological profiles. Depending on the specific antipsychotic, the adverse experiences and drug interactions may involve impairment of the CNS, the cardiovascular system, or and the autonomic nervous system. Hyperprolactinemia, tardive dyskinesia, and neuroleptic malignant syndrome (see Table 15–5) may also occur with this group to a variable degree. Some also may cause blood dyscrasias (clozapine), cholestatic jaundice (phenothiazines), and photosensitivity (phenothiazines).[29, 41] Some of these drugs are metabolized by cytochrome P450 enzymes (see Table 15–1). Examples of adverse experiences and drug interactions for the antipsychotics are found in Table 15–5.

PSYCHOSTIMULANTS

The *psychostimulants* include amphetamine, methylphenidate, and pemoline.[42–44] They have a propensity to alter motor adeptness and cause dependency, and they are subject to potential abuse by patients. Each may produce variable cardiovascular and CNS stimulation with attendant elevation in blood pressure, psychic excitation, and lowering of seizure thresholds. Therefore, many of these psychostimulants should be avoided in persons who have underlying clinically significant symptomatic arteriosclerosis, cardiovascular or psychotic disease states, motor tics, Tourette's syndrome, glaucoma, hypertension, hyperthyroidism, agitation, or drug abuse potential. Psychostimulants should not be used within at least 14 days of MAOI administration, because hypertensive crises may occur. Pemoline has only minimal sympathomimetic activity, but it should not be given to persons with hepatic impairment.[42] Methylphenidate may act as an enzyme inhibitor and impede the biotransformation of drugs such as phenobarbital, phenytoin, and phenylbutazone.[44] The psychostimulants can cause a variety of adverse experiences, but of particular note is their inclination to cause anorexia, tachycardia, hypertension, dizziness, nervousness, insomnia, and suppression of growth in children.

Summary

Examples of adverse experiences and drug interactions with selected systemically administered oral antifungal, antibiotic, hormone or hormone-modifying, and psychotherapeutic medications that may be used to treat hair and nail disorders have been reviewed. Recognition of patients' inherent risk factors and relevant pharmacological profiles can help reduce or avoid iatrogenic drug-induced consequences associated with therapeutic intervention in hair or nail disorders.

REFERENCES

1. Gillum JGG, Israel DS, Polk RE: Pharmacokinetic drug interactions with antimicrobial agents [review]. Clin Pharmacokinet 25:450–482, 1993.
2. Katz HI, Gupta AK: Oral antifungal drug interactions. Dermatol Clin 15:535–544, 1997.
3. Spatzenegger M, Jaeger W: Clinical importance of hepatic cytochrome P450 in drug metabolism. Drug Metab Rev 27:397–417, 1995.
4. Kerremans AL: Cytochrome P450 isoenzymes: importance for the internist. Neth J Med 48:237–243, 1996.
5. Preskorn SH: Clinically relevant pharmacology of selective serotonin reuptake inhibitors. Clin Pharmacokinet 32:1–21, 1997.
6. Black DJ, Kunze KL, Wienkers LC, et al: Warfarin-fluconazole: II. A metabolically based drug interaction: in vivo studies. Drug Metab Dispos 24:422–428, 1996.
7. Lamisil tablet (terbinafine) [package insert]. East Hanover, NJ: Novartis Pharmaceuticals Corporation; 1997.
8. Personal communication, V. Fischer, PhD, Novartis Pharmaceuticals, East Hanover, NJ, 1999.
9. van der Kuy P-HM, Hooymans PM: Nortriptyline intoxication by terbinafine. Br Med J 316:441, 1998.
10. Keftab (cephalexin) [package insert]. Indianapolis, IN: Eli Lilly & Company; 1997.
11. Cipro (ciprofloxacin) [package insert]. West Haven, CT: Bayer Corporation Pharmaceutical Division; 1998.
12. Biaxin (clarithromycin) [package insert]. North Chicago, IL: Abbott Laboratories; 1997.
13. Shenfield GM: Oral contraceptives: are drug interactions of clinical significance? Drug Saf 9:21–37, 1993.
14. Epstein ME, Amodio-Groton M, Sadick NS: Antimicrobial agents for the dermatologist: 1. beta-lactam antibiotics and related compounds. J Am Acad Dermatol 37:149–165, 1997.
15. Horn JR, Hansten PD: Drug interactions with antibacterial agents. J Fam Pract 41:81–90, 1995.
16. Zithromax (azithromycin) [package insert]. New York, NY: Pfizer Labs Division; 1997.
17. Dicloxacillin [package insert]. Philadelphia, PA: Wyeth-Ayerst; 1995.
18. Acromycin V (tetracycline) [package insert]. Pearl River, NY: Lederle Pharmaceutical Division; 1997.
19. Minocin (minocycline) [package insert]. Pearl River, NY: Lederle Pharmaceutical Division; 1993.
20. Deltasone (prednisone) [package insert]. Kalamazoo, MI: The Upjohn Company; 1995.
21. Methylprednisolone [package insert]. North Chicago: IL: Abbott Laboratories; 1991.
22. Katz HI: Corticosteroids. In: Katz HI (ed): Guide to Adverse Treatment Interactions for Skin, Hair and Nail Disorders, Philadelphia, Lippincott-Raven Publishers, 1998, pp 51–54.
23. Androcur (cyproterone acetate) [package insert]. In: Gillis MC (ed): Compendium of Pharmaceuticals and Specialties, 1996 ed. Ottawa, Canada, Canadian Pharmaceutical Association, 1996, pp 81–82.
24. Estrogen [package insert]. Philadelphia, PA: Wyeth-Ayerst; 1993.
25. Propecia (finasteride) [package insert]. West Point, PA: Merck and Company, 1997.
26. Eulexin (flutamide) [package insert]. Kenilworth, NJ: Schering Corporation; 1997.
27. Lupron (leuprolide) [package insert]. Deerfield, IL: TAP Pharmaceuticals, Inc; 1998.
28. Aldactone (spironolactone) [package insert]. Chicago, IL: G. D. Searle & Company; 1996.
29. Clozaril (clozapine) [package insert] East Hanover, NJ: Novartis Pharmaceuticals Corporation; 1998.
30. Prozac (fluoxetine) [package insert]. Carolina, Puerto Rico: Dista Products Company; 1997.
31. Xanax (alprazolam) [package insert]. Kalamazoo, MI: Pharmacia and Upjohn, Inc; 1997.
32. Valium (diazepam) [package insert]. Nutley, NJ: Roche Laboratories Inc; 1997.
33. Stoudemire A. New antidepressant drugs and the treatment of depression in the medically ill patient. Psychiatr Clin North Am 19:495–514, 1996.

34. BuSpar (buspirone) [package insert]. Princeton, NJ: Mead Johnson Pharmaceuticals; 1998.

35. Nardil (phenelzine) [package insert]. Morris Plain, NJ: Parke-Davis; 1998.

36. Luvox (fluvoxamine) [package insert]. Marietta, GA: Solvay Pharmaceuticals; 1998.

37. Elavil (amitriptyline) [package insert]. Wilmington, DE: Zeneca Pharmaceuticals; 1998.

38. Haloperidol [package insert]. Columbus, OH: Roxane Laboratories, Inc; 1994.

39. Orap (pimozide) [package insert]. Sellersville, PA: Gate Pharmaceuticals; 1997.

40. Risperdal (risperidone) [package insert]. Titusville, NJ: Janssen Pharmaceutica; 1998.

41. Thorazine (chlorpromazine) [package insert]. Philadelphia, PA: Smith Kline Beecham; 1995.

42. Cylert (pemoline) [package insert]. North Chicago, IL: Abbott Laboratories; December 1996.

43. Adderall (amphetamine, dextroamphetamine) [package insert]. Florence, KY: Shire Richwood Inc; 1998.

44. Ritalin (methylphenidate) [package insert]. East Hanover, NJ: Novartis Pharmaceutical Corporation; February 1998.

c h a p t e r

16

Aging

PHILIP R. COHEN

—

RICHARD K. SCHER

▌Nails

CLINICAL FEATURES

Changes and disorders occur in the nails with aging. As people age, the color, contour, histology, growth, surface, and thickness of the nail unit changes (Table 16–1).[1] Aging-associated disorders include brittle nails, faulty biomechanics and trauma-induced onychodystrophies, infections, onychauxis, onychoclavus, onychocryptosis, onychogryphosis, onychophosis, splinter hemorrhages, subungual exostosis, and subungual hematomas (Table 16–2).[2]

Changes

Color

As a person ages, the color of the nail plate may change. The nails appear dull and opaque, and their color can vary from yellow to gray (Fig. 16–1). Also, in older people, the lunula is frequently decreased or absent[3] (Fig. 16–2).

Neapolitan nails were observed in almost 20% of fingernails and toenails of persons older than 70 years of age. There was a loss of the lunula, with a white appearance of the proximal portion of the nail, a more normal pink band, and an opaque free edge of the nail.[4] These color changes were referred to as "Neapolitan

TABLE 16-1 ■ Nail Changes Associated with Aging

Characteristics	Change
Color	Yellow to gray with a dull, opaque appearance
	"Neapolitan" nails: nails with a loss of the lunula and a white proximal portion, a normal pink central band, and an opaque distal free edge
Contour	Increased transverse convexity
	Decreased longitudinal curvature
Histology	Nail plate keratinocytes
	Increased size
	Increased number of pertinax bodies (keratinocyte nuclei remnants)
	Nail bed dermis
	Thickening of the blood vessels
	Degeneration of elastic tissue
Linear growth	Decreased
Surface	Increased friability with splitting and fissuring
	Longitudinal furrows that are superficial (onychorrhexis) and deep (ridges)
Thickness	Variable: normal, increased, or decreased

Adapted from Cohen PR, Scher, RK: Geriatric nail disorders: diagnosis and treatment. J Am Acad Dermatol 26:521–531, 1992.
© 1992, Mosby–Year Book, St. Louis, MO.

TABLE 16-2 ■ Aging-Associated Nail Disorders

Nail Disorder	Clinical Features
Brittle nails	Excessive longitudinal ridging, horizontal layering (lamellar separation) of the distal nail plate, roughness (trachyonychia) of the nail plate surface, and irregularity of the distal edge of the nail plate
Faulty biomechanics and trauma-induced onychodystrophies	Manifests as onychauxis, onychoclavus, onychocryptosis, onychrogryphosis, onychophosis, splinter hemorrhages, subungual exostosis, subungual hematoma, or subungual hyperkeratosis
Infections	Onychomycosis: distal subungual, white superficial, proximal subungual, and *Candida*
	Paronychia: acute (the nail fold is red, tender, and contains pus) or chronic (the cuticle is absent and the nail fold is swollen and uncomfortable)
Onychauxis	Localized hypertrophy of the entire nail plate characterized by a hyperkeratotic, discolored, nontranslucent nail plate
	Subungual keratosis and debris are often present
Onychoclavus (subungual heloma, subungual corn)	A sometimes painful, hyperkeratotic process most commonly located under the distal nail margin of the great toenail
Onychocryptosis (ingrown nail)	The nail plate pierces the lateral nail fold and causes inflammation with or without accompanying granulation tissue, tender at rest, and pain on ambulation or with pressure to the digit
Onychogryphosis	An exaggerated, oyster- or ram's horn–like nail plate enlargement primarily involving only the great toenails
Onychophosis	Localized or diffuse hyperkeratotic tissue of varying degree that develops on the lateral or proximal nail folds, in the space between the nail folds and the nail plate, or subungually
Splinter hemorrhages	Idiopathic or trauma-induced lesions, black, located in the middle or distal third of the nail
Subungual exostosis	A benign tender bony proliferation, most commonly on the great toe; usually produced hypertrophy of the entire nail bed so that the appearance of the nail is an inverted U with incurvation of the medial and lateral aspects of the nail plate
Subungual hematomas	Acute: recent hemorrhage may be red and painful
	Chronic: older lesions with residual hematoma may appear dark blue and are usually nontender

Adapted from Cohen PR, Scher RK: Nail changes in the elderly. Geriatric Dermatol 1:45–53, 1993. © 1993, Health Management Publications, Inc.

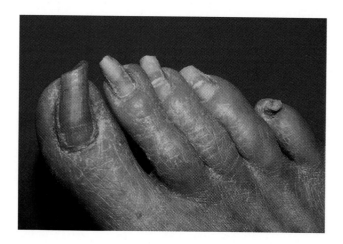

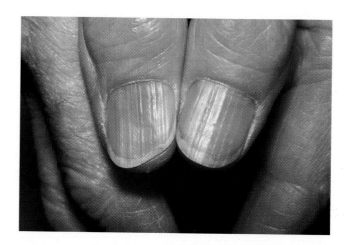

FIGURE 16–1 ■ The great toenail is yellow and thickened. The transverse convexity is increased, and there are early changes of onychogryphosis. (Reprinted with permission from Cohen PR, Scher RK: Nail changes in the elderly. J Geriatr Dermatol 1:45–53, 1993. © 1993, Health Management Publications, Inc.)

FIGURE 16-2 ■ Age-associated absence of the lunula and "sausage-shaped" ridges on the thumb nails of a 69-year-old man. The subungual erythema is secondary to osteoarthritis.

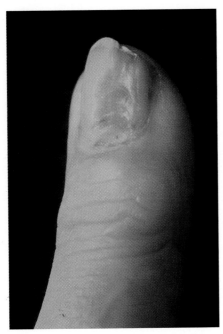

FIGURE 16–3 ■ The normal fingernail contour is altered by focal mucinosis (a myxoid cyst), which presses against the proximal nail matrix and results in a groove in the nail plate. (Reprinted with permission from Cohen PR, Scher RK: Nail changes in the elderly. J Geriatr Dermatol 1:45–53, 1993. © 1993, Health Management Publications, Inc.)

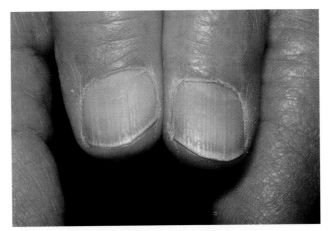

FIGURE 16–4 ■ Age-related superficial longitudinal striations (onychorrhexis) and deeper longitudinal lines (ridging) on the thumb nails of a 77-year-old man.

nails" because there were three distinct color bands on the nails, analogous to those of Neapolitan ice cream.[3]

Contour

A smooth surface and a double curvature (longitudinal and transverse) are present in the normal nail plate. In elderly persons, the transverse convexity is increased and the longitudinal curvature is decreased. Other changes in the nail plate contour include flattening of the nail plate (platyonychia), spooning of the nail plate (koilonychia), and clubbing of the digit (Fig. 16–3). Primarily restricted to the great toenails, a "ram's horn" deformity (onychogryphosis) may also occur.[1–3]

Linear Growth

The average growth rate of the fingernails is 0.1 mm/day, or 3.0 mm/mo. Toenails grow at one half to one third the rate of fingernails: 0.3 mm/day to 1.0 mm/mo. Hence, it takes approximately 6 months for a fingernail and 12 to 18 months for a toenail to grow from the matrix to the distal free edge.

The rate of linear nail growth decreases with age. The linear nail growth of thumbnails is most rapid in the first three decades of life and decreases steadily thereafter. Specifically, the linear growth rate decreases approximately 0.5% per year from 25 to 100 years of age.[1–3]

Surface

Friability, splitting, fissuring, and superficial longitudinal striations (onychorrhexis) of the nail plate frequently develop with advancing age. These surface changes may be localized or diffuse. The deeper longitudinal lines (ridg-

ing) have been described as "sausage-shaped" or "sausage-link" ridges[1–3] (Figs. 16–4 through 16–6; see Fig. 16–2).

Thickness

The thickness of the nail plate is determined by the length of the nail matrix; it varies with the sex of the individual and with each digit. The nail plate is approximately 0.6 mm thick in men and 0.5 mm thick in women. The nail plate of the thumb is the thickest, followed by that of the index finger, middle finger, and ring finger. The nail plate of the little finger is the

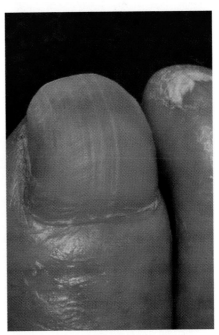

FIGURE 16–5 ■ Multiple deep longitudinal ridges on a nail plate that also has increased longitudinal curvature. (Reprinted with permission from Cohen PR, Scher RK: Nail changes in the elderly. J Geriatr Dermatol 1:45–53, 1993. © 1993, Health Management Publications, Inc.)

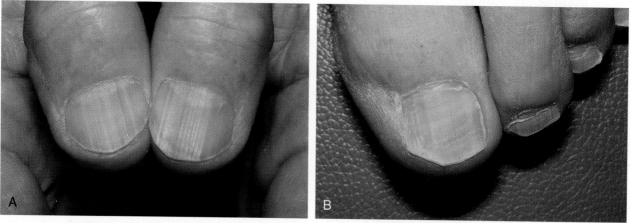

FIGURE 16–6 ■ Age-associated longitudinal superficial striations (onychorrhexis) and deeper lines (ridging) on the thumbnails (*A*) and toenails (*B*) of a 72-year-old Caucasian man. The horizontal ridges on the toenails are secondary to repeated trauma of the nails contacting the inside of his sneakers.

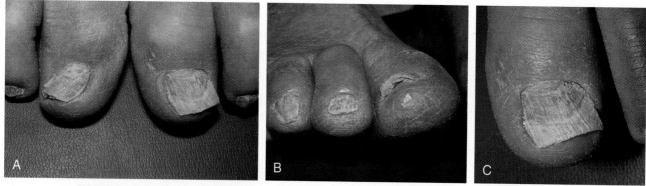

FIGURE 16–7 ■ Toenails of a 77-year-old man. There is congenital malalignment of the right great toenail, with secondary early hemionychogryphosis (*A*) and nail plate hypertrophy (onychauxis) (*B*). There is distal subungual onychomycosis of both great toenails (*A*, *B*, and *C*).

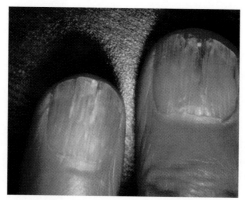

FIGURE 16–8 ■ Onychorrhexis and trachyonychia with irregularity and lamellar separation of the distal nail plate are noted on these brittle fingernails. (From Cohen PR, Scher RK: Geriatric nail disorders: diagnosis and treatment. J Am Acad Dermatol 26:521–531, 1992. © 1992, Mosby–Year Book, St. Louis, MO.)

thinnest. The relation between nail plate thickness and aging is variable: thickness may be unchanged, increased, or decreased with advancing age.

Onychauxis describes localized nail plate hypertrophy, and pachyonychia refers to thickening of the entire nail plate (Fig. 16–7). Onychauxis and pachyonychia may be found as idiopathic, age-associated nail plate changes. It is important to differentiate thickened nail plates from subungual hyperkeratosis, which can also occur in elderly patients.[1-3]

Disorders

Nail disorders that may occur in older persons are summarized in Table 16–2.[2]

Brittle Nails

Excessive longitudinal ridging, horizontal layering (lamellar separation) of the distal nail plate, roughness (trachyonychia) of the nail plate surface, and irregularity of the distal edge of the nail plate clinically characterize brittle nails (Fig. 16–8). Brittle nails may be observed in elderly persons. Repetitive hydration and dehydration cycles or excessive use of dehydrating agents such as nail enamels, nail enamel removers, and cuticle removers can be the cause of acquired brittle nails in aging patients.

Nail plate hardness is related to its state of hydration. The normal water content of the nail plate is approximately 18%, varying between 10% and 30%. Brittle nails appear when the water content decreases below 16%, and softness of the nail plate occurs when the water content is greater than 25%.[1-3]

Faulty Biomechanics and Trauma

Onychodystrophy can result from acute trauma to the nail unit. The nail changes may be temporary or permanent. Faulty biomechanics can result in chronic trauma to the nail unit (Figs. 16–9 and 16–10). Other causes of chronic trauma to the nail unit in elderly persons

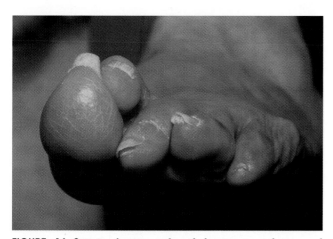

FIGURE 16–9 ■ Overlapping and underlapping toes that caused faulty ambulatory biomechanics and subsequent onychauxis. (From Cohen PR, Scher RK: Geriatric nail disorders: diagnosis and treatment. J Am Acad Dermatol 26:521–531, 1992. © 1992, Mosby–Year Book, St. Louis, MO.)

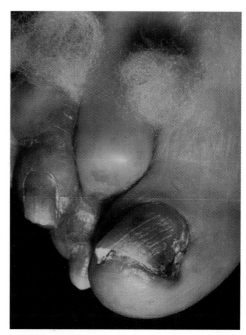

FIGURE 16–10 ■ Onychocryptosis, subungual hematoma, and subungual hyperkeratosis that resulted from altered pedal function secondary to bony deformities of the toes. (From Cohen PR, Scher RK: Geriatric nail disorders: diagnosis and treatment. J Am Acad Dermatol 26:521–531, 1992. © 1992, Mosby–Year Book, St. Louis, MO.)

include self-induced habits such as onychotillomania, onychophagia, and habit tic deformity. Shoe-induced biomechanical abnormalities can also result in trauma to the toenails and subsequent onychodystrophy (see Fig. 16–6).[1-3]

Infections

The nail structures may be the target of a primary acute or chronic bacterial infection, a viral infection (most commonly, herpes simplex virus or human papillomavirus), or one caused by fungal (Figs. 16–11 and 16–12; see Fig. 16–7), mite (*Sarcoptes scabiei*) (Fig. 16–13), mycobacterial (leprosy), or spirochetal (syphilis) organisms. In other cases the nail structures are secondarily involved in an infectious process localized to that area.[1-3]

Onychauxis

Onychauxis refers to localized hypertrophy of the nail plate, whereas *pachyonychia* refers to thickening of the entire nail plate. Hyperkeratosis, discolored nails, and loss of translucency of the nail plate clinically characterize onychauxis (see Fig. 16–7). Subungual hyperkeratosis and debris are often present also. Aging may be associated with idiopathic onychauxis. Local complications of onychauxis include distal onycholysis, increased susceptibility to onychomycosis, pain, subungual hemorrhage, and subungual ulceration.[1-3]

Onychoclavus

Onychoclavus (also referred to as a subungual heloma and a subungual corn) is a hyperkeratotic process in the nail area. It is most commonly located under the distal

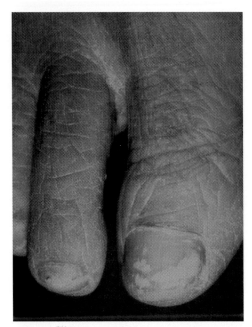

FIGURE 16–11 ■ White superficial onychomycosis located on the surface of the toenails. (From Cohen PR, Scher RK: Geriatric nail disorders: diagnosis and treatment. J Am Acad Dermatol 26:521–531, 1992. © 1992, Mosby–Year Book, St. Louis, MO.)

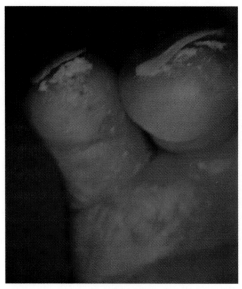

FIGURE 16–13 ■ *Sarcoptes scabiei* mites were present in the subungual hyperkeratotic debris from this elderly patient living in a nursing home. (From Cohen PR, Scher RK: Geriatric nail disorders: diagnosis and treatment. J Am Acad Dermatol 26:521–531, 1992. © 1992, Mosby–Year Book, St. Louis, MO.)

nail margin and results from either an anatomical abnormality or a mechanical change in foot function. An epidermoid cyst, a foreign body, a subungual melanoma, or a subungual exostosis can clinically mimic an onychoclavus (Fig. 16–14).[1–3]

Onychocryptosis

Onychocryptosis refers to ingrown nails and results from the nail plate's piercing the lateral nail fold (Fig. 16–15; see Fig. 16–10). Improper cutting of the nails and external pressure from poorly fitting footwear are the most common causes of onychocryptosis. Clinical features of onychocryptosis are inflammation, tenderness at rest, and pain on ambulation or with pressure to the digit. Granulation tissue may be present at the lateral nail fold.[1–3]

Onychogryphosis

Onychogryphosis, an exaggerated enlargement of the nail plate, most often involves only the great toenails (Fig. 16–16; see Fig. 16–1). The onychogryphotic nail appears "oysterlike" or "ram's horn–like." The nail plate is uneven, thickened, and brown to opaque, with multiple transverse striations. The underlying nail bed is often hypertrophic.

Hemionychogryphosis, a potential complication in elderly patients in whom a congenital malalignment of the great toenails persists into adulthood, clinically mimics

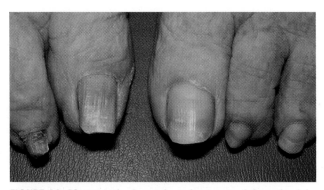

FIGURE 16–12 ■ Distal subungual onychomycosis of the nails of the right great toe and second toe in a 67-year-old woman.

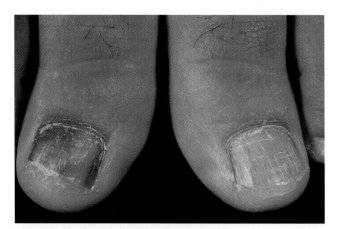

FIGURE 16–14 ■ Although the distal subungual hyperkeratosis mimicked an onychoclavus, the melanocytic pigmentation of the proximal nail fold (positive Hutchinson's sign) prompted a biopsy, which revealed a subungual malignant melanoma. (From Cohen PR, Scher RK: Geriatric nail disorders: diagnosis and treatment. J Am Acad Dermatol 26:521–531, 1992. © 1992, Mosby–Year Book, St. Louis, MO.)

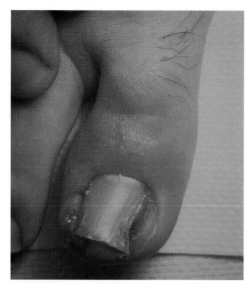

FIGURE 16–15 ■ Recurrent onychocryptosis with subsequent periungual inflammation and granulation tissue. (From Cohen PR, Scher RK: Geriatric nail disorders: diagnosis and treatment. J Am Acad Dermatol 26:521–531, 1992. © 1992, Mosby–Year Book, St. Louis, MO.)

onychogryphosis. In hemionychogryphosis, the abnormal nail growth is initially in a lateral direction. In contrast, in onychogryphosis, the hypertrophic nail initially grows upward before its lateral deviation.[1–3]

Onychophosis

Onychophosis mainly involves the first and fifth toes, results from repeated minor trauma to the nail plate, and is characterized by the localized or diffuse hyperkeratotic tissue that can develop on the lateral or proximal nail folds, in the space between the nail folds and the nail plate, and even subungually. In elderly persons, conditions that predispose to the development of ony-

chophosis include nail fold hypertrophy, onychocryptosis, onychomycosis, and xerosis.[1–3]

Splinter Hemorrhages and Subungual Hematomas

The main cause for splinter hemorrhages in older persons is trauma to the nails. In these patients, idiopathic or trauma-induced lesions are typically black and located distally. In contrast, splinter hemorrhages in patients with underlying systemic disorders are usually red and are found on the proximal third of the nail plate.

Subungual hematomas have variable clinical appearance and symptoms, depending on the age of the lesion. A recent hemorrhage is typically red and painful, whereas an older lesion often appears dark blue and is usually nontender (see Fig. 16–7). Although idiopathic hemorrhage under the nail plate has been observed in older persons, trauma to the fingernail or toenail is the most common cause in these patients.[1–3]

Subungual Exostosis

A subungual exostosis is typically an acquired solitary tumor arising after local trauma to the involved digit. It most commonly occurs on the medial surface of the distal great toe as a reactive hyperkeratotic nodule with secondary onychodystrophy of the overlying nail plate (Fig. 16–17). Symptoms related to alteration of the surrounding soft tissue (pain, paronychia, a pyogenic granuloma, or a callus) often prompt the patient to seek medical attention.[1–3]

PATHOLOGY

With advancing age, thickening of the subungual blood vessels and degeneration of the nail bed elastic tissue

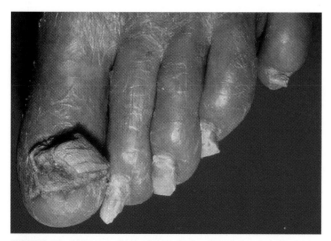

FIGURE 16–16 ■ Onychogryphosis of the great toenail is characterized by an opaque, thickened nail plate with subungual hyperkeratosis and transverse striations in which there has been exaggerated growth in an upward and lateral direction. (From Cohen PR, Scher RK: Geriatric nail disorders: diagnosis and treatment. J Am Acad Dermatol 26:521–531, 1992. © 1992, Mosby–Year Book, St. Louis, MO.)

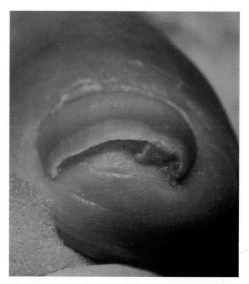

FIGURE 16–17 ■ Radiographic examination confirmed that the incurvature of the medial and lateral aspects of this elderly patient's great toenail was caused by a subungual exostosis. (From Cohen PR, Scher RK: Geriatric nail disorders: diagnosis and treatment. J Am Acad Dermatol 26:521–531, 1992. © 1992, Mosby–Year Book, St. Louis, MO.)

occur. These changes in elastic tissue are more pronounced in the nail bed than in the adjacent paronychial skin. The alteration of elastic tissue is most severe in the dermis beneath the pink nail bed, less marked beneath the lunula, and absent in the matrix area beneath the proximal nail fold.[1-4]

The keratinocyte morphology of the human nail plate varies with age. As nail plate growth decreases, the size of keratinocytes from the nail plate surface increases. Also, there is an increased number of pertinax bodies (remnants of keratinocyte nuclei) within the nail plate keratinocytes of older persons.[1-3]

TREATMENT

Treatments are available for some of the nail changes that occur in elderly persons and for each of the age-associated nail disorders[2] (Table 16–3).

Changes

Onychorrhexis and Ridging

Longitudinal striations (onychorrhexis) and deeper longitudinal lines (ridging) may be of cosmetic concern for the elderly person. Daily buffing of the nail plates is a practical and safe treatment. Buffing powders, pastes,

and creams contain waxes for enhancing nail surface gloss and finely ground pumice as an abrasive. A chamois-covered buffer is used to polish each nail plate until it shines after the buffing agent has been applied.[1-3]

Onychauxis and Pachyonychia

Daily buffing may improve the cosmetic appearance of thickened nail plates. Alternatively, the superficial surface of the nail plate can be mechanically thinned with the use of an abrasive disk attached to an electric drill. Mechanical or chemical avulsion of the nails may be required if there is severe nail plate thickening. To prevent recurrences, concurrent destruction of the nail matrix may be necessary.[1-3]

Disorders

Brittle Nails

Elimination of exacerbating factors is the initial treatment of brittle nails. Inauguration of local measures to rehydrate the nail plate, cuticle, and surrounding nail folds is the next intervention. After the nails have been soaked for 10 to 20 minutes in lukewarm water, a moisturizer should be applied. The use of nail enamel may be helpful in extreme cases or when preliminary measures are unsuccessful. When used, the nail enamel

TABLE 16-3 ■ Treatment of Aging-Associated Nail Disorders

Nail Disorder	Treatment
Brittle nails	Eliminate exacerbating factors and rehydrate the nail plate, cuticle, and surrounding nail folds; oral biotin may be useful; weekly applications of nail enamel may be helpful when preliminary measures are unsuccessful or in extreme cases
Faulty biomechanics and trauma-induced onychodystrophies	Treatment of the underlying limb function or gait cycle abnormality, correction of the associated bony deformity, or use of a molded shoe or an orthotic insert
Infections	Onychomycosis: medical (topical or systemic antifungals) or surgical (nail avulsion)
	Paronychia: acute (lancing, warm soaks, oral or topical antibiotics) or chronic (keeping the nail fold dry and applying topical antifungal or antiseptic agents
Onychauxis	Periodic partial or total debridement of the thickened nail plate: nail thinning using electric drills and burs; nail avulsion chemically (40% urea paste) or surgically; if necessary, matricectomy chemically (phenol) or surgically
Onychoclavus (subungual heloma, subungual corn)	Removal of the lesion, and prevention of recurrence by modifying footwear and using protective pads or tube foam to eliminate the causative pressure
Onychocryptosis (ingrown nail)	Correct predisposing factors and proper nail trimming
	Elevate the lateral nail border by placing a small wisp of cotton beneath the edge of the nail plate
	Provide local care consisting of warm soaks and topical antibiotics
	Surgically remove the nail plate with or without partial or total ablation of the nail matrix, or
	Use alternative modalities such as liquid nitrogen spray cryotherapy or an orthonyx technique using a stainless steel wire nail brace
Onychogryphosis	Proper nail plate trimming and foot care by filing the thickened nail plate using an electric drill and bur and removal of the subungual hyperkeratosis
	Nail avulsion with or without ablation of the nail matrix
Onychophosis	Initially, debride the hyperkeratotic tissue
	Additional management may also include thinning of the nail plate, packing of the nail, or surgical intervention similar to that described for onychocryptosis
Splinter hemorrhages	Avoidance of trauma
Subungual exostosis	Nail plate avulsion and aseptic removal of the excess bone
Subungual hematomas	Acute: a roentgenogram if a fracture of the underlying phalanx is suspected, and piercing the nail plate with a needle or electric drill to relieve the underlying pressure
	Chronic: if the patient cannot remember an associated traumatic incident, it may be necessary to rule out a pigmented lesion (melanoma) with microscopic evaluation of the nail plate and a biopsy specimen from the underlying nail matrix and/or nail bed

Adapted from Cohen PR, Scher RK: Nail changes in the elderly. Geriatric Dermatol 1:45–53, 1993. © 1993, Health Management Publications, Inc.

should not be removed and reapplied more often than once a week. Oral biotin has also been used successfully to manage brittle nails.[1–3]

Faulty Biomechanics and Trauma

The management of onychodystrophy resulting from biomechanical abnormalities should address both the underlying bony abnormality and the elderly patient's foot care and footwear. Instead of laced shoes, footwear with Velcro closures may be used. A molded shoe or an orthotic insert may be useful in the nonsurgical management of bony deformities. A less expensive, although less optimal, footwear alternative is soft shoes or sneakers.[1–3]

Onychauxis

Periodic partial or total debridement of the thickened nail plate is the treatment for onychauxis. Electric drills and burs can be used to thin the nail plate. Urea paste can be used for partial or complete chemical avulsion of the nail in older persons. Alternatively, the hyperkeratotic nail plate can be removed surgically. Permanent ablation with either chemical (phenol) or surgical matricectomy may be necessary when onychauxis is recurrent or associated with significant morbidity and local complications.[1–3]

Onychoclavus

Treatment of onychoclavus involves removal of the lesion and prevention of recurrence. Enucleation of the onychoclavus can be performed by removing the corresponding section of nail plate and excising the hyperkeratotic tissue. If there is an associated underlying bony abnormality, the osseous lesion must also be corrected. Elimination of the causative pressure by modifying the footwear and using protective pads or tube foam may be useful to prevent recurrence.[1–3]

Onychocryptosis

Prophylactic measures to prevent onychocryptosis include correction of predisposing factors and proper nail trimming. The distal nail plate should be cut straight across to allow the corners of the nail plate to extend beyond the distal edge of the lateral nail folds. Placing a small wisp of cotton beneath the free edge of the lateral nail plate is a conservative treatment for onychocryptosis. In addition, warm soaks and topical antibiotics are helpful. If a secondary infection is present, systemic antibiotics are indicated.

Complete or partial avulsion of the ingrown nail and excision of the involved adjacent tissue may be necessary for severe onychocryptosis or if the preliminary therapeutic measures have been unsuccessful. Other treatment alternatives include a stainless steel wire nail brace to flatten the nail plate and cryotherapy.[1–3]

Onychogryphosis

Onychogryphosis can be prevented with proper nail plate trimming and foot care. Filing of the thickened nail plate with an electric drill and bur and removal of the subungual hyperkeratosis are conservative treatments for onychogryphosis; subsequently, the dystrophic nail should periodically be clipped and trimmed. Nail avulsion (with or without ablation of the nail matrix) is an aggressive approach to the management of this condition.[1–3]

Onychophosis

Wearing comfortable shoes and relieving any pressure exerted by the nail on the surrounding soft tissue are precautionary measures to prevent the development of onychophosis. Debridement of the hyperkeratotic tissue with keratolytics is the initial treatment once onychophosis is present. To maintain hydration and lubrication, emollients may also be helpful. To reduce further trauma to the nail, thinning of the nail plate, packing of the nail, and surgical intervention similar to that described for onychocryptosis are additional options.[1–3]

Subungual Exostosis

Once the diagnosis of subungual exostosis has been confirmed radiographically, treatment involves aseptic removal of the excess bone.[1–3]

Hair

CLINICAL FEATURES

The quantity and quality of hair changes with age; the number, rate of growth, and diameter of the individual hairs decline. In addition to intrinsic, aging-associated hair loss, localized hypertrichosis occurs in elderly men and women. There is graying of the hair. The concentration of several metals and the activity of certain enzymes are decreased in the hair of older persons. Also, there are changes in the physical properties of the hair.[5–18]

There is a decline in the activity of hair follicles with aging. These changes result in a reduction of the density of scalp hairs (number of hairs per unit area) and a deterioration in the quality of the scalp hair. Specifically, reduction in the duration of hair growth and in the diameter of hair shafts (most evident in the thickest hairs) and slower cycling time of the hair, with a shorter anagen (growing) phase and a prolongation of the interval separating the loss of a hair in telogen and the emergence of a replacement hair in anagen, have been observed in scalp hair.[5–8]

Tensile strength of hair also diminishes. Up to the age of 20 years, the breaking strength of hair increases; afterward, it decreases with advancing age. Both the percent extension at breaking and the amount of energy required to break the hair increase up to the age of 15 years; subsequently, both of these measures of tensile strength of hair decline gradually with aging.[5–8]

Changes in Number of Hairs

Hair Loss

There is a general decrease in the absolute number of hair follicles in elderly persons, not only on the scalp but also on the body. Furthermore, the size of the

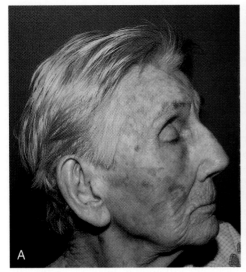
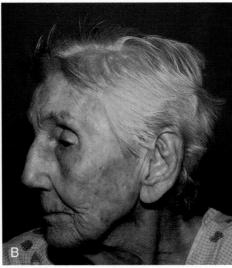

FIGURE 16–18 ■ Right (*A*) and left (*B*) views of an 85-year-old woman. Age-related thinning of the hair is most readily observed on her left scalp. There is also age-associated graying of the hair.

FIGURE 16–19 ■ Anterior (*A*) and lateral. (*B*) views of androgenetic alopecia in a man.

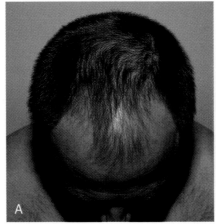
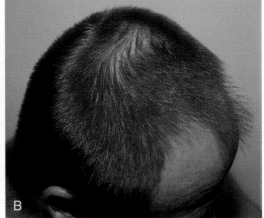

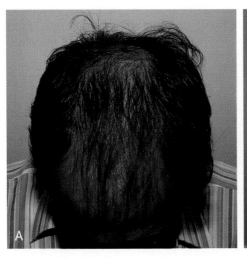
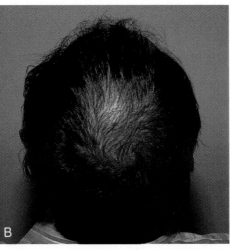

FIGURE 16–20 ■ Anterior (*A*) and posterior (*B*) views of androgenetic alopecia in another man.

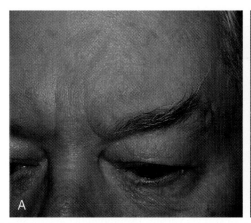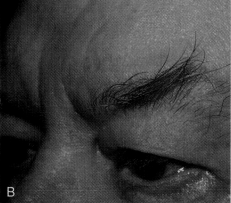

FIGURE 16–21 ■ Anterior (A) and lateral (B) views of age-related increased hair growth on the eyebrows of a 72-year-old man. Age-associated graying of the hair is also present.

residual hairs on the scalp is decreased, contributing to the appearance of diffuse hair loss (Fig. 16–18). There is also atrophy and fibrosis of the hair follicles. In addition to the intrinsic hair loss that accompanies aging, some older persons have hereditary hair loss, which is known as patterned, androgenic, or androgenetic alopecia. In contrast to age-related hair loss, which is primarily caused by a decrease in the number of follicles, androgenetic balding results from a change in the type of hair follicle, from terminal to vellus.[5–8]

Androgenetic alopecia is more likely to occur in men; however, women may also be affected. In men, this condition begins in the frontal and temporal regions of the scalp as a recession of the hairline (the so-called bitemporal recession or "widow's peak") (Fig. 16–19). Subsequently, there is thinning over the vertex; later, the process may spread to include most of the crown, resulting in the typical "billiard ball" appearance (Fig. 16–20). In women, the hair loss is most marked on the vertex of the scalp.[5–8]

Hair Gain

Paradoxically, as scalp hair thins with advancing age, unwanted hairs begin to appear in other areas because of a conversion of the pale, fine, vellus hairs to dark, coarse, terminal hairs. This is observed in both sexes, but in different anatomical sites. In men, these unsightly long terminal hairs are seen on the nose, in the nasal vestibules, on the eyebrows, on the outer ridges of the ears, and in the external auditory canals (Fig. 16–21). In postmenopausal women, these coarse, pigmented, terminal hairs develop above the upper lip and on the chin.[5–8]

Changes in Hair Color

Graying

Graying (also referred to as *canities*) is a physiological manifestation of the aging process. Heredity also plays a role in this change of hair color. Premature graying may be an important risk marker for osteopenia. However, premature graying has not been shown to be a marker for premature morbidity, mortality, or cause of death.[11–13]

The age at onset of graying is similar for men and women. Although it begins earlier in dark-haired persons, the rate at which the pigment decreases is independent of the hair's initial color. Complete graying of the hair occurs earlier in fair-haired than in dark-haired people.

Graying starts around the temples and sideburns in men (Fig. 16–22; see Fig. 16–21). In contrast, women start to gray in the 2 inches around the hairline (see

FIGURE 16–22 ■ Anterior (A) and lateral (B) views of graying in a 63-year-old man.

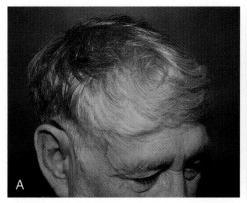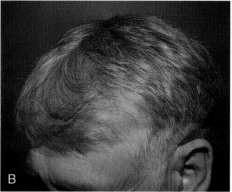

TABLE 16-4 ■ Aging-Associated Chemical Changes in Hair

Decreased Metal Concentration or Enzyme Activity	No Change in Metal Concentration or Enzyme Activity
Metals	Metals
Cadmium	Chromium
Copper	Iron
Zinc	Manganese
Strontium	
Enzymes	Enzymes
γ-Glutamyl transpeptidase	Glutathione peroxidase
Glucose-6-phosphate dehydrogenase	
Glutathione reductase	
Glutathione-S-transferase	

Fig. 16–18). The gray area gradually extends throughout the hair (see Figs. 16–18 and 16–22).

Gray hair may be thinner and sparser than pigmented hair, but it is not weaker. Some elderly persons find gray hair to be brittle and unmanageable.

After sympathectomy, delay of physiological graying has been observed on the sympathectomized side of the body; the mechanism for this is unknown. Temporary repigmentation of gray hair has also been noted; the darkening of the hair has occurred after an inflammatory process such as a furuncle or an exudative dermatosis.[5–13]

PATHOLOGY

In elderly persons there are age-associated changes in the chemical composition and histology of the hair. Changes in the concentration of metals and activity of enzymes within the hair are summarized in Table 16–4.[14–18] In the epidermis of the scalp, the stratum granulosum is reduced to either zero or one cell layer; however, the stratum corneum may actually be thickened owing to a slower rate of desquamation.[9–10]

The number of grouped hair follicles is also affected by aging. Normally, new follicles grow from existing ones and subsequently form additional single and grouped follicles. Involution, predominantly of the grouped hair follicles, occurs with aging. Also, age-related atrophy of the papillary body develops; this begins around the hair follicles and gradually spreads peripherally.[9, 10]

Hair Loss

In older persons, there is an increase in the number of hair follicles that are in the telogen (resting) phase of the hair cell cycle. The hair follicles are also smaller and are seated more shallowly in the skin. In addition, with aging, the hairs are smaller and have narrower hair shaft diameters.

A cyclical pattern is established in androgenetic alopecia. As a response to circulating androgens, the hair follicles in certain areas undergo a shortening of their growing phase. Subsequently, there is increased shedding of resting hairs (club hairs). Thinning of individual hairs follows. Hence, the coarse, pigmented terminal hairs that were originally present are eventually replaced by fine, nonpigmented vellus hairs.[9, 10] Separating aging effects from androgen-mediated effects on the hair follicle can be difficult.

Graying

With advancing age, melanocytes are lost from the hair bulbs. Graying results from the replacement of fully pigmented hairs by hairs that contain progressively decreased amounts of pigment. Gray hairs do contain melanocytes; some of the melanocytes have large vacuoles in their cytoplasm. However, the majority of the melanosomes within the melanocytes of gray hair are not fully melanized. Also, there are fewer melanin granules in the hair matrix and hair shaft. Melanocytes are no longer seen in hair papillae and are rare in the hair shafts as the hair turns white.[9–11]

TREATMENT

Changes in Number of Hairs

Hair Loss

Nonmedical and surgical modalities are available for the management of scalp alopecia caused by aging. In addition, there are medical treatments that can be used in the elderly patient with androgenetic alopecia.

Cosmetic approaches for alopecia of the scalp include the following:

- Not parting the hair, because this makes the hair lie flat and look thinner.
- Cutting the hair in layers, because this makes the hair appear thicker.
- Shampooing the hair frequently, because this gives the hair a fluffy, thicker appearance.
- Having a permanent wave, because this gives the hair more body; however, too tight a curl can make a woman look much older—especially a woman in her seventies or eighties.

Spironolactone, at oral doses of 50 to 200 mg/day, has been used for androgenetic alopecia. Twice-daily application of topical 2% minoxidil has also been used successfully by both men and women to treat androgenetic alopecia. Topical 5% minoxidil has also been successfully used to treat male androgenetic alopecia.[19] A minimum trial of 4 months with topical minoxidil is necessary, and lifelong treatment is required to maintain hair growth.

Dihydrotestosterone is the primary hormone that triggers androgenetic alopecia in men. Finasteride inhibits the conversion of testosterone to dihydrotestosterone. Significant increases in hair counts and clinical improvement from baseline were observed in men with androgenetic alopecia taking oral finasteride (1 mg/day) for 12 months.[20]

Hair transplantation and scalp reduction are potential surgical approaches for the management of scalp alopecia.[21, 22]

Hair Gain

Facial bleaches, depilatories, tweezing, shaving, electrolysis, lasers, and waxing are available modalities to eliminate cosmetically compromising facial hairs in elderly persons.

Changes in Hair Color

Graying

It may not be necessary to treat gray hair. Gray hair may be attractive for those elderly patients with a pink, bright complexion. Older patients with gray hair and sallow complexions may choose to change their makeup foundation or blush; alternatively, they may elect to whiten their gray hair.

Removal of the gray hairs may be considered for those patients whose hair is less than 10% gray. In men whose graying is restricted to the sideburns, short trimming allows the gray to disappear. However, removal or close trimming of gray hairs is a temporary solution that works for only 1 or 2 years, until the graying progresses and begins to involve more of the scalp hairs.

Highlighting (bleaching) or coloring (darkening) some of the gray hairs may give the hair a more natural or sophisticated appearance. Applying blond streaks to the hair lightens its appearance. Alternatively, because hair that is all of one shade may look artificial, darkening some of the gray hair gives it a more natural look.

Complete coloring of the gray hair is another option. Temporary hair coloring (using a textile dye), gradual hair coloring (using dyes consisting of metallic salts of lead acetate and silver nitrate), semipermanent hair coloring (using low-molecular-weight dyes), and permanent hair coloring (using paraphenylenediamine dyes) are available alternatives.[21]

REFERENCES

1. Cohen PR, Scher RK: Geriatric nail disorders: diagnosis and treatment. J Am Acad Dermatol 26:521–531, 1992.
2. Cohen PR, Scher RK: Nail changes in the elderly. J Geriatric Dermatol 1:45–53, 1993.
3. Cohen PR, Scher RK: The nail in older individuals. In: Scher RK, Daniel CR III (eds): Nails: Therapy, Diagnosis, Surgery. Philadelphia, WB Saunders 1997, pp 127–150.
4. Cohen PR: The lunula. J Am Acad Dermatol 34:943–953, 1996.
5. Courtois M, Loussouarn G, Hourseau C, Grollier JF: Ageing and hair cycles. Br J Dermatol 132:86–91, 1995.
6. Naruse N, Fujita T: Changes in the physical properties of human hair with age. J Am Geriatr Soc 19:308–314, 1971.
7. Turner ML: Skin changes after forty. Am Fam Physician 29:173–181, 1984.
8. Fenske NA, Lober CW: Structural and functional changes of normal aging skin. J Am Acad Dermatol 15:571–585, 1986.
9. Smith L: Histopathologic characteristics and ultrastructure of aging skin. Cutis 43:414–424, 1989.
10. Kurban RS, Bhawan J: Histologic changes in skin associated with aging. J Dermatol Surg Oncol 16:908–914, 1990.
11. Cline DJ: Changes in hair color. Dermatol Clin 6:295–303, 1988.
12. Rosen CJ, Holick MF, Millard PS: Premature graying of hair is a risk marker for osteopenia. J Clin Endocrinol Metab 79:854–857, 1994.
13. Glasser M: Is early onset of gray hair a risk factor? Med Hypotheses 36:404–411, 1991.
14. Gross SB, Yeager DW, Middendorf MS: Cadmium in liver, kidney, and hair of human, fetal through old age. J Toxicol Environ Health 2:153–167, 1976.
15. Shapcott D, Cloutier D, Demers P-P, Vobecky JS, Vobecky J: Hair chromium at delivery in relation to age and number of pregnancies. Clin Biochem 13:129–131, 1980.
16. Kermici M, Pruche F, Roguet R, Prunieras M: Evidence for an age-correlated change in glutathione metabolism enzyme activities in human hair follicle. Mech Ageing Dev 53:73–84, 1990.
17. Liu X, Su B, Yin F, Han Q, Hu Z: Relationship between age and hair strontium in a population from the Dalian district of China [letter]. Clin Chem 40:2324–2325, 1994.
18. Sturaro A, Parvoli G, Doretti L, Allegri G, Costra C: The influence of color, age, sex on the content of zinc, copper, nickel, manganese, and lead in human hair. Biol Trace Elem Res 40:1–8, 1994.
19. Pharmacia & Upjohn, Kalamazoo, MI. ROGAINE Extra Strength for Men (5% minoxidil topical solution) for nonprescription use. Data presented at FDA Non-prescription Drug Advisory Committee Meeting, July 16, 1997.
20. Kaufman KD, Olsen EA, Whiting D, et al and the Finasteride Male Pattern Hair Loss Study Group: Finasteride in the treatment of men with androgenetic alopecia. J Am Acad Dermatol 39:578–589, 1998.
21. O'Conoghue MN: Cosmetics for the elderly. Dermatol Clin 9:29–34, 1991.
22. Sawaya ME: Clinical updates in hair. Dermatol Clin 15:37–43, 1997.

Forensic and Medicolegal Issues

DIANA GARSIDE

—

BRUCE A. GOLDBERGER

For many years, blood and urine specimens have been used routinely for the detection and measurement of therapeutic drugs and drugs of abuse. With increased concern regarding the widespread societal abuse of drugs, in combination with recent analytical developments in immunological and chromatographic techniques, the use of alternative biological specimens, including hair and nails, for drug detection has gained popularity.[1]

Research in this specialized area of drug monitoring began in the 1950s with the initial discovery of barbiturates in hair. Since then, studies have demonstrated the presence of many therapeutic drugs and drugs of abuse in hair. To date, several hundred scientific papers regarding hair analysis have been published. In addition, two books[2, 3] and three complete volumes of a prominent forensic science journal[4–6] have been devoted to hair analysis. Research in the area of nail analysis began in the 1980s and is currently limited to the analysis of a few therapeutic drugs and drugs of abuse.

Anatomy and Physiology

Hair and nails are derived from the same cells as the epidermis and consist of hard, dead keratinous cells. Hair grows in alternating cycles from a follicle in which the hair bulb is imbedded, whereas nails grow continuously from the germinal matrix.

A single hair consists of three layers: cuticle, cortex, and medulla. The cuticle forms a protective sheath around the hair shaft and consists of overlapping scales pointing toward the distal end of the hair. Within the cuticle is the cortex, which contains the melanin (pigment granules) that gives hair its color. The canal running through the center of the hair is known as the medulla. Not all hair strands have a medulla, or the medulla may be fragmented. Figure 17–1 illustrates the anatomy of a hair.

Each nail has a free edge and a body, which are the visible portions, and a root that is imbedded within the finger or toe in the region known as the germinal matrix. The thick proximal skinfold is known as the cuticle. A modified epidermis, known as the nail bed, extends beneath the nail. Nails are almost colorless but appear pink except for a white crescent called the lunula. The variation in coloration is caused by differences in the blood supply in the underlying dermis. Figure 17–2 illustrates the anatomy of a nail.

Hair grows at an average rate of 0.35 mm/day, or about 1 cm/mo. However, hair from different anatomical regions grows at differing rates and exhibits differing morphology from head hair. For example, head hair is generally circular in cross-section, whereas beard hair is triangular and grows more slowly than head hair. Nails

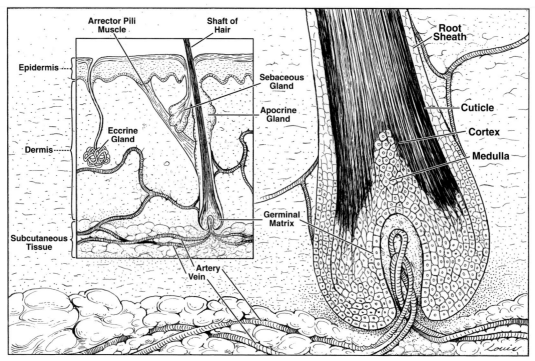

FIGURE 17-1 ■ Anatomy of hair.

grow about three times more slowly than hair, at an average rate of 0.1 mm/day, or about 3 mm/mo. Fingernails grow several times faster than toenails, and each digit grows at a slightly different rate. The middle fingernail grows the fastest of all the digits, and the thumbnail the slowest.

There are many factors that influence the growth of hair and nail. For example, growth is affected by age, sex, anatomical site, ethnicity, pregnancy, climate, nutri-

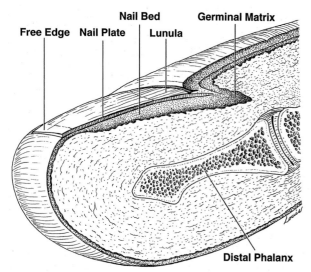

FIGURE 17-2 ■ Anatomy of nail. (From Garside D, Ropero-Miller JD, Goldberger BA, Hamilton WF, Maples WR: Identification of cocaine analytes in fingernail and toenail specimens. J Forensic Sci 43: 974–979, 1998. Copyright ASTM. Reprinted with permission.)

tion, and disease state. These factors must be taken into account during interpretation of a drug test result.

Drug Incorporation

Data regarding the precise mechanism of incorporation of drugs and drug metabolites into hair and nails are limited. The majority of studies described in the literature are based primarily on the analysis of hair obtained from known drug users and are epidemiological in nature. In these studies, important clinical data such as drug dose, time and frequency of drug administration, and plasma drug concentration are often unknown. Other studies of drug incorporation into hair have used animal models, in vitro models, and transplantation of human hair onto athymic mice.[7]

It is assumed that the dividing cells responsible for hair and nail formation also incorporate drug analyte into the growing matrix. Studies have shown that the distribution of analyte across membranes into the hair and nail matrix is facilitated by high lipid solubility and physiochemical factors that favor the nonionized form of the drug analyte. Nonpolar analytes, such as heroin and cocaine, readily cross membranes and enter hair- and nail-forming cells, whereas polar analytes, such as benzoylecgonine (a cocaine metabolite), are less likely to cross membranes.[7–9]

Based on a compilation of data, the following mechanisms of drug incorporation into hair have been proposed: (1) passive diffusion of the analyte from the blood supply to the hair follicle and hair cells; (2) diffusion of the analyte from skin to hair; (3) exposure of

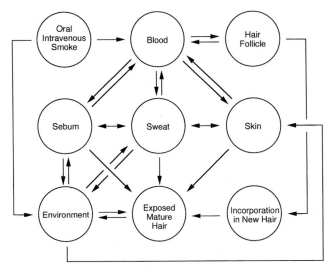

FIGURE 17-3 ■ Model of drug deposition in hair. (From Cone EJ: Mechanisms of drug incorporation into hair. Ther Drug Monit 18: 438–443, 1996.)

hair follicles and maturing hair fibers to eccrine, sebaceous, and apocrine gland secretions; and (4) exposure of the hair fibers to the external environment including drug vapor and drug residue.[7-9] A model of drug deposition in hair illustrating the various routes of incorporation is shown in Figure 17–3.

The physical binding of analyte to hair is influenced by the chemical nature of hair and the analyte and presumably involves electrostatic forces, van der Waals attraction, and other mechanisms. For example, analytes that are positively charged (cationic) at physiological pH are incorporated to a greater extent than those that are noncationic. Presumably, the cationic forms are attracted to anionic sites present on matrix proteins such as melanin and keratin.[7-9]

The proposed mechanisms of drug incorporation into nails are similar to those for hair and include (1) passive diffusion of the analyte from the blood supplying the dividing cells at the lunular germinal matrix as the nail plate grows distally; (2) incorporation through continuous nail production by cornification of the nail bed; (3) diffusion of analyte from the blood along the nail bed to the ventral portion of the nail plate; (4) exposure of the nail to body fluids such as sweat, sebum, saliva, and urine; and (5) exposure of the nail to the external environment including drug vapor and drug residue.

Drug Analysis

The analysis of drugs in hair and nails involves the following steps: (1) sample preparation to facilitate ease of handling and release of drug analytes; (2) decontamination of the surface of the matrix through washing; (3) release of drug analytes from the matrix; (4) extraction and purification of drug analytes; and (5) identification of drug analytes by an immunochemical or chromatographic technique. Current instrumentation is exceed-

TABLE 17-1 ■ Methods of Analysis of Drugs in Hair and Nail

Specimen Preparation

Collection
Storage
Cut and weigh
Decontamination

Drug Isolation

Base hydrolysis
Acid hydrolysis
Methanolic extraction
Enzymatic digestion

Purification of Hair Extracts

Liquid-liquid extraction
Solid-phase extraction
Solid-phase microextraction
Supercritical fluid extraction

Drug Identification by Immunochemical Techniques

Enzyme immunoassay
Fluorescence polarization immunoassay
Radioimmunoassay

Drug Identification by Chromatographic Techniques

Capillary electrophoresis
Gas chromatography
Gas chromatography/mass spectrometry
Gas chromatography/mass spectrometry/mass spectrometry
High-performance liquid chromatography
Liquid chromatography/mass spectrometry
Thin-layer chromatography

ingly sensitive and specific, capable of detecting minute traces of drug analytes in hair and nails.[10, 11] The methods of analysis of drugs in hair and nails are summarized in Table 17–1.

Hair is usually obtained by cutting a small lock, about the thickness of a pencil, from the vertex or crown of the head. The hair should be cut as close as possible to the scalp, and its orientation (distal to proximal) should be maintained for appropriate laboratory sampling or segmentation. If head hair is not available, hair specimens from other areas of the body (e.g., arm, chest, pubic regions) may be collected. Nail specimens (distal segments) are usually obtained with the use of cosmetic nail clippers. As an alternative, nail scrapings may be obtained with a scalpel or curette.

As little as 10 to 50 mg of either matrix is required for drug analysis. Once collected, both hair and nail specimens should be stored at room temperature in a dry, sealed container such as a paper envelope. Unlike the usual body fluids, hair and nail specimens are generally not susceptible to degradation, although they must be handled with care to avoid contamination. Also, in forensic applications, a strict chain-of-custody document must be maintained to ensure the integrity of the specimen and the scientific reliability of the drug test result.

Before analysis, the hair and nail specimens are cut into small pieces or pulverized in a ball mill so as to yield increased surface area for optimal drug analyte extraction. The specimen is washed to remove dirt, body secretions, and external drug contamination. A variety of decontamination techniques have been used; they generally are performed at room temperature by soaking, gently shaking, or sonicating the specimen for a brief period in one or more solvents or aqueous solutions, ranging from methanol and other organic solvents to water and soap solutions. Wash solutions are usually retained for analysis of drug content. Some laboratories have optimized their wash procedures as a means of distinguishing environmental contamination from internally incorporated drug.[3, 11]

Before drug analysis, the analytes must be released from the matrix. This is done by chemical hydrolysis of the matrix using dilute or strong acid or base, by solvent extraction of the analytes using methanol or chemically modified (e.g., acidified) methanol, or by enzyme digestion of the hair or nail using proteolytic enzymes (e.g., proteinase K). Supercritical fluid extraction has also been used with limited success.[3, 11]

The analyte sought must be carefully considered before an appropriate method of release is chosen because some drug analytes are not stable under certain conditions. For example, the severe conditions of strong base

hydrolysis cause cocaine and heroin to hydrolyze. Also, after digestion or hydrolysis, the crude isolate may require pretreatment before analysis. For example, before immunoassay analysis, the pH of an isolate prepared with strong acid or base must be neutralized.[11, 12]

The most cost-effective technique to identify presumptive positive specimens is immunoassay. Usually, the crude isolate or a slightly modified isolate can be analyzed directly by the immunoassay. All presumptively positive specimens should be subjected to confirmation using a more specific chromatographic technique.

Purification of isolates for chromatographic analysis is accomplished with either liquid-liquid or solid-phase extraction. After extraction, the purified analytes are usually analyzed by gas chromatography/mass spectrometry or gas chromatography/mass spectrometry/mass spectrometry. Other less commonly used chromatographic methods of analysis include thin-layer chromatography, high-performance liquid chromatography, gas chromatography with flame ionization detection or nitrogen phosphorus detection, liquid chromatography/mass spectrometry, and capillary electrophoresis. A typical selective ion chromatogram (gas chromatography/mass spectrometry) of a hair extract obtained from a subject who self-administered both cocaine and heroin and a laboratory-prepared comparison standard are shown in Fig. 17-4.

The cost of hair and nail analysis is considerably higher than blood and urine analysis and is often prohibitive. Depending on the analyses requested, the fee per specimen may range from $50 to $500. An over-the-counter hair collection kit is now available at pharmacies throughout the United States. With the kit, hair is sent directly to a commercial laboratory for confidential analysis.

FIGURE 17-4 ■ Selective ion chromatogram recordings of hair and standard extracts. *A,* An extract of hair from a user of cocaine and heroin. *B,* An extract of drug-free control hair with cocaine, heroin, and metabolites added. D3-, D6-, and D9- refer to the isotopically labeled drug that was used as an internal standard. COC, cocaine; BE, benzoylecgonine; EME, ecgonine methyl ester; CE, cocaethylene; NBE, norbenzoylecgonine; NCOC, norcocaine; NCE, norcocaethylene; COD, codeine; MOR, morphine; 6AM, 6-acetylmorphine; NCOD, norcodeine; NMOR, normorphine; HER, heroin. (Adapted from Cone EJ, Darwin WD, Wang W-L: The occurrence of cocaine, heroin and metabolites in hair of drug abusers. Forensic Sci Int 63:55–68, 1993, with permission of Elsevier Science.)

Drugs Identified

All common drugs of abuse, including amphetamines, cannabinoids, cocaine, heroin, and phencyclidine, have been identified in hair. In addition, many therapeutic drugs have been identified in hair, including antibiotics, antidepressants, antipsychotics, barbiturates, benzodiazepines, methylxanthines, opioids, and steroids. Only a few drugs have been identified in nail to date. Complete listings of therapeutic drugs and drugs of abuse found in hair and nail are shown in Tables 17–2 and 17–3, respectively.

Interpretation of Data

Hair and nail analyses lend themselves to the long-term detection of drug exposure. Unlike conventional specimens such as blood and urine, in which drugs have a limited lifetime, hair and nail provide a retrospective, long-term measure of drug exposure that is directly related to the life span of the matrix. In addition, it is

TABLE 17-2 ■ Therapeutic Drugs and Drugs of Abuse Found in Hair

Opioids	Methamphetamine	Nordiazepam
	Methylenedioxyamphetamine (MDA)	Oxazepam
Acetylcodeine	Methylenedioxymethamphetamine (MDMA)	Others
Buprenorphine	Cocaine analytes	Meprobamate
Codeine	Anhydroecgonine methyl ester	Methaqualone
Dextromoramide	Benzoylecgonine	
Dihydrocodeine	Cocaine	**Others**
Ethylmorphine	Cocaethylene	
Fentanyl	Ecgonine methyl ester	Antidepressants
Heroin analytes	Ecgonine ethyl ester	Amitriptyline and nortriptyline
Heroin	Norbenzoylecgonine	Clomipramine
6-Acetylmorphine	Norcocaethylene	Doxepin and nordoxepin
Morphine	Norcocaine	Imipramine and desipramine
Hydromorphone	Methylxanthines	Anti-epileptic
L-α-Acetylmethadol	Caffeine	Carbamazepine
Methadone	Theobromine	Anti-infectious
Morphine	Theophylline	Chloroquine
Pentazocine	Nicotine and cotinine	Ofloxacin
Pholcodine		Fluconazole
Zipeprol	**Sedative/Hypnotics**	Temafloxacin
	Barbiturates	Cardiovascular drugs
Hallucinogens	Amobarbital	Atenolol
	Phenobarbital	Betaxolol
Cannabinoids	Secobarbital	Digoxin
Δ⁹-Tetrahydrocannabinol	Thiopental	Propranolol
Δ⁹-Tetrahydrocannabinol-carboxylic acid	Benzodiazepines	Sotalol
Lysergic acid diethylamide	Alprazolam	Neuroleptics
Phencyclidine	Diazepam	Chlorpromazine
	Flunitrazepam	Clozapine
Stimulants	Lorazepam	Haloperidol
	Nitrazepam	Thioridazine
Amphetamines		
Amphetamine		
Fenfluramine		

possible to perform sectional analyses of hair in order to estimate the pattern of drug use, including chronicity and periods of abstinence.

The interpretation of hair and nail drug test results, positive or negative, must be performed with caution because the precise mechanism of incorporation of drug

TABLE 17-3 ■ Therapeutic Drugs and Drugs of Abuse Found in Nail

Stimulants

Amphetamines
  Amphetamine
  Methamphetamine
  Methylenedioxyamphetamine (MDA)
  Methylenedioxymethamphetamine (MDMA)
Cocaine analytes
  Anhydroecgonine methyl ester
  Benzoylecgonine
  Cocaine
  Cocaethylene
  Ecgonine methyl ester
  Ecgonine ethyl ester
  Norbenzoylecgonine
  Norcocaethylene

Antipsychotics

  Haloperidol

Anti-infectives

  Itraconazole
  Ketoconazole
  Terbinafine

and drug metabolite is not known. For example, a negative drug test result cannot be used to rule out drug exposure because the incorporation of drug in hair and nails has not been fully characterized. This characterization includes the determination of the time course of drug appearance in hair and nail and the minimum dose required to result in a positive drug test result. In addition, there are many confounding chemical, biological, and other factors that clearly influence the incorporation of drug and drug metabolite in hair and nails. Further, many laboratory techniques cannot adequately differentiate environmental contamination from internal incorporation of drug and some drug metabolites.

Despite these limitations, the presence of specific analytes can be informative and may reveal the route of drug administration. In addition, the presence of certain drug metabolites can eliminate the possibility of environmental contamination. For example, detection of cocaethylene indicates the simultaneous ingestion of ethanol and cocaine, whereas the presence of anhydroecgonine methyl ester (a pyrolysis product of cocaine) indicates exposure to "crack" cocaine. Similarly, the detection of 6-acetylmorphine (a unique heroin metabolite) establishes heroin use and could not be explained by the legitimate use of other opiates, including morphine and codeine.[3, 10]

Deposition of drug and drug analyte in hair has been shown to be susceptible to selective accumulation by specific hair types, leading to a potential color bias. For example, it has been shown that heavily black–pigmented hair tends to accumulate more cocaine than does blond or brown hair. Although there is no specific explanation, results of several studies suggest that the ultrastructure, morphology, and protein structure of the hair may be responsible for these differences. A number of specific hair characteristics have been suggested, including the degree of pigmentation (amount of melanin) and the permeability of the hair fibers. Although it has yet to be determined, it is suspected that nail analysis is not prone to color bias because nails contain little or no pigment.

Other factors that can affect the results of drug analysis of hair and nail are personal hygiene, color and cosmetic treatments of hair (including permanents and bleaching), and nail treatments. In addition, variations in growth rates and exposure to the environment and to sweat, based on the anatomical location of the specimen, must be taken into consideration when interpreting the results of an analysis. For example, pubic hair is less likely to be contaminated through environmental exposure but more likely to be bathed in sweat and urine than head hair. In the same way, toenails are less exposed to the environment but are more exposed to sweat than fingernails are.

Potential Applications

Historically, elemental analysis has dominated the field of hair and nail analysis, particularly in the area of heavy metals in clinical and environmental applications and arsenic, cadmium, lead, and mercury in forensic cases. More recently, the analysis of hair and nails for drugs has been used in a variety of applications, including workplace drug testing (both pre-employment and random testing), drug treatment programs, therapeutic drug monitoring, determination of prenatal drug exposure, and forensic investigations including criminal justice, epidemiological studies, and research.[12] In the United States, hair analysis results have been used as scientific evidence in child custody and adoption cases, military courts-martial, probation revocation proceedings, and unemployment compensation cases.[3]

Because drugs remain in hair and nails for the life span of the matrix, hair and nail analyses are commonly used in epidemiological studies as a means to obtain an accurate representation of a subject's drug use history independent of self-report and other less accurate data. Short-term abstinence commonly leads to negative blood and urine drug test results, but hair analyses are not affected.

Hair and nail analyses have also been used in anthropological studies as a means to assess lifestyles and habits of deceased persons, including ancient Egyptian and Peruvian mummies, the poet John Keats, and the outlaw Jesse James.

Advantages and Disadvantages

The principal advantage of hair and nail analysis is the ability to provide a long-term measure of drug exposure potentially representing several months to years. Other advantages of hair and nail analysis are that (1) samples are readily obtainable and are relatively noninvasive to collect; (2) samples are easy to handle and store, and once incorporated, the analytes are presumably stable; (3) the potential for donor manipulation (adulteration) of the sample to alter the test result is minimal; and (4) similar samples can be obtained for reanalysis. In addition, hair analysis can potentially provide useful data regarding the time and magnitude of drug exposure through sectional analysis.

Disadvantages of hair and nail analysis include (1) the limited research in this relatively new, evolving area of forensic toxicology; (2) the lack of standardization among toxicology laboratories, including collection techniques, analytical procedures, targeted analytes, and cut-off concentrations; (3) the inability to readily detect recent drug use; (4) the potential for environmental contamination leading to false-positive test results; and (5) the limited number of laboratories that offer hair and nail analysis.

Finally, legal issues regarding the applicability of hair analysis (especially in the workplace) must be resolved before hair and nails are accepted as appropriate alternative tissues for drug analysis.

REFERENCES

1. Pichini S, Altieri I, Zuccaro P, Pacifici R: Drug monitoring in nonconventional biological fluids and matrices. Clin Pharmacokinet 30:211–228, 1996.
2. Cone EJ, Welch MJ, Babecki MBG (eds): Hair Testing for Drugs of Abuse: International Research on Standards and Technology. Rockville, Maryland, National Institute on Drug Abuse, 1995.
3. Kintz P (ed): Drug Testing in Hair. Boca Raton, FL, CRC Press, 1996.
4. Forensic Science International, Volume 63, Numbers 1–3, December 1993.
5. Forensic Science International, Volume 70, Numbers 1–3, January 1995.
6. Forensic Science International, Volume 84, Numbers 1–3, January 1997.
7. Rollins DE, Wilkins DG, Gygi SP, Slawson MH, Nagasawa PR: Testing for drugs of abuse in hair: experimental observations and indications for future research. Forensic Sci Rev 9:23-36, 1997.
8. Henderson GL: Mechanisms of drug incorporation into hair. Forensic Sci Int 63:19–29, 1993.
9. Cone EJ: Mechanisms of drug incorporation into hair. Ther Drug Monit 18:438–443, 1996.
10. Inoue T, Seta S, Goldberger BA: Analysis of drugs in unconventional samples. In: Liu RH, Goldberger BA (eds): Handbook of Workplace Drug Testing. Washington, DC, AACC Press, 1995, pp 131–158.
11. Chiarotti M, Strano-Rossi S: Preparation of hair samples for drug analysis. Forensic Sci Rev 8:111–128, 1996.
12. Höld KM: Drug testing in hair. Ther Drug Monit Toxicol 17:311–318, 1996.

Psychiatric Issues

ELIZABETH REEVE

Androgenetic Alopecia

Although many practitioners have anecdotal evidence that male pattern baldness affects the lives of their patients, the literature suggests that this impact may be more significant than previously understood. Although most persons voice concerns about physical attractiveness, self-esteem, and aging, others experience their hair loss in a more pathological manner. One study of 116 patients who sought medical help at an outpatient dermatology clinic revealed that 76.3% were diagnosed with at least one personality disorder as defined by the *Diagnostic and Statistical Manual of Mental Disorders, Third Edition, Revised.*[1] This rate was considerably higher than the 10% rate found in the general public. In this study, no difference was found between men and women in the rate of personality disorders. However, the patient population in this study may not represent the "typical" patient in that the subjects were seeking medical help for their baldness. Most persons with baldness accept their condition as a normal part of life and do not seek medical consultation. Those who seek medical treatment may represent a population subset that has more significant baldness, more difficulty with psychological adjustment to their condition, or a combination of both. Personality disorders are well-developed personality patterns that are established by early adulthood. The presence of a pre-existing personality disorder may influence a subject's adjustment to baldness. It is not likely that the presence of the baldness is the cause of the personality disorder.

Women with androgenetic alopecia deserve separate consideration. It is hypothesized that women have more difficulty coping with this disorder because of the smaller number of women affected and the cultural differences between the sexes related to physical attractiveness. Although research in this area is limited, it has been suggested that the impact for women with androgenetic alopecia is greater than for men. In one study, women were twice as likely as men to be characterized as "very" or "extremely" upset by their hair loss.[2]

No data exist regarding the effectiveness of either psychological support or individual therapy for persons with androgenetic alopecia. Long-term studies are needed to determine whether poor psychological adjustment affects either the course of hair loss or the results expected from treatment.

Telogen Effluvium

The diffuse hair loss of telogen effluvium is associated with several stressors, including childbirth, fever, chronic medical illness, crash dieting, surgery, medications, and severe psychological trauma.[3] Treatment may be as simple as removal of the precipitating event or factor. The hair loss in this disorder is typically reversible and self-limited. No published studies have discussed the relation between mental health and telogen effluvium. Although "severe psychological stress" is commonly listed as a precipitating cause of the disorder, no specific clarification is provided. (Compare alopecia areata and stress in a later section.)

Many persons with telogen effluvium become anxious because of self-doubt about whether they are "really" losing hair. Patients may have been told by health care providers or others that "nothing is wrong" with their hair and "it looks fine." This worsens their underlying worry and concern. Reassurance and understanding are necessary to help these patients identify the true cause of their hair loss.

Hair Loss Related to Chemotherapy

Although hair loss related to chemotherapy may seem to be an insignificant issue in the presence of a potentially fatal illness, many patients view their hair loss as catastrophic. Hair loss in the context of chemotherapy may carry unique significance. Baldness may emphasize patients' lack of control over their illness and may symbolize their vulnerability. The baldness may also serve as a visible public reminder of the presence of disease, a fact that may elicit either sympathy or fear in others. Studies in the past have investigated methods to prevent hair loss associated with chemotherapy. The use of scalp hypothermia and scalp tourniquets to prevent hair loss have proved to be controversial because studies show conflicting results.

Research in the area of chemotherapy and hair loss is limited to very few studies. Many of these are anecdotal case reports without the necessary controls and designs to ensure the statistical significance of the findings. One study specifically addressed the social and cultural dimensions of hair loss in women who underwent therapy for breast cancer.[4] Extensive face-to-face, semistructured interviews of 10 women were conducted. Hair loss for these women caused a variety of feelings, including a diminished self-concept, a sense of loss of privacy, and feelings of personal and societal failure. Other research showed that perceptions of body image differed significantly between persons who experienced alopecia from chemotherapy and those who did not. Those who experienced alopecia had an overall more negative body image. Patients did not seem to become accustomed to seeing themselves without hair.[5]

Onchyophagia

Nail biting is commonly found in children and adults. The literature suggests that nail biting prevalence may be as high as 50% during childhood, peaking between the ages of 10 and 18 years.[6] Usually it represents a benign condition, but at times of increased personal stress, nail biting, like most habits, may increase. Chronic, pathological nail biting may result in medical complications such as infection, periungual warts, inflammation, or loss of the nail due to damage to the nail bed. There is no clear relation between nail biting and specific psychological or psychiatric disorders. The early literature suggested associations with "anxiety" or "stress," but few systematic or controlled studies exist. One study that focused primarily on treatment systematically assessed subjects and found them to be free of major psychiatric disturbances.[6]

Treatment of nail biting usually is initiated when medical complications such as infection develop. The most effective treatments are behavioral. Habit reversal, negative practice, response prevention, hypnosis, and relaxation therapies are behavioral techniques that have been used successfully in the treatment of pathological nail biting. One study systematically assessed the treatment response of pathological nail biters to two medications, desipramine and clomipramine. Clomipramine showed a modest superior efficacy in reducing the nail biting. This response is intriguing, because clomipramine is one of the currently available drugs that is useful in treating obsessive-compulsive disorder (OCD). Although it may be reasonable to initiate a medication trial for severe cases of nail biting with medical complications, behavioral treatment should be considered as the first treatment for uncomplicated cases in both children and adults.

Alopecia Areata

Unlike many other aspects of dermatology, considerable literature exists regarding the potential role of psychological factors in alopecia areata. The bulk of the literature is divided into two areas: the interaction of psychological stress with the onset of symptoms and course of illness, and the rates of psychopathology in patients with this condition. Two publications have offered concise reviews of the literature relating to the overlap between alopecia areata, stress, and mental health diagnoses.[7, 8]

ALOPECIA AREATA AND STRESS

The early literature offers a variety of opinions as to whether stress is causally related to alopecia areata. In one of the largest clinical samples studied, Muller and Winkelmann concluded that chronic psychological difficulties and acute emotional stress are more likely to be trigger events for other, unknown factors than to be primary etiological factors.[9] In this retrospective study of 736 patients, 12% identified an acute emotional stress (e.g., death in the family) as occurring before the hair loss. No relation was found between the degree of hair loss and the severity of the stressor.

More recently, Perini and colleagues assessed the impact of life events on alopecia areata in a comprehensive study, using a structured interview to assess recent life events.[10] Adult patients with alopecia areata were compared with patients with fungal infections and patients with common baldness. The authors found that patients with alopecia areata experienced a significantly greater number of life events in the 6 months preceding the onset of alopecia than did the other subjects. These included events with negative impact as well as events that were viewed as socially desirable. However, because the study was done retrospectively, it is possible that those patients with alopecia areata were more likely to recall past events in an attempt to explain their symptoms, thus allowing for potential bias. When Van Der Steen and associates asked 178 patients with alopecia areata whether they could attribute their first attack of hair loss to a particular event that took place at that time (i.e., within the previous 6 months), only 6.7% answered that a significant stressor had preceded the alopecia, suggesting little relation between stress and the onset of symptoms.[11] Finally, a third study found that 12 of 31 subjects identified "stress" as an etiological factor in their alopecia.[8] Details of the specific stressors were not reported.

To date no published study has prospectively correlated the course of alopecia areata with ongoing and newly arising life stressors. Because of the difficulty in monitoring and measuring everyday stressors, such a study would be difficult to complete. Nevertheless, because of the current recognized relation between stress and changes in immune function, it is increasingly important to understand the role of stress in immunologically mediated disorders such as alopecia areata.

ALOPECIA AREATA AND COMORBID PSYCHIATRIC DIAGNOSES

The presence of associated mental health psychopathology in persons with alopecia areata has been systematically assessed in both children and adults.[7, 8] Early literature implied a relation between psychopathology and alopecia areata, but the terminology used to describe the associated mental health disorders was vague and nonspecific, and the symptoms were poorly documented. Diagnoses such as "psychoneurotic," "nerves," and "neuroses" were used descriptively but provide very little meaningful information to practitioners.

In a 1991 study, Colon and colleagues[8] used structured and semistructured interviews to assess adults with alopecia areata who presented to a dermatology clinic for participation in a drug treatment study. These patients were not in need of acute psychiatric care. Of the 31 subjects, 23 (74%) had at least one lifetime psychiatric diagnosis. The two most common lifetime diagnoses were major depression and generalized anxiety disorder, with a prevalence of 39% each. The expected lifetime prevalences of these disorders in the general population are 8% to 15% and 5%, respectively.[12] No relation was found between lifetime psychiatric diagnoses and the number of episodes of alopecia. Subjects with one or more episodes of patchy alopecia were more likely to have had a diagnosis of generalized anxiety disorder at some time. Of particular interest was a finding of a higher than expected rate of anxiety and mood disorders, as well as substance use disorders, among first-degree relatives with alopecia areata. The authors speculated that the immunological and neuroendocrine changes associated with psychiatric disorders "may predispose or facilitate the development of alopecia areata or its course."

Reeve and associates assessed 12 children referred to a comprehensive dermatology clinic for evaluation and treatment of their alopecia areata.[7] Participants underwent a structured psychiatric interview and completed rating scales assessing anxiety, depression, and self-esteem. Five of the 12 children met criteria for an anxiety disorder (excluding simple phobia). No subjects met criteria for major depression, although one did have dysthymia. Subjects' rating scales measuring depression and anxiety were not elevated. Measures of self-esteem showed the subjects to have a high positive self-concept, in the 93rd percentile. The authors reported that although the subjects had a higher than expected rate of anxiety disorders on structured interview, they did not self-endorse anxiety or depression symptoms on rating scales. They also reported no difficulties with self-esteem. The disparity between the structured interview results and the rating scale responses may indicate that although some symptoms existed they did not significantly impair the children.

In summary, both children and adults with alopecia areata appear to have a higher rate of anxiety disorders than the general population, and adults also have increased rates of depression. Although subject samples have been small and results cannot be generalized, it is important to identify the potential for increased psychiatric illness in this population so that appropriate therapy can be initiated for persons with psychiatric diagnoses. Anxiety and depression in both adults and children respond well to appropriate medications or psychotherapy, or both.

Trichotillomania

CLINICAL DESCRIPTION

Trichotillomania, the pulling out of one's hair with resulting hair thinning or baldness, has been identified in both children and adults. Historically the disorder was thought to be relatively rare. Although there is no current epidemiological study of the general population, a 1994 review by Christenson and Mackenzie indicated that early prevalence was less than 1%, and current estimates indicate that a range of 2% to 4% is more likely.[13] By *Diagnostic and Statistical Manual of Mental Disorders, Fourth Edition*, the criteria for the diagnosis of trichotillomania requires that subjects experience tension before the pulling of their hair, or a sense of relief after pulling their hair, or both. Clinically, many subjects do not report experiencing tension or relief. This seems to be particularly true in children and adolescents, who more frequently report that they "just catch themselves" pulling their hair. Practitioners are encouraged to recognize hair pulling as significant regardless of whether the patient meets strict psychiatric criteria for the disorder.

Chronic hair pulling is reported more frequently in women than in men, except in very young children, where a more equal distribution may exist. It is speculated that the available gender information represents a biased sample. Women may be more motivated, because of the significant social implications of hair loss, to seek psychiatric consultation about their hair pulling. It is also possible that men more readily explain their hair loss from trichotillomania as normal "male baldness."

Trichotillomania can begin at any age, although most patients report an onset in early adolescence. It is unknown whether the age at onset of the disorder has implications for the prognosis, although persons who have pulled their hair for more than 6 months are more likely to have a chronic course than those who have done so for a shorter period. It is possible that a population of childhood hair pullers has time-limited pulling that does not progress into later years. However, when a young patient presents with hair pulling, it is not possible to predict whether the course will be progressive or time limited.

Most persons who pull their hair pull from more than one site on their body. Although any hair on the body can be pulled, including pubic hair, the most common sites for hair pulling are the scalp and the eyebrows or eyelashes. Although most hair pulling is restricted to one's own body, pulling of pet hair, hair of other persons, or hair from dolls or other toys is possible. Associated rituals are frequently reported after pulling out hair. These rituals commonly include rubbing the hair between the fingers or around the mouth, examining or biting off the hair bulb, or ingesting the entire hair. Although ingestion of significant amounts of hair is relatively rare, it must be considered in all hair pullers, because the consequence of ingesting large amounts of hair (trichobezoar) is medically significant. Hair pulling most often occurs when a person is engaged in quiet activities, such as watching television, driving, lying in bed before falling asleep, talking on the telephone, reading, or doing homework.[13, 14] Children also report an increase in their pulling behavior when they are alone. The presence of another person may be a strong deterrent and can be useful in setting up a treatment strategy (see later discussion).

Hair regrowth in persons with trichotillomania is often described as "different" from the hair that was pulled. The regrown hair is described as being thicker, more coarse, or more kinky or curly than the original hair. Color changes may also occur with the newly grown hair. These factors may precipitate further pulling for some persons, because it is the quality of "difference" of a specific hair that makes it attractive to pull.

In cases where the patient has trouble acknowledging the hair-pulling behavior, a scalp biopsy can distinguish trichotillomania from other disorders such as alopecia areata.

ETIOLOGY

Although there are numerous theories to explain hair pulling, recent literature is behaviorally and biologically focused. Past theories suggested that rupture of the mother-infant bond, maternal deprivation in early life, oedipal conflicts, or castration wishes explained the development of hair pulling. Stress has also been implicated as a causal factor. In numerous case reports, subjects have identified specific stressors preceding the development of hair pulling. Many of these stressors involved loss or separation of some type, including death of a family member or close friend, divorce, a change of schools or move, or hospitalization of a child or parent. For child and adolescent hair pullers, academic concerns are a commonly identified stressor, including upcoming examinations and perceived strictness of teachers. Many of these identified stressors are common life occurrences that are prevalent in today's society. Therefore, it is difficult to believe they can be the sole etiological factor for hair pulling. It is more likely that a multifactorial etiology exists and that a significant stressor serves as an initiating factor in a population already vulnerable to the development of hair pulling.

Dysregulation of serotonin, a neurotransmitter thought to play a role in OCD, has also been studied as a possible etiological factor in hair pulling. Hair pulling is considered by some to belong to the spectrum of obsessive-compulsive behaviors, which includes such entities as nail biting, neurotic excoriation, body dysmorphic disorder, pedophilia, pathological shopping, and gambling. Although some evidence indicates that persons with hair pulling are similar to persons with OCD, there is no agreement within the scientific community about this subject. Some of the similarities between people with trichotillomania and people with OCD include family psychiatric history and the positive response that some trichotillomania subjects have to medications typically effective for the treatment of OCD. The argument against a relation between the two disorders points to the lack of other obsessions and compulsions in most hair pullers.

For many persons with hair pulling, the behavior is best described as a habit with little or no cognitive component (e.g., obsessional thinking, tension or relief with pulling). Others have a behavior that may best be described as a motor tic that occurs in isolation or in conjunction with other motor and vocal tics such as Tourette's syndrome.

PSYCHIATRIC COMORBIDITY

There is a significant degree of psychiatric comorbidity in both children and adults with trichotillomania.[15] As with alopecia areata, there appears to be an increased prevalence of associated mood and anxiety disorders. The presence of a comorbid psychiatric diagnosis is significant in that it affects the choice of treatment for an individual patient. For instance, a medication can be chosen that treats anxiety or depression and may also lessen the "urge to pull" (see later discussion).

TREATMENT

The available literature is inconclusive about the best approach to treating and managing this disorder. Most studies are focused on behavioral treatment strategies, and there seems to be doubt as to the efficacy of such methods in the treatment of hair pulling in both children and adults. In the largest study of behavioral therapy for trichotillomania, habit reversal was found to be an effective treatment.[16] Habit reversal is a process that uses monitoring of behaviors, relaxation techniques, and competing response training to eliminate a behavior. In this study, habit reversal decreased hair pulling by 99% after 1 day of treatment and maintained a decrease of 87% at follow-up 22 months later. Although habit reversal has been used successfully in other protocols, there is some indication that most subjects need more than a single visit to eliminate trichotillomania.

Although behavioral therapy can be highly successful for both adults and children, many patients lack the insight, motivation, or perseverance to make use of behavioral therapy. Above all other criteria for success is the need for a motivated patient. This becomes particularly evident with adolescents, who may view therapy as a means of control by their parents, resulting in increased family tension and conflict. Young children need the involvement of a parent to achieve success with behavioral therapy.

Pharmacotherapeutic strategies for treatment of hair pulling have shown inconsistent results and less promise. There are numerous case reports in children and adults documenting the success of a large variety of medications, including lithium, tricyclic antidepressants, selective serotonin reuptake inhibitors, antipsychotics, naltrexone, methylphenidate, buspirone, and monoamine oxidase inhibitors. Much of the case report literature depicts patients with multiple comorbid diagnoses and is therefore difficult to interpret.

Controlled research studies in adults using serotonin reuptake inhibitors have shown mixed results, including positive results with clomipramine and negative findings with fluoxetine.[13] There are no controlled studies of medications in children with hair pulling. Anecdotally, medications seem to have little benefit in decreasing hair pulling in children.

There are several unique medication circumstances to be considered for young hair pullers. Many children report that most of their hair pulling occurs while they are lying in bed at night trying to fall asleep. In this subgroup of children, medication specifically targeting the insomnia may significantly decrease the hair pulling. Although there are numerous medications that could be used for this purpose, trazodone and clonidine can be effective for most children in inducing sleep. The possibility of hair pulling manifesting as a motor tic should also be considered in all children. Hair pulling may be successfully treated with medications appropriate for use in tic disorders, although the risk of medication side effects (particularly from neuroleptics) needs to be carefully considered.

There have been some reported successes with hypnotic therapies for trichotillomania. Treatment protocols using hypnosis have not been part of controlled studies and are difficult to compare because of the variety of different hypnotic and relaxation techniques used.

In conclusion, treatment for trichotillomania must be individualized to be successful. For most patients, it is reasonable to initiate treatment with behavioral therapy. Caution must be taken to choose a therapist experienced in the behavioral treatment of hair pulling. Therapists not familiar with this disorder may focus on seeking a psychodynamic cause for the hair pulling rather than initiating behavioral therapy. A thorough psychiatric assessment for the presence of comorbid mental health problems is essential, and treatment for comorbid problems should be initiated. It is reasonable to treat comorbid problems with medications that have the potential to decrease hair pulling. For example, although supportive data are limited, selective serotonin reuptake inhibitors may be useful in treating trichotillomania and are also beneficial in treating some anxiety and depressive disorders. Caution should be exercised in prescribing medications to a patient who is not participating in behavioral therapy. Although there is anecdotal evidence that treatment with medications alone may be helpful, the patient may also develop an inappropriate sense of optimism if medications are the only treatment prescribed and behavioral or supportive therapy is not also used.

Summary

Numerous disorders of hair and nails have been shown to be associated with unique mental health issues. It is imperative that the practitioner dealing with this interesting subgroup of patients be aware of the potential interplay between the dermatological disorder and psychiatric difficulties so that comprehensive, appropriate, and effective treatment is offered.

REFERENCES

1. Maffei C, Fossati A, Rinaldi F, Riva E: Personality disorders and psychopathologic symptoms in patients with androgenetic alopecia. Arch Dermatol 130:868–872, 1994.
2. Cash TF, Price VH, Savin RC: Psychological effects of androgenetic alopecia on women: comparisons with balding men and with female control subjects. J Am Acad of Dermatol 29:568–575, 1993.
3. Headington JT. Telogen effluvium, new concepts and review. Arch Dermatol 129:356–363, 1993.
4. Freedman TG: Social and cultural dimensions of hair loss in women treated for breast cancer. Cancer Nurs 17:334–341, 1994.
5. Pickard-Holley S: The symptom experience of alopecia. Semin Oncol Nurs 11:235–238, 1995.
6. Leonard HL, Lenane MC, Swedo SE, Rettew DC, Rapoport JL: A double-blind comparison of clomipramine and desipramine treatment of severe onychophagia (nail biting). Arch Gen Psychiatry 48:821–827, 1991.
7. Reeve ER, Savage TA, Bernstein GA: Psychiatric diagnoses in children with alopecia areata. J Am Acad Child Adolesc Psychiatry 35:1518, 1996.
8. Colon EA, Popkin MK, Callies AL, Dessert NJ, Hordinsky MK: Lifetime prevalence of psychiatric disorders in patients with alopecia areata. Compr Psychiatry 32:245–251, 1991.
9. Muller SA, Winkelmann RK: Alopecia areata: an evaluation of 736 patients. Arch Dermatol 88:290–297, 1963.
10. Perini GI, Veller Fornasa C, Cipriani R, Bettin A, Zecchino F, Peserico A: Life events and alopecia areata. Psychother Psychosom 41:48–52, 1984.
11. Van Der Steen P, Boezeman J, Duller P, Happle R: Can alopecia areata be triggered by emotional stress? An uncontrolled evaluation of 178 patients with extensive hair loss. Acta Derm Venereol 72:279–280, 1992.
12. American Psychiatric Association: Diagnostic and Statistical Manual of Mental Disorders, 4th ed. Washington, DC, APA, 1994, pp 618–621.
13. Christenson GA, Mackenzie TB: Clinical presentation and treatment of trichotillomania. Directions in Psychiatry 12(February 24): 1–8, 1994.
14. Reeve E: Hairpulling in children and adolescents. In: Stein DJ, Christenson GA, Hollander E (eds): Trichotillomania. Washington, DC, American Psychiatric Press, 1999, pp 201–224.
15. Christenson GA, Mackenzie TB, Mitchell JE: Characteristics of 60 adult chronic hair pullers. Am J Psychiatry 148:365–370, 1991.
16. Azrin NH, Nunn RG, Frantz SE: Treatment of hairpulling (trichotillomania): a comparative study of habit reversal and negative practice training. J Behav Ther Exp Psychiatry 11:13–20, 1980.

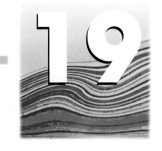

Molecular Basis of Inherited Hair and Nail Diseases

PETER B. CSERHALMI-FRIEDMAN

WASIM AHMAD

ANGELA M. CHRISTIANO

Molecular genetic approaches to the study of human diseases have yielded unexpected insights into the pathophysiology of many dermatologic disorders. This large body of evidence has provided the foundation for achieving the two major goals of management of a genetic disease: prevention when it is possible, and treatment when it is not. In genetic disorders, prevention has taken the form of DNA-based prenatal and preimplantation diagnoses, and it is anticipated that future treatments for many of these disorders will include gene-based therapies. Neither of these approaches would be possible without a fundamental understanding of the genes that underlie the respective genodermatoses and how mutations in those genes give rise to the phenotype.

More recently, the advances in molecular genetics have begun to extend to inherited disorders of the hair and nail as well. In this review, we illustrate the power of these approaches through their application to two rare inherited disorders: papular atrichia and pachyonychia congenita. It is anticipated that these insights will lead to effective, rationally designed genetic therapies for these disfiguring and frequently devastating disorders.

Molecular Basis of Papular Atrichia

ETIOLOGY

Papular atrichia is a rare, recessively inherited form of total alopecia that results from failure to initiate the first adult catagen. Affected individuals are born with hair that falls out and never regrows.[1] To understand the molecular basis of inherited congenital atrichia, we studied 10 families from Pakistan, Ireland, and Israel with congenital atrichia segregating as a single abnormality without associated defects.[2–4] In the affected individuals, who ranged in age from 8 months to 60 years, hair was absent from the scalp, axillae, pubis, and other parts of the body, and eyebrows and eyelashes were sparse. Natal hairs were present at birth but began shedding within 1 month and completely disappeared by 3 months of age. Scalp skin biopsies showed the complete absence of mature hair follicles. In affected patients, numerous keratin-filled follicular cysts developed over extensive areas of the skin, usually between the ages of 5 and 10 years. These papular lesions were most numerous on the cheeks, scalp, arms, forearms, thighs, and shins. A wide variability in the number of papules and their distribution on the body was observed and was not age related. Papules were not detected in unaffected normal members of the families, and the mode of inheritance of the disease was clearly autosomal recessive. We have described elsewhere the involvement of the human homologue of mouse hairless gene in this rare form of congenital hair loss.[2–4]

The phenotype of patients with congenital atrichia resembles that of hairless and rhino mice, with the rhino phenotype representing a more severe manifestation of the hairless mutation.[5] The hairless and rhino mutations are autosomal recessive allelic mutations that map to mouse chromosome 14.[6] These mice develop a normal first pelage up to the age of about 14 days, at which time they begin to lose their hair. The hair loss is normally complete in 1 week, and then the animals remained entirely naked. In the rhino mouse the skin becomes progressively thick, loose, and redundant with age, forming rhinoceros-like folds and flaps. This expansion of the surface is caused by development of utriculi containing horny cells, which are apparent at the age of 6 months. The mature rhino mouse usually weighs more than its haired littermates, mainly because of the large masses of skin, and the muscles and subcutaneous tissue regress.[5] One to two rows of horn-filled cysts of variable size occupy the lower dermis and arise from epithelial cells of imperfectly grown hair bulbs, fragmented and disoriented hair follicles with no ducts to the surface.

The rhino mutation is maintained on a number of different genetic backgrounds, such as BALB/c and RHJ/LeJ. Three other mouse alleles with the rhino phenotype (hr^{rh7J}, hr^{rh8J}, and hr^{rh9J}) have been found among breeding mouse stocks maintained in The Jackson Laboratory, Bar Harbor, Maine.[5] The molecular basis of the hairless mouse was demonstrated earlier to be a provirus insertion in intron 6 of the hairless (hr) gene, which is thought to interfere with messanger RNA splicing.[7] We also have identified a series of nonsense mutations in different alleles of rhino mice.[8–10]

At the cellular level in a normal hair, when the follicles enter catagen, elongation ceases and the follicle regresses because the hair matrix cells stop proliferating. During catagen, the dermal papilla remains intact but undergoes several remodeling events, including degradation of the elaborate extracellular matrix that is deposited during anagen. At the close of catagen, the hair is only loosely anchored in a matrix of keratin, with the dermal papilla just below. Finally, the follicle enters a quiescent phase known as telogen, during which the hair is usually shed. At the end of the resting phase, the dermal papilla migrates toward the epidermal stem cells located in the bulge region of the outer root sheath and recruits them to form the hair matrix, and a new cycle of growth is initiated.[11]

In patients with papular atrichia and in hairless and rhino mice, there are several well-defined morphological changes that lead to the failure of the next hair cycle.[5] Specifically, the hair matrix cells undergo a premature and massive apoptosis, together with a concomitant decline in *Bcl-2* expression, a loss of neural cell adhesion molecule positivity, and a disconnection with the overlying epithelial sheath essential for the movement of the dermal papilla.[12] As a consequence, the hair bulb and dermal papilla remain stranded in the dermis, and indispensable messages between the dermal papilla and stem cells in the bulge are not transmitted, so no further hair growth occurs. In hairless mice and humans with congenital atrichia, it appears that the absence of hairless protein initiates a premature and abnormal catagen due to abnormalities in the signaling that normally controls catagen-associated hair follicle remodeling.[5–12] These findings suggest that the hairless gene product plays a crucial role in maintaining the delicate balance between cell proliferation, differentiation, and apoptosis in the hair follicle as well as in the interfollicular epidermis.

CLINICAL FEATURES

There are many common forms of human hair loss that are collectively known as alopecias and that affect millions of people. In addition, there are several rare forms of hereditary alopecia that occur as a single gene disorder segregating in a classic autosomal recessive pattern. As reviewed by Feinstein and colleagues,[13] alopecia may occur alone or in association with various defects such as abnormalities of teeth and nails, microcephaly, cataracts, retinitis pigmentosa, epilepsy, mental retardation, pyorrhea, and total or partial anodontia.

Congenital atrichia (MIM 209500) is a rare form of total hair loss from the body that is inherited in an autosomal recessive pattern. Cases resembling this disease from Pakistan, with loss of hair over the entire body, have been reported under the name *alopecia universalis* (MIM 203655)[2, 14]; however, *congenital atrichia with papules* (MIM 209500) may be a more precise description of the phenotype resulting from mutations in the human hairless gene. Affected individuals show no growth or developmental delay; normal hearing, teeth, and nails; and no abnormalities in sweating.

As early as the 1950s, this rare human disease was named *atrichia with papular lesions* and was characterized as normal hair formation at birth followed by hair loss associated with the formation of comedones and follicular cysts.[1, 15, 16] In 1989, the human disease was first proposed to be a homologue of the hairless mouse mutation.[17]

PATHOLOGY

Congenital atrichia is the only form of alopecia for which the molecular basis has been described thus far. In persons affected with this form of hair loss, hairs are typically absent from the scalp, and patients are completely devoid of eyebrows, eyelashes, axillary hair, and pubic hair, once shedding of the natal hair occurs shortly after birth (Fig. 19–1). A scalp skin biopsy reveals the absence of hair follicles with sparsely distributed sebaceous glands. Variations in the structure and shape of hair follicle remnants have been reported in patients with congenital atrichia. These include short-

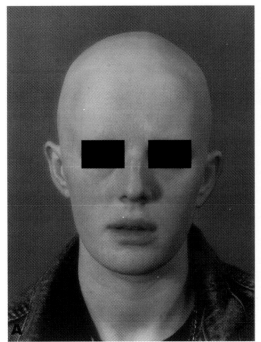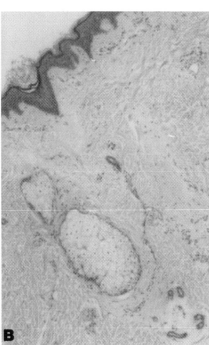

FIGURE 19–1 ■ Clinical and histopathological findings in congenital atrichia. *A,* Phenotypic appearance of an affected woman at approximately 25 years of age. Note the complete absence of hair on the scalp, eyebrows, and eyelashes. *B,* A scalp biopsy from the same woman reveals complete absence of hair follicle structures. A sebaceous gland and some hair follicle remnants are visible in the dermis. (Hematoxylin and eosin, magnification 150×). (From Ahmad W, Irvine AD, Lam H, et al: A missense mutation in the zinc-finger domain of the human hairless gene underlies congenital atrichia in a family of Irish travellers. Am J Hum Genet 63:984–991, 1998.)

ened hair follicles containing horny plugs and a reduced number of pilosebaceous units containing malformed hairs without cuticles.[18] Histologically, the skin biopsy samples show the absence of normal hair follicle structures with the formation of cysts and/or utriculi, which are skin surface–connected ampuliform structures with a hyperkeratotic epithelium.

DIAGNOSIS AND DIFFERENTIAL DIAGNOSIS

The most striking feature of congenital atrichia is the complete hair loss soon after birth. Affected patients have the additional characteristic features of grouped cystic and milia-like lesions on the skin. Clinically, atrichia is virtually indistinguishable from alopecia universalis; therefore, a scalp biopsy is necessary. However, if one obtains a history of complete nonresponsiveness to steroid injections and no regrowth of hair at all, the differential diagnosis of atrichia should be kept in mind for all cases of alopecia universalis. Based on the population frequency of atrichia, we estimate that a small percentage of children with total alopecia may have one of the mendelian forms of hair loss. Making the diagnosis early could spare these children painful and unnecessary steroid injections.

TREATMENT

There are currently no treatments available for this rare genetic disorder. However, discovery of the genes directly implicated in the pathogenesis of inherited hair loss will have far-reaching implications for affected persons. The genes will provide targets for transgenic and knockout mice in addition to hairless and rhino mice,

which would be essential for testing novel, rationally designed therapeutic pharmacological or genetic therapies in the future.

Molecular Basis of Pachyonychia Congenita

ETIOLOGY

Pachyonychia congenita (PC) represents a group of inherited disorders characterized by hypertrophic nail dystrophy and hyponychial keratosis.[19] The classification of these disorders is difficult and is based entirely on the clinical findings that are present in conjunction with the nail changes. Most authors agree on the existence of two major subgroups, but classification of the remainder of the cases remains somewhat controversial. Once genotype-phenotype correlations between the clinical findings and the underlying mutations are more completely understood, a DNA-based classification system can be established.

The two main subtypes of PC, Jadassohn-Lewandowsky syndrome (PC-1) and Jackson-Lawler syndrome (PC-2), are inherited in an autosomal dominant fashion and their clinical appearance is similar. The numerous possible skin and extracutaneous manifestations can serve as diagnostic criteria for minor subgroups, usually defined as PC-3 and PC-4.[19]

Among the members of the cytokeratin subfamily of intermediate filament proteins, keratin 17 (KRT17) is remarkable in that it is normally expressed in the basal cells of complex epithelium but not in stratified or simple epithelium. Synthesis of KRT17 seems to be a marker of basal cell differentiation in complex epithelium and is therefore believed to indicate a certain type of epithelial "stem cell."[20] KRT17 was considered a candidate gene for PC on the basis of its restricted tissue distribution.

In a large Scottish kindred with many individuals affected by PC-2, linkage of the disease locus was established with the use of markers mapping within the type I keratin gene cluster at 17q12-q21. Maximum locus of disease scores for linkage of the disease to a KRT10 polymorphism and to D17S800, a chromosomal marker known to be very tightly linked to KRT10, were 4.51 and 7.73, respectively, with no recombination.[21] A heterozygous missense mutation (Asn92→Asp) in the helix initiation motif of KRT17 was subsequently found to cosegregate with the disease.[22] In a second family, in which five individuals in three generations had PC, Smith and coworkers described a missense mutation caused by an A-to-G transition in KRT17, producing the predicted Asn92→Ser amino acid change at the same amino acid position.[23] The identical mutation was found in three sporadic cases. Heterozygous KRT17 missense mutations in the same conserved domain have been reported in five additional PC-2 families. Heterozygous missense mutations in KRT17 also were found in two families previously diagnosed as having steatocystoma multiplex. On review, mild nail changes were observed in some, but not all, of these patients.[23] The authors concluded that phenotypic variation is observed with KRT17 mutations, as is the case with other keratin disorders.

In a three-generation British Caucasian family, Covello and associates[24] found the same Asn92→Ser mutation in the KRT17 gene as the cause of PC-2. The 18-year-old proband presented with rough skin, caused by follicular keratoses, and thickened nails, and plantar skin. Although she did not have clinically obvious cysts and had mild hyperkeratosis of the buccal mucosa, other family members had abnormal nails, blistering of the feet, and multiple cysts. Her mother had a history of painful keratoses and blistering on the feet, with thickened nails, yellowish cysts on the trunk and limbs, and recurrent flexural abscesses. She also had multiple milia. A lesion excised from the labium majus proved to be an epidermoid cyst.[24]

Other candidate genes for PC include the KRT16, a type I keratin, which is mapped to chromosome 17.[25] The helix initiation motif of KRT16 is a short sequence of about 20 amino acids at the start of the central α-helical rod domain whose sequence is conserved in all type I or acidic keratins. Most strongly dominant-negative mutations in keratins have been found to be missense (or occasionally in-frame deletion) mutations in this sequence or in the equivalent sequence at the end of the rod domain, the helix termination motif. In a sporadic case of the Jadassohn-Lewandowsky type of PC, McLean and colleagues[22] identified a heterozygous missense mutation (Leu130→Pro) in the helix initiation peptide of KRT16. The known expression patterns of this keratin in epidermal structures also correlated with the specific abnormalities observed in PC. It is customary to refer to the mutations by the number of the amino acid affected in the 1A helical domain. Therefore, the first mutation to be identified in KRT16 can alternatively be designated Leu130→Pro or Leu15→Pro.

In a Slovenian family, Bowden and colleagues[26] reported PC-1 in three generations, including a grandfather, a father, and a daughter. The father and daughter had classic changes with thickened nails, palmoplantar keratoderma, and leukokeratosis of the tongue. The grandfather had only minor nail changes and mild keratoderma, raising the possibility of somatic and germ-line mosaicism. No mutation was found in KRT16 or KRT17, in contrast to other patients with PC. Instead, there was a heterozygous 3-bp deletion (AAC) in exon 1 of the KRT6A gene, which removed a highly conserved asparagine residue from position 8 of the 1A helical domain. Therefore, mutations in either of three genes, KRT6A, KRT16, or KRT17, can underlie PC.[22, 23, 26]

CLINICAL FEATURES

The most typical clinical sign is the severe wedge-shaped thickening of the fingernails and toenails, sometimes together with unguis incarnatus–like changes at the edges of the nail plate.[19] In certain instances, the clinical appearance can resemble onychogryphosis with dark discoloration of the nails. Under the thickened nail plate, an extensive, firm keratotic mass can sometimes be found. The typical skin finding that occurs together with the nail disorder in PC-1 is a patchy or sometimes striated, nonepidermolytic hyperkeratosis of the palms, less often of the soles, and hyperhidrosis.

PC-2 consists of the nail and skin symptoms of PC-1 in addition to involvement of the oral and nasopharyngeal mucous membranes. White plaques can be observed on the buccal mucosa, on the tongue, less often on the nasal and pharyngeal mucosa, and rarely on the larynx. PC-2 reportedly also occurs together with steatocystoma multiplex, natal teeth, and pili torti.

The much rarer subtype, PC-3, is a combination of the symptoms described in PC-1 with keratosis or cataracts, and sometimes natal teeth. Some authors separate another subtype, PC-4, that includes cases with atypical skin findings, such as macular pigmentation and blistering, and extracutaneous symptoms, such as osteodysmorphogensis or mental retardation. In all forms, follicular or patchy hyperkeratosis can be present, usually on the trunk, elbows, and knees, and less often on the genital area or the axillae.

PATHOLOGY

There are no characteristic histological signs that are pathognomonic for PC. Histological examination can show hyperkeratosis, acanthosis, and focal dyskeratosis. Mild epidermal edema usually is present, and the basal keratinocytes show irregular arrangement. The dermis is either normal or with signs of minor inflammation in the upper dermis.

DIAGNOSIS AND DIFFERENTIAL DIAGNOSIS

The main diagnostic criteria are the characteristic nail and skin findings that are usually present from neonatal age or appear in young adulthood. The family history is also important because of the dominantly inherited nature of the disorder. The nail changes can be very similar to those of severe onychomycosis or onychogryphosis, but in these cases the other findings are missing and the subungual mass is soft and easily removable, whereas in PC the keratotic mass under the nail plate is hard. The nail findings can be minimal in certain cases, with a predominance of the palmoplantar hyperkeratosis or steatocystoma multiplex. Palmoplantar psoriasis with psoriatic nail dystrophy can resemble PC, but the typical characteristics of the psoriatic nail dystrophy (e.g., Beau's points) can usually be easily distinguished, or histology of the skin lesions can confirm the diagnosis. The involvement of the oral mucosa and the tongue can be very similar to lichen planus, but the presence of the associated skin findings helps to establish the diagnosis. It also can be difficult to exclude other keratinization disorders that are accompanied by nail changes, such as ichthyoses or Olmsted's syndrome.

TREATMENT

Topical keratolytic treatment is recommended for the palmoplantar hyperkeratosis, and also the physical removal of the dystrophic nails may be necessary. In severe cases, systemic retinoid therapy can help to achieve moderate to significant improvement. As with many other genodermatoses, it is anticipated that insights gained through molecular genetics will provide a foundation for the eventual treatment of these disorders with gene-based therapies.

REFERENCES

1. Fredrich HC: Zur kenntnis der kongenitale hypotrichosis. Dermatol Wochenschr 121:408, 1950.
2. Ahmad W, ul Haque MF, Brancolini V, et al: Alopecia universalis associated with a mutation in the human hairless gene. Science 279:720, 1998.
3. Ahmad W, Irvine AD, Lam H, et al: A missense mutation in the zinc-finger domain of the human hairless gene underlies congenital atrichia in a family of Irish travellers. Am J Hum Genet 63: 984, 1998.
4. Zlotogorski A, Ahmad W, Christiano AM: Congenital atrichia in five Arab Palestinian families resulting from a deletion mutation in the human hairless gene. Hum Genet 103:400, 1998.
5. Panteleyev AA, Paus R, Ahmad W, et al: Molecular and functional aspects of the hairless gene in laboratory rodents and humans. Exp Dermatol 7:249, 1998.
6. Sundberg JP: The hairless (*hr*) and rhino (*hr*^rh) mutations, chromosome 14. In: Sundberg, JP (ed): Handbook of Mouse Mutations with Skin and Hair Abnormalities: Animal Models and Biomedical Tools. Boca Raton, Florida, CRC Press, 1994, p 241.
7. Cachon-Gonzalez MB, Fenner S, Coffin JM, et al: Structure and expression of the hairless gene of mice. Proc Natl Acad Sci U S A 91:7717, 1994.
8. Ahmad W, Panteleyev A, Sundberg JP, et al: Molecular basis for the rhino (*hr*^rh-8J) phenotype: a nonsense mutation in the mouse hairless gene. Genomics 53:383, 1998.
9. Ahmad W, Panteleyev A, Henson-Apollnio V, et al: Molecular basis for a novel rhino phenotype: a nonsense mutation in the mouse hairless gene. Exp Dermatol 7:298, 1998.
10. Panteleyev A, Ahmad W, Malashenko AM, et al: Molecular basis for the rhino Yurlovo (ht rhY) phenotype: severe skin abnormalities and female reproductive defects associated with an insertion in the hairless gene. Exp Dermatol 7: 281, 1998.
11. Hardy M: The secret life of the hair follicle. Trends Genet 8:55, 1992.
12. Panteleyev AA, Botchkareva NV, van der Veen C, et al: Pathobiology of the the hairless phenotype: dysregulation of hair follicle apoptosis and topobiology during the initiation of follicle cycling. J Invest Dermatol 110:577, 1998.
13. Feinstein A, Engelberg S, Goodman RM: Genetic disorders associated with severe alopecia in children: a report of two unusual cases and a review. J Craniofac Genet Dev Biol 7:301, 1973.
14. Ahmad M, Abbas H, ul Haque S: Alopecia universalis as a single abnormality in an inbred Pakistani kindred. Am J Med Genet 46: 369, 1993.
15. Damste J, Prakken JR: Atrichia with papular lesions: a variant of congenital ectodermal dysplasias. Dermatologica 108:114, 1954.
16. Landes E, Langer I: Ein beitrag zur hypotrichosis congenita. Hautzart 7:413, 1956.
17. Sundberg JP, Dunstan RW, Compton JG: Hairless mouse, HRS/J hr/hr. In: Jones TC, Mohr U, Hunt RD (eds): Monographs on Pathology of Laboratory Animals. Integument and Mammary Glands. Heidelberg, Springer-Verlag, 1989, pp 192.
18. Porter PS: Genetic disorders of hair growth. J Invest Dermatol 60: 493, 1973.
19. Gorlin RJ, Pindborg JJ, Cohen MM: Syndromes of the Head and Neck, 2nd ed. New York: McGraw-Hill, 1976, p. 600.
20. Troyanovsky SM, Leube RE, Franke WW: Characterization of the human gene encoding cytokeratin 17 and its expression pattern. Eur J Cell Biol 59:127, 1992.
21. Munro CS, Carter S, Bryce S, et al: A gene for pachyonychia congenita is closely linked to the keratin gene cluster on 17q12-q21. J Med Genet 31:675, 1994.
22. McLean WHI, Rugg EL, Lunny DP, et al: Keratin 16 and keratin 17 mutations cause pachyonychia congenita. Nat Genet 9:273, 1995.
23. Smith FJD, Corden LD, Rugg EL, et al: Missense mutations in keratin 17 cause either pachyonychia congenita type 2 or a phenotype resembling steatocystoma multiplex. J Invest Dermatol 108: 220, 1997.
24. Covello SP, Smith FJD, Sillevis-Smitt JH, et al: Keratin 17 mutations cause either steatocystoma multiplex or pachyonychia congenita type 2. Br J Dermatol 138:475, 1998.
25. Rosenberg M, RayChaudhury A, Shows TB, et al: A group of type I keratin genes on human chromosome 17: characterization and expression. Mol Cell Biol 8:722, 1988.
26. Bowden PE, Haley JL, Kansky A, et al: Mutation of a type II keratin gene (K6a) in pachyonychia congenita. Nat Genet 10:363, 1995.

INDEX

Note: Page numbers in *italics* refer to illustrations; page numbers followed by the letter t refer to tables.